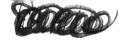

The Clinical Handbook for
# Surgical
# Critical Care

THE CLINICAL HANDBOOK SERIES

# The Clinical Handbook for
# Surgical Critical Care

**Kenneth W. Burchard, MD**
Dartmouth-Hitchcock Medical Center, New Hampshire

**Donald S. Gann, MD, and Charles E. Wiles, MD**
University of Maryland, Maryland

**The Parthenon Publishing Group**
International Publishers in Medicine, Science & Technology

NEW YORK                                    LONDON

Published in the USA by
The Parthenon Publishing Group Inc.
One Blue Hill Plaza
PO Box 1564, Pearl River
New York 10965, USA

Published in the UK and Europe by
The Parthenon Publishing Group Limited
Casterton Hall, Carnforth
Lancs., LA6 2LA, UK

**Library of Congress Cataloging-in-Publication Data**
The clinical handbook for surgical critical care / Kenneth W. Burchard, Donald S. Gann
and Charles E. Wiles.
    p.   cm.-(The clinical handbook series)
    Includes bibliographical references and index.
    ISBN 1-85070-633-6
    1. Surgical intensive care—Handbooks, manuals, etc.  2. Critical care medicine—
Handbooks, manuals, etc. I. Gann, Donald S., 1932–. II. Wiles, Charles E. III. Title.
IV. Series.
    [DNLM: 1. Critical Care handbooks.  2. Surgical Procedures, Operative handbooks.
WO 39 B947c 1998]
    RD51.5.B87   1998
    617'.919—dc21
    DNLM/DLC
    for Library of Congress                             98-22291
                                                  CIP

**British Library Cataloguing in Publication Data**
Burchard, Kenneth W.
    The clinical handbook for surgical critical care. - (The clinical handbook series)
    1. Surgical intensive care
    I. Title   II. Gann, Donald   III. Wiles, Charles E.   IV. Surgical critical care
    617.9'19

ISBN 1-85070-633-6

Typeset by Speedlith Photo Litho Ltd, Manchester, UK
Printed by J. W. Arrowsmith Ltd., Bristol, UK

# CONTENTS

# FOREWORD

Critical care has emerged as a well-defined specialized area within general surgery only in the last decade. Yet, despite its relatively recent appearance, there are already several large multi-authored textbooks in the field, as well as a few handbooks. The information and therapeutic suggestions that some of these books contain is both established and currently useful. Accordingly, anyone contemplating a new book in the area must identify an approach to the field that is distinct and will fill a need. It is in this spirit that we have undertaken the present volume. In our view, critical care must be rendered in the context of a clear understanding of the underlying pathophysiological processes and their interrelations. Although it is essential to consider organ systems in isolation in order to be clear about their functioning, malfunctioning and the treatments required to correct the latter, one must always have in mind the interrelations that are essential for coordinated functioning of the organism, and ultimately survival. In this manual, we present the normal physiology with respect to each system, together with prominent features to be found on physical examination and laboratory analysis, especially physiological monitoring. *The Clinical Handbook for Surgical Critical Care* deals with disease states, examining first the pathophysiology that underlies them and then the results of physical examination, monitoring and laboratory results that lead to a diagnosis. Finally, we deal with appropriate management in terms of the deranged physiology and supporting evidence.

In one sense, surgery itself may be regarded as a set of interventions designed to correct anatomical or physiological derangements. In that context, one may regard surgical critical care as a set of treatment interventions that may on the one hand prepare the patient to undergo surgery successfully, or on the other, to facilitate the patient's recovery from surgical intervention. We thus view surgical critical care as an integral part of surgical practice and as a set of therapeutic maneuvers designed to complement surgical interventions themselves.

Donald S. Gann

vii

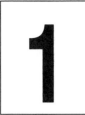

# BASIC PRINCIPLES

'Those who cannot remember the past are condemned to repeat it.'

George Santayana (1863–1952)

## HISTORIC CONCEPTS OF SHOCK

'The theory with the strongest support is that of a toxin causing increased capillary permeability and escape of plasma into the tissues...According to this theory, there might be no essential difference between the effects of toxins given off by damaged tissues and of toxins resulting from the activity of bacteria.'

Walter B. Cannon, 1923

'No conclusive evidence exists that development of an irreversible circulatory state is due to cellular damage which manifests itself by reduced oxygen utilization...There is little evidence of total body leaky capillaries.'

Wiggers, 1950

Over the last one hundred years modern concepts of critical surgical illness have evolved primarily from theories applied to the clinical condition called 'shock'. At the turn of the century severe impairment of the circulation (e.g. hypotension, severe vasoconstriction, thready pulse) was the primary clinical manifestation of shock. Despite recognition that shock appeared to be characteristically a circulatory disorder, etiologies different from hypovolemic or cardiogenic states were considered possible, including disorders of the nervous and endocrine systems and toxemia.

During the first half of the 20th century these theories were extensively investigated by such renowned physiologists as Ernest Starling, George Crile, Walter Cannon, Alfred Blalock and Carl Wiggers. By 1950, two theories were predominant and characterized by the quotes of Cannon and Wiggers above. Cannon argued that shock was associated with a process which resulted in continuing alterations of homeostasis after the circulation was initially restored and suggested that this was secondary to toxins. For instance, Cannon's concept of toxin-induced increased capillary permeability was used to explain ongoing hypovolemic hypoperfusion. Wiggers argued that severe shock resulted primarily in impairment of both the macro- and microcirculation which would continue despite restoration of intravascular volume. This was a disorder of the heart or vascular tree (plugging, etc.) and not secondary to continuing loss of intravascular volume.

Clearly, both Cannon and Wiggers focused attention on the circulatory alterations common to 'shock' as clinically recognized during their respective eras. However, obvious marked impairment of the circulation is not necessarily coexistent with evidence of cellular and organ injury in today's critical care environments. For example, severe inflammation can result in the malfunction of many organs remote from the primary inflammatory site despite an increase in cardiac output and total body oxygen delivery. Therefore, today shock may be more broadly defined as a disease which results in total body cellular malfunction. Using this broader concept of shock Cannon and Wiggers can be considered early advocates of two prevalent and often competing theories of cellular and organ damage in critical care today:

(1) The cells are not receiving enough oxygen – Wiggers;

(2) The cells are suffering from toxic injury – Cannon.

**CURRENT CONCEPTS**

The last several years of experimental and clinical investigation have demonstrated that both inadequate oxygen supply and toxic injury are present in most forms of shock. The primary toxins are not exogenous, but endogenous – the products of tissue injury and inflammation. In essence, both theories about cellular and organ injury are correct and coexistent. Inadequate oxygen delivery begets inflammation and inflammation begets hypoperfusion (Table 1).

The effects of inadequate oxygen delivery (usually from a poor circulation) and severe inflammation on cellular function can be very similar. For instance, both can result in an elevated level of lactic acid and the production of a circulating protein which interferes with cellular function sufficiently to cause membrane depolarization. Therefore, trying to separate these processes is artificial and is like trying to argue that light is either a particle or a wave. As a consequence, the best understanding and management of critical illness – disease that can cause cellular malfunction, organ malfunction and death – requires knowledge and knowledge-based manipulations of both the circulatory and inflammatory manifestations of the disease.

Unfortunately, these manifestations are often complex and difficult to understand and manipulate. This is particularly true of inflammation,

## TABLE 1   RELATIONSHIP BETWEEN INADEQUATE OXYGEN DELIVERY AND INFLAMMATION – EXAMPLES

*Inadequate oxygen supply begets inflammation*
Ischemia/reperfusion
Activated PMNs during hemorrhagic shock
Elevated IL-1, TNF after hemorrhagic shock

*Inflammation begets hypoperfusion*
Decreased vascular volume
Venous vasodilatation
Myocardial depression
Microvascular alterations

PMN, polymorphonuclear cells; IL, interleukin; TNF, tumor necrosis factor

since inflammation has both beneficial/physiological effects (e.g. removal of dead tissue, defense against microorganisms, healing wounds) and detrimental/pathological effects (impaired circulation, organ malfunction). The clinician must direct efforts for each critically ill patient which attempt to overcome these difficulties and in essence strive to provide an excellent circulation and treat pathological inflammation.

## THE SURGEON IN CRITICAL CARE

### The surgical trainee in critical care
The trainee in surgical critical care characteristically proceeds through three phases in achieving competence in the primary goals of surgical critical care listed above. The first phase is exemplified by the question 'where is the hole?'. This refers to the early encounters of a trainee with a patient who is usually suddenly ill and trainee efforts are undertaken to define the primary, sometimes life-threatening, organ alteration which needs immediate attention (Table 2). For instance, sudden hypotension after major abdominal surgery might prompt questions about hypovolemia, anesthetics and myocardial infarction.

The next trainee question is 'how do I plug the hole?' (Table 2). Asking this the trainee who has decided that the hypotension is from hypovolemia questions the type and amount of intravenous fluid to administer.

The third and most important question is 'why is the hole there?' (Table 2). This question is best answered when knowledge of the surgical disease and surgical procedure(s) is present and, therefore, is often a question that has an impact on surgical decision making. Is there an anastomotic leak?

## TABLE 2   THE SURGICAL TRAINEE IN CRITICAL CARE
## EXAMPLES OF QUESTION-RELATED PROBLEMS

*Where is the hole?*
Hypotension
Respiratory distress
Oliguria
Fever
Mental status change

*How do I plug the hole?*
Intravenous fluid
Packed red blood cells
Inotropes
Ventilator
Diuretics
Sedatives

*Why is the hole there?*
Bleeding
Infection
Missed intra-abdominal injury
Anastomotic leak
Pulmonary embolism
Myocardial infarction

Is there an ischemic left colon? Attention to questions like these, more than the supportive measures encompassed by 'where is the hole?' and 'how do I plug the hole?', is the most important determinant of outcome for surgical patients.

### The practicing surgeon

In essence every practicing surgeon is faced with managing disease in keeping with the primary goals of surgical critical care. Trauma, burns, intestinal hemorrhage, intestinal perforation and pancreatitis are common examples of disease states for which providing an excellent circulation and treating pathological inflammation are crucial for good outcome. The fundamentals of good surgical care – resuscitation of the circulation, debridement of dead tissue, drainage of infection and minimizing surgical trauma all diminish the risk of cellular injury and organ malfunction.

However, it is often difficult for practicing surgeons to maintain current knowledge of advances in monitoring and technology which provide more information and sometimes enhanced management of the 'how do I plug the hole?' issues of critical care. In addition, the practicing surgeon may not encounter critically ill patients with sufficient frequency immediately to recognize how a problem with the circulation or respiration may relate to the underlying surgical disease or procedure. In essence, the practicing surgeon may have difficulty answering 'why is the hole there?' for some of his/her patients.

### The Clinical Handbook for Surgical Critical Care

The purpose of this guide is to assist the surgical/critical care trainee as well as the practicing surgeon with all three questions related to surgical critical care and to emphasize the question 'why is the hole there?'. This guide is not designed to be a cook book or quick reference for dosing of medicines or the technical aspects of critical care (i.e. line placement, fine tuning ventilator therapy). Rather, this guide should be used to review and contrast organ physiology during normal and pathological states. This is a guide for the recognition of pathophysiological states which relate to surgical disease and procedures, a guide to help answer 'why is the hole there?'.

Since much of surgical critical illness is secondary to either an inadequate circulation or pathological inflammation, or both, these topics will begin the guide and will be given special consideration in each subsequent Chapter, as appropriate. Particular attention will be given to the recognition of an inadequate circulation and pathological inflammation associated with particular disease states.

At the close of the 20th century there has been a melding of concepts of shock which allow for consolidation rather than continuing separation of theories. Yes, history is being repeated, but critical care physicians and surgeons should not feel condemned but rather optimistic that this consolidation will lead to better understanding of disease and patient outcome.

# 2

# THE CIRCULATION

## CARDIOVASCULAR PHYSIOLOGY

### Oxygen delivery and consumption

Oxygen delivery to cells is vital for most cell survival and constitutes the major function of the cardiopulmonary organ system. Oxygen demands are often increased in critical surgical illness. Before discussing the cardiovascular component of oxygen delivery, a description of oxygen movement at the capillary and cellular level as well as oxygen affinity for hemoglobin will be presented.

*Blood flow and diffusion*

Capillaries are so readily permeable to oxygen that movement of oxygen across the capillary is limited only by the rate of perfusion rather than diffusion. Oxygen enters the capillary at a $Po_2$ and hemoglobin saturation close to arterial levels (some is lost in arterioles) and diminishes exponentially as the distance along the capillary lengthens. The drop in $Po_2$ and saturation is dependent upon the length of the capillary and the rate of oxygen extraction by the cells supplied by the capillary.

The diffusion of oxygen from the capillaries to the cells is indirectly proportional to the distance of the cells from the capillaries. Therefore, an increase in the interstitial space may diminish oxygen concentration at the cellular level. However, mitochondria can function with a $Po_2$ in excess of only 0.1 mmHg ($Po_2$ is the partial pressure of oxygen in a solution or in a gas). Thus, mitochondrial hypoxia is more likely a function of little oxygen getting to capillaries (diminished perfusion) rather than diminished diffusion.

At the capillary level oxygen release from hemoglobin is an important aspect of oxygen transfer to the interstitium and, subsequently, to the cells. The relationship between hemoglobin saturation and oxygen tension is described by the oxyhemoglobin saturation curve (Figure 1). The position of the oxyhemoglobin dissociation curve along the horizontal axis is described by the $P_{50}$ value, the oxygen tension necessary to saturate 50% of the hemoglobin (normal 27 mmHg). The shape of the curve illustrates that little oxygen is released when $Po_2$ drops at the higher level (60–100 mmHg), but much is released at levels which develop in the capillary circulation (30–50mmHg). A shift of the oxyhemoglobin curve to the right (an increase in the $P_{50}$) results in more oxygen release (less oxygen affinity), whereas a shift to the left results in less oxygen release.

Factors which cause right and left shift are listed in Table 1. 2,3-diphosphoglycerate, a product of erythrocyte glycolysis, is a major determinant and is directly proportional to hemoglobin–oxygen affinity.

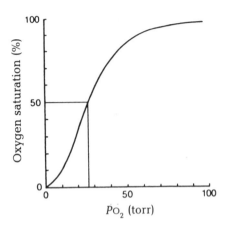

**Figure 1** Characteristic oxyhemoglobin saturation curve ($P_{50}$ = 26.6 torr)

**TABLE 1   FACTORS ALTERING HEMOGLOBIN–OXYGEN AFFINITY (adapted from Sibbald WJ. Myocardial function in the critically ill: factors influencing left and right ventricular performance in patients with sepsis and trauma. *Surg Clin N Am* 1985;65:867–93)**

| *Decreased affinity* | *Increased affinity* |
| --- | --- |
| Decreased pH | Increased pH |
| Increased temperature | Decreased temperature |
| Increased $P_{CO_2}$ | Decreased $P_{CO_2}$ |
| Increased 2,3-diphosphoglycerate | Decreased 2,3-diphosphoglycerate |
| thyroid hormone | hypothyroidism |
| increased organic phosphate | decreased organic phosphate |
| red cell age (young) | red cell age (old) |
| cortisol | |
| Aldosterone | Carboxyhemoglobin |
| | Methemoglobin |

2,3-diphosphoglycerate is diminished in stored red blood cells and more than 24 h may be needed before transfused blood regains normal levels. Low serum inorganic phosphate levels result in 2,3-diphosphoglycerate depletion. Importantly, hypothermia and metabolic alkalosis, commonly seen in critically ill surgical patients, increase hemoglobin oxygen affinity.

Therefore, the use of fresh red cells, providing inorganic phosphate intravenously, reversing hypothermia and correcting metabolic alkalosis may all improve oxygen delivery to the cells.

The main function of the cardiovascular system is to deliver oxygen to the capillaries. The determinants of total body oxygen delivery are listed with other commonly measured or calculated hemodynamic variables in Table 2. The pulmonary component is limited to providing adequate arterial oxygen saturation ( $\geq$ 90% at $Pao_2$ >60 mmHg). This is usually readily achieved with modern respiratory therapy. Hemoglobin is frequently increased with transfusion. Often the most difficult component to treat is cardiac output. The determinants of cardiac output can be organized both by the variables which affect ventricular function and the variables which affect venous return. Depending on clinical circumstances, the logical application of one such physiology ('physiologic') may be more suitable than the other, as described below.

**Ventricular physiology**
The major determinants of ventricular performance are preload, afterload, contractility and heart rate. Preload represents the magnitude of myocardial stretch, the stimulus to muscle contraction described by the Frank–Starling mechanism (Figure 2) whereby increased stretch leads to increased contraction until the muscle is overstretched. Preload is most appropriately measured as end-diastolic volume (EDV). Since volume is not easily measured clinically, the direct proportion between ventricular volume and ventricular end-diastolic pressure (EDP) allows pressure measurement to estimate volume. However, the pressure–volume relationship (compliance) may change and make pressure measurements difficult to interpret (see Confounding variables; page 18).

Ventricular afterload is determined primarily by the resistance to ventricular ejection present in either the pulmonary (pulmonary vascular resistance – PVR) or systemic arterial tree (systemic vascular resistance – SVR). With constant preload increased afterload diminishes ventricular ejection, decreased afterload augments ejection (Figure 3).

Contractility represents the force of contraction under conditions of a predetermined preload and/or afterload. Factors which increase contractility include catecholamines, inotropic drugs, increased preload and decreased afterload. Factors which decrease contractility include catecholamine depletion/receptor malfunction, $\alpha$- and $\beta$-blockers, calcium channel blockers, decreased preload, overstretching of myocardium, increased afterload and severe inflammation and/or ischemia. A change in

**TABLE 2   HEMODYNAMIC AND OXYGEN DELIVERY VARIABLES**

| | Definition | Normal |
|---|---|---|
| Central venous presure (CVP) | CVP = RAP; in the absence of tricuspid valve disease, CVP = RVEDP | 5–15 mmHg |
| Left atrial pressure (LAP) | in the absence of mitral valve disease, LAP = LVEDP | 5–15 mmHg |
| Pulmonary capillary wedge pressure (PCWP) | PCWP = LAP, except sometimes with high PEEP levels | 5–15 mmHg |
| Mean arterial pressure (MAP) | $MAP = DP + \frac{1}{3}(SP - DP)$ | 80–90 mmHg |
| Cardiac index (CI) | $CI = CO/m^2$ BSA | $2.5–3.5$ l min$^{-1}$ m$^{-2}$ BSA |
| Stroke index (SI) | $SI = SV/m^2$ BSA | $35–40$ ml beat$^{-1}$ m$^{-2}$ BSA |
| Systemic vascular resistance (SVR) | $SVR = \dfrac{(MAP - CVP) \times 80}{CO}$ | 1000–1500 dyne-sec/cm$^5$ |
| Pulmonary vascular resistance (PVR) | $PVR = \dfrac{(MAP - PCWP) \times 80}{CO}$ | 100–400 dyne-sec/cm$^5$ |
| Arterial oxygen content (Ca$o_2$) | $Cao_2 = 1.39 \times Hgb \times Sao_2 + (Pao_2 \times 0.0031)$ | 20 vol% |
| Mixed venous oxygen content (C$\bar{v}o_2$) | $C\bar{v}o_2 = 1.39 \times Hgb \times S\bar{v}o_2 + (P\bar{v}o_2 \times 0.0031)$ | 15 vol% |
| Arterial venous oxygen content difference C(a – $\bar{v}o_2$) | $C(a - \bar{v})o_2 = Cao_2 - C\bar{v}o_2$(vol%) | 3.5–4.5 vol% |
| Oxygen delivery (O$_2$D) | $O_2D = CO \times Cao_2 \times 10$; 10 = factor to convert ml O$_2$/100 ml blood to ml O$_2$/l blood | 900–1200 ml/min |
| Oxygen consumption (O$_2$C) | $O_2C = (Cao_2 - C\bar{v}o_2) \times CO \times 10$ | 250 ml/min 130–160 ml min$^{-1}$ m$^{-2}$ |

BSA, body surface area (m$^2$); CO, cardiac output; DP, diastolic pressure; Hgb, hemoglobin (g/dl); LVEDP, left ventricular end-diastolic pressure; Pa$o_2$, arterial P$o_2$ (mmHg); P$\bar{v}o_2$, mixed venous P$o_2$ (mmHg); PEEP, positive end-expiratory pressure; RAP, right atrial pressure; RVEDP, right ventricular end-diastolic pressure; Sa$o_2$, arterial oxygen saturation (%); S$\bar{v}o_2$, mixed venous oxygen saturation; SP, systolic pressure; SV, stroke volume; PCWP also called pulmonary artery occlusion pressure (PAOP)

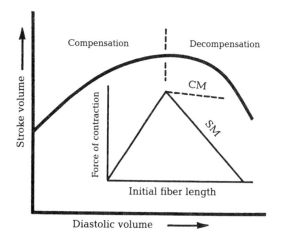

**Figure 2** Schematic diagram of Starling's law of the heart – the cardiac function curve. The inset demonstrates the difference between cardiac muscle (CM) and skeletal muscle (SM), where CM does not decompensate as rapidly with increasing stretch. Reproduced with permission from Burton, AC. *Physiology and Biophysics of the Circulation: An Introductory Text*, edn. 2. Chicago; Year Book Medical Publishers Inc., 1972

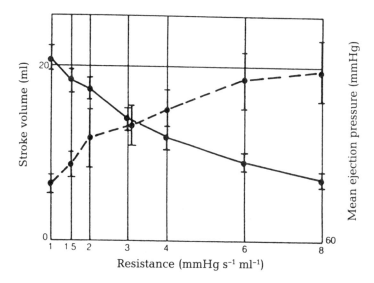

**Figure 3** The decrease in stroke volume (solid line) develops secondary to an increase in resistance (dashed line). Reproduced with permission from Rankin JC. Hemodynamics Management. In Wilmore DW, Cheung LY, Harken AH, *et al.*, eds. *Scientific American Surgery*. New York: Scientific American, Inc., 1988

contractility, like a change in afterload, will result in a different cardiac function curve (Figure 4). The combined influence of increasing contractility and decreasing afterload to improve ventricular function is illustrated in Figure 5.

Heart rate is directly proportional to cardiac output (not cardiac muscle mechanics *per se*) until rapid rates diminish ventricular filling during diastole.

### Right and left ventricular differences

The differences in the structure and position of the right and left ventricles can influence the relative importance of each of the determinants of ventricular function listed above. For instance, the thin-walled more compliant right ventricle has less contractile reserve than the left. When confronted with increased afterload the right ventricle more easily dilates and increasingly depends upon preload to augment function. If this continues, the right ventricle eventually fails (output decreases as preload increases) and the left ventricle may consequently suffer from diminished preload from poor right ventricular output and diminished volume from leftward shift of the interventricular septum.

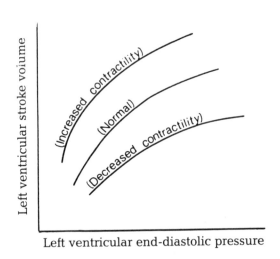

Left ventricular end-diastolic pressure

**Figure 4** Schematic representation of the cardiac function curve with different contractility states. Reproduced with permission from Willis Hurst J, Schlant RC, eds. *The Heart, Arteries and Veins*, 7th edn. New York: McGraw-Hill Information Services Co., Health Professions Division, 1990

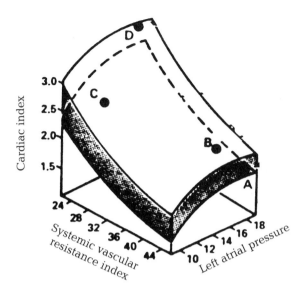

**Figure 5** Schematic representation of the effects of inotrope (dopamine) administration and afterload reduction (nitroprusside) on cardiac index. Note that afterload reduction also reduced preload and that augmentation of preload further increased cardiac index. A, control; B, dopamine; C, dopamine and nitroprusside; D, dopamine and nitroprusside and preload restoration. Reproduced with permission from Miller DC, *et al.* Postoperative enhancement of left ventricular performance by combined inotropic-vasodilator therapy with preload control. *Surgery* 1980;88:108–16

### Vascular resistance

The relationship between cardiac output and circulatory pressure is described by the formulae for systemic and pulmonary vascular resistance shown in Table 2. Resistance to flow in the systemic and pulmonary artery systems resides mostly in the arteriolar region. This is distinctly different from the venous system where resistance is primarily located in the large veins in the thorax and abdomen.

Arterial vascular resistance is the most common afterload against which the right and left ventricles must eject. As will be illustrated in further sections, calculation and manipulation of vascular resistance can greatly assist hemodynamic management in critically ill surgical patients. Common conditions which increase systemic vascular resistance include hypovolemia, congestive heart failure (CHF), cardiogenic shock, very severe inflammation, hypocapnia and vasoconstrictors. Those which decrease systemic vascular resistance include inflammation, spinal shock, anaphylaxis, hypercapnia and vasodilators. Factors which increase pulmonary vascular resistance include hypoxia, hypercapnia, chronic obstructive pulmonary disease (COPD), bronchospasm, pulmonary edema, inflammation, pulmonary embolism, pulmonary contusion, pneumonia, pneumothorax and positive end-expiratory pressure (PEEP). Vasodilators decrease pulmonary vascular resistance. It should be noted that disease may have variable effects upon the systemic circulation but almost always increases pulmonary resistance.

**Venous return**
While the term venous return is used commonly in clinical medicine, the determinants of venous return are rarely understood despite descriptions dating back to Starling in 1897. More recently Guyton has documented the physiological principles of venous return. As will be emphasized, in surgical patients the 'physio-logic' of augmenting venous return may be more frequently applicable for improving cardiac output than the physiological approach to improving ventricular function.

Venous return (VR) is described by the following formula:

$$VR = \frac{MSP - CVP}{RV + RA/19}$$

where MSP is mean systemic pressure, CVP is central venous pressure (right atrial pressure), RV is venous resistance and RA is arterial resistance. MSP is not mean arterial pressure. MSP is the pressure in small veins and venules which must be higher in the periphery than CVP so that blood can flow from the periphery to the thorax. Venous resistance is located primarily in the large veins in the abdomen and thorax. Arterial resistance is located mostly in the arterioles. Factors that alter venous return variables are listed in Table 3. It is evident from this list that surgical patients frequently have diseases or therapeutic interventions which may inhibit venous return.

**Physical examination of the circulation**
For the surgeon, examination of the cardiovascular system (observing or measuring the parameters listed in Table 4) is used primarily to assess total body and regional blood flow as well as the most likely etiology of diminished perfusion, when present.

## TABLE 3   FACTORS ALTERING VENOUS RETURN VARIABLES

*Increased venous return*
Increased MSP
   increased vascular volume
   increased vascular tone
   external compression
   Trendelenburg position (increased MSP in lower extremities and
      abdomen)
Decreased CVP
   hypovolemia
   negative pressure respiration
Decreased venous resistance
   decreased venous constriction
   negative pressure respiration

*Diminished venous return*
Decreased MSP
   hypovolemia
   vasodilatation
Increased CVP
   intracardiac
      CHF
      cardiogenic shock
      tricuspid regurgitation
      right heart failure
   extracardiac
      positive pressure respiration
      PEEP
      tension pneumothorax
      cardiac tamponade
      increased abdominal pressure
Increased venous resistance
  increased thoracic pressure
     positive pressure respiration
     PEEP
     increased abdominal pressure
     tension pneumothorax
  increased abdominal pressure
     ascites
     bowel distension

*(continued over)*

### TABLE 3 (continued)

tension pneumoperitoneum
intra-abdominal hemorrhage
retroperitoneal hemorrhage

MSP, mean systemic pressure; CVP, central venous pressure; CHF, congestive heart failure; PEEP, positive end-expiratory pressure

### TABLE 4   CARDIOVASCULAR PHYSICAL EXAMINATION

*Assessment of total body perfusion*
Blood pressure
Pulse
Mentation
Skin color and temperature
Neck veins
Heart examination
Urine output

*Assessment of regional (extremity) perfusion*
Pulse
Color
Temperature
Pain
Movement

*Total body perfusion*
Low blood pressure usually indicates hypoperfusion. However, blood pressure may be normal or elevated in the face of hypoperfusion with such conditions as hypovolemia, CHF, hypothermia and in patients with underlying hypertension. In addition, hypotension may be present in the face of normal or augmented perfusion such as occurs in severe inflammation or spinal cord injury. Tachycardia is a more sensitive indicator of hypoperfusion but is less specific and can be present from a variety of other causes (i.e. anxiety, pain, temperature elevation). With mild to moderate hypoperfusion patients often become restless and agitated, pulling at restraints, intravenous lines and nasogastric tubes. With severe hypoperfusion obtundation and coma may result. Most commonly hypoperfusion stimulates a neuroendocrine response which results in peripheral vasoconstriction and consequently pale to cyanotic and cold extremities. Skin covering the patella is particularly sensitive to hypoperfusion and vaso-

constriction and resulting 'purple knee caps' may be an early clinical sign. Distended neck veins usually indicate significant impairment of cardiac function, but not always CHF or cardiogenic shock. Central venous pressure may be elevated by pressure exerted outside the lumen of the right atrium (tension pneumothorax, pericardial tamponade).

Examination of the heart should focus on the quality of heart sounds (diminished sounds may represent pericardial fluid or shift of the mediastinum) and presence or absence of a gallop. Distinguishing an S3 gallop from an S4 may be difficult, especially with tachycardia. The distinction is important, however, since an S4 is common in patients aged 50 years and over and an S3 is quite specific but not very sensitive for a failing left ventricle. Urine output greater than 0.5 ml/kg/h is usually considered an indication of adequate total body perfusion. Unfortunately, as described in the 'Confounding variables' section of this Chapter, even this clinical tool must be evaluated with caution. Examination of the lungs and the extremities for evidence of edema is not specific for cardiac dysfunction. As will be emphasized later, in critical surgical illness total body salt and water excess are commonly associated with normo- or hypovolemia. Under these circumstances relying on the lung or the periphery to make decisions about cardiac function can be dangerously misleading.

*Regional perfusion*
Physical examination evidence of regional hypoperfusion is limited primarily to the extremities. A painful, pale, pulseless, paralyzed and cold extremity with paraesthesias is diagnostic of acute arterial insufficiency. Chronic arterial insufficiency demonstrates loss of pulse, hair loss, dependent rubor and sometimes loss of muscle mass. Acute venous obstruction, particularly in the iliofemoral region, may also cause decreased extremity perfusion. The lower extremity may be edematous and white (phlegmasia alba dolens) with little arterial compromise, or edematous and blue (phlegmasia cerulea dolens) with increased muscular pressure sufficient to diminish arterial circulation and cause tissue necrosis, often resulting in skin with fluid-filled bullae.

Physical examination alone is rarely sufficient to evaluate precisely other types of regional hypoperfusion (cerebral, gastrointestinal) but can contribute greatly to the overall clinical evaluation. For instance, evidence of sudden neurological deficit consistent with middle cerebral artery occlusion or an unremarkable abdominal examination coexistent with severe abdominal pain may lead to the diagnosis of cerebral and intestinal infarction, respectively.

## HEMODYNAMIC MONITORING

The purpose of hemodynamic monitoring is to measure the cardiovascular variables which help assess the adequacy of the circulation, the etiology of an inadequate circulation, and the effect of therapeutic interventions. In this section emphasis will be placed on the fundamentals of commonly used hemodynamic monitors, the confounding variables which make a monitor difficult to interpret, methods of reducing confusion, complications of monitoring equipment, and selection of patients for increasing complexity of hemodynamic monitoring. No technical details of monitor placement or use will be presented, except as related to complications.

### Physical examination

Hemodynamic monitoring begins with the basic physical examination described above. Usually some common clinical parameter (e.g. hypotension, tachycardia, vasoconstriction, agitation, diminished urine output) is the first clue that the circulation is inadequate.

### Continuous electrocardiographic (ECG) monitoring

Continuous ECG monitoring to record heart rate and indicate arrhythmias is the simplest and most frequently used hemodynamic monitor after non-invasive blood pressure and pulse determinations.

### Measurement of arterial pressure

Arterial catheterization is often used to supplement non-invasive blood-pressure cuff measurements allowing constant monitoring and ease of blood sampling. Under normal conditions the aortic pressure pulse is altered as the aortic root pressure is transmitted to the peripheral arteries, producing a small increase in systolic pressure and decrease in diastolic pressure. Most often the radial and femoral arteries are used, more rarely the dorsalis pedis arteries, and result in a lower pressure measurement than the aortic root. This may be less so with femoral cannulation, but severe vasoconstriction impeding peripheral pulses is hardly of less concern if a higher pressure is recorded in a larger vessel.

Usually cannulation is accomplished percutaneously, but occasionally a cutdown is required. While radial artery cannulation is most common, femoral artery cannulation appears to be safe and provide accurate information.

## Measurement of venous pressures

The measurement of central venous and pulmonary venous pressure is commonly used to estimate right and left atrial pressure, respectively. In the absence of obstruction (superior vena cava syndrome) superior vena cava pressure (CVP) equals mean right atrial pressure (RAP) which, in the absence of tricuspid valve disease, equals right ventricular end-diastolic pressure (RVEDP). Similarly, in the absence of pulmonary venous obstruction (high alveolar pressure with PEEP, pulmonary veno-occlusive disease) the pressure obtained by inflating the balloon on the end of a flow directed pulmonary artery catheter (Figure 6), referred to as the pulmonary artery occlusion pressure (PAOP) or pulmonary capillary wedge pressure (PCWP), equals mean left atrial pressure (LAP), which in the absence of mitral valve disease equals left ventricular end-diastolic pressure (LVEDP). Therefore, in most patients CVP and PAOP measure right and left ventricular filling pressures. As described in 'Ventricular physiology' these pressures are directly proportional to end-diastolic volume (EDV) and, therefore, provide an indirect measure of ventricular preload and a direct measure of the pressure within the lumen of the superior vena cava and pulmonary capillaries. Ranges of normal and representative abnormal values for CVP and PAOP are presented in Table 5.

In patients with normal cardiac function CVP and PAOP are equal and equivalent to LAP. However, acute and chronic heart and pulmonary disease may not only interfere with the relationship of atrial pressures to VEDP but can also make CVP and PAOP unequal, sometimes changing in opposite directions. Disease likely to manifest a LAP not equal to CVP includes:

(1) Acute left-sided myocardial infarct;

(2) Disease with an ejection fraction of <50%;

(3) Mitral or tricuspid regurgitation;

(4) Pulmonary embolism;

(5) Tension pneumothorax;

(6) Early pericardial tamponade.

Thus in patients with known significant cardiac or pulmonary disease simultaneous measurement of right and left ventricular filling pressure is most useful and is usually achieved by placing the flow directed pulmonary artery catheter percutaneously.

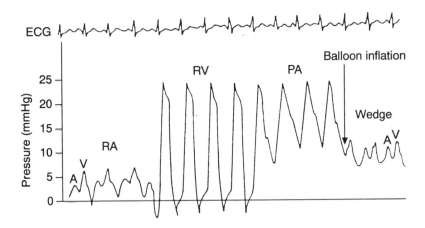

**Figure 6** A representation of the pressure tracing as a balloon-tipped pulmonary artery catheter is passed from the right atrium (RA), through the right ventricle (RV) and into the pulmonary artery (PA). Further advancement results in the 'wedge' or PA occlusion pressure waveform depicted. Note that this wave is not flat, but with atrial and ventricular contraction will exhibit an 'A' and a 'V' wave. Adapted with permission from Voyce SJ, Rippe JM. Pulmonary artery catheters: an update. *J Intens Care Med* 1990;5:175–92

### TABLE 5   REPRESENTATIVE VALUES OF VENOUS PRESSURES (mmHg)

|  | *CVP* | *LAP (PAOP)* |
|---|---|---|
| Normovolemia | 5–15 | 5–15 |
| Hypovolemia | <5 | <5 |
| Hypervolemia | >18 | >18 |

CVP, central venous pressure; LAP, left atrial pressure; PAOP, pulmonary artery occlusion pressure

### Cardiac output measurement

Cardiac output can be easily measured using the same pulmonary artery catheter which measures pulmonary artery pressures and PAOP. The principle of indicator dilution is used in a similar fashion to that used to measure static physiological volumes (blood volume, extracellular fluid volume) except that cardiac output is a time-dependent variable which must, then, include time in the measurement. For example, to measure a static volume (V) a known amount of indicator (I) can be mixed in the volume and the concentration of I (C) measured. V then equals I/C = I/I/V. In a time-dependent system a known amount of I, such as indocyanine green or temperature, is mixed into a time dependent volume, Q(t), and results in a time-dependent concentration, C(t). The measurement of concentration of the indicator as a function of time is depicted in Figure 7 where the indicator is a change in temperature. To calculate Q the mean of the measured concentration must be determined by the mean value theorem such that:

$$\text{mean } C(t) = \frac{\text{the integral of } C(t) \text{ dt from time 0 to time T}}{T}$$

$$Q(t) = I/\text{mean } C(t)$$

The same concept is used with the thermodilution technique. Therefore, using an 'amount' of cold injected into the right atrium which mixes with the blood in the right ventricle and pulmonary artery, the 'concentration' of cold is measured by the thermistor at the end of the pulmonary artery catheter. The integration of this time-dependent concentration and division into the amount of cold is automatically accomplished by the computer supplied with the pulmonary artery catheter. The correlation between thermodilution cardiac output and indocyanine green indicator dilution is excellent ($r = 0.99$).

### Measurement of oxygen delivery and utilization
Placement of a pulmonary artery catheter not only allows measurement of cardiac output, but also of mixed venous blood gases, which along with

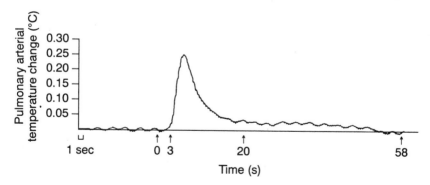

**Figure 7** A typical indicator dilution curve which can be used to calculate cardiac output. Adapted with permission from Weisel RD, Berger RL, Hechtman HB. Current concepts: measurement of cardiac output by thermodilation. *N Engl J Med* 1975;292:682–4

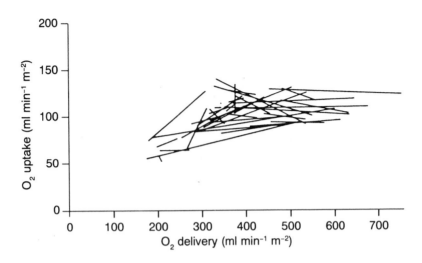

**Figure 8** The relationship between oxygen consumption and delivery is plotted here, demonstrating the variety of results possible in individual patients. Patients with increasing consumption as delivery increases may be considered to require more oxygen delivery. Patients who demonstrate no increase or a decrease in oxygen consumption as delivery increases do not require more oxygen delivery. Adapted with permission from Shibutani K, *et al.* Critical level of oxygen delivery in anesthetized man. *Critical Care Med* 1983;11:641

arterial blood gases and hemoglobin allow for calculation of oxygen delivery and oxygen consumption (Table 2). Since many disease states either diminish oxygen delivery or increase oxygen consumption, a plot of the relationship between delivery and consumption may be a more useful indication of the need for further hemodynamic interventions than the absolute value of these variables (Figure 8). Optimization of oxygen delivery may be considered present when an increase in oxygen delivery results in no further oxygen use. This concept has resulted in considerable controversy in patient management.

*Continuous measurement of mixed venous oxygen saturation*
Continuous measurement of mixed venous oxygen saturation (venous oximetry, $S\bar{v}o_2$) with a photometric sensor on the end of a pulmonary artery catheter has been described as an indicator of the interaction of oxygenation by the lungs, perfusion by the heart and total body oxygen

consumption. Therefore, a significant fall in $S\bar{v}o_2$ could occur from a deterioration in lung and/or cardiac function, or an increase in oxygen consumption. Most studies demonstrate that decreased $S\bar{v}o_2$ is secondary to diminished cardiac output. However, in critically ill surgical patients $S\bar{v}o_2$ appears to correlate best with the ratio of oxygen consumption to oxygen delivery, the 'oxygen utilization coefficient', rather than cardiac output. Since critical surgical illness is frequently associated with increased oxygen consumption (trauma and severe inflammation) as compared to medical illness (heart and lung disease), which more commonly produces decreased delivery, the importance of oxygen use as a determinant of $S\bar{v}o_2$ in surgical patients is easily comprehended.

### Non-invasive tissue $Po_2$ monitoring

Except for standard vital sign measurements and physical examination, the hemodynamic monitors described above are all invasive. Non-invasive monitoring is preferred, especially if as useful as the invasive devices.

Since development in 1954, the polarographic $Po_2$ electrode has been most useful in the transcutaneous measurement of skin $Po_2$ ($Ptco_2$) and conjunctival $Po_2$ ($Pcjo_2$). Skin and conjunctival $Po_2$ is, in general, determined by two variables: skin perfusion and arterial $Po_2$. Skin perfusion is dependent on the total body perfusion, body temperature, regional perfusion and degree of cutaneous vasoconstriction. $Ptco_2$ requires a heated sensor to penetrate the effects of keratinized skin and must be repositioned periodically to prevent burns. In addition, 10 min are needed for stabilization of the device. For this reason $Pcjo_2$ has been used where the lack of keratin allows oxygen tension measurement without heating and delay. $Ptco_2$ is more useful for assessing regional hypoperfusion (i.e. pre- and postoperative monitoring of vascular reconstruction, assessing traumatic vascular injury). Since the face is usually well perfused, $Pcjo_2$ appears useful as a measure of total body perfusion and parallels tissue oxygen tension in brain, kidney, intestine and skin.

Similar to measuring mixed venous oxygen saturation, the determinants of $Ptco_2$ and $Pcjo_2$ may differ depending on the experimental study or patient population evaluated. For instance, in graded experimental hemorrhage $Pcjo_2$ diminished significantly before a significant drop in oxygen delivery. In critically ill patients, however, $Ptco_2$ correlated best with arterial $Po_2$ and showed less dependence on oxygen delivery.

In summary, the multitude of variables which affect non-invasive measurement of skin or conjunctival oxygen tension relegates these instruments to early warning devices which can also assess the response to therapy. However, they cannot predict precisely which physiological parameter needs adjustment.

*Non-invasive arterial oxygen saturation measurement*
Pulsed oximetry is a non-invasive method of measuring arterial oxygen saturation ($Sao_2$). Rather than measure $Po_2$ with an electrode, as in $Ptco_2$ measurements, the percentage of oxygen saturation is measured by photometric techniques. After empirical calibration with the saturation from an arterial sample the oximeter has been shown to predict well $Sao_2$ in hemodynamically stable patients and critically ill children. The relationship of non-invasive oximetry to changes in hemodynamics has been variable, with one study demonstrating a relationship to blood pressure rather than cardiac output.

As with $Ptco_2$ determination, pulsed oximetry is primarily useful as an early warning device for hypoxemia but cannot precisely distinguish the etiology.

**Confounding variables**
Each of the hemodynamic monitors described above can provide misleading information because of improper technique, inadequate experience with the device, or because of physiological changes which make the information difficult to interpret. This section will cover the common confounding variables in hemodynamic monitoring and suggest methods to diminish confusion.

*Physical examination*
In critical illness, physical examination and other clinical information are often inadequate to predict measured hemodynamic variables. For instance, a common error is to misinterpret the physical examination information suggesting total body salt and water excess (evidence of peripheral and pulmonary edema and weight gain) as evidence that intravascular volume is in excess (i.e. presence of CHF). Therefore, other monitoring techniques are often used to assess the circulation. Unfortunately, just like physical examination, these tools are not immune to artifacts or misinterpretation.

*Arterial pressure monitoring*
As mentioned previously, severe peripheral vasoconstriction may lower pressures measured in the radial or dorsalis pedis arteries compared to pressures measured in the femoral or more proximal vessels. Even if the

more proximal pressure is higher, vasoconstriction of this magnitude usually denotes significant hypoperfusion which requires intervention. Such physiological reasons for a significant discrepancy between aortic pressure and more peripheral pressures are rare and a normal arterial pressure tracing sufficiently well understood that artifactual alterations in a pressure tracing (e.g. plugged catheter, position related dampening of the signal) are usually readily recognized by the critical care team.

### Venous pressure monitoring

In contrast to arterial pressure monitoring, venous pressure monitoring (CVP, PAOP) is subject to many confounding variables, including: the lack of recognition of proper waveform, disregard for unphysiological relationship between monitored variables, diminished ventricular compliance and increased intrathoracic pressure (Table 6).

*Lack of recognition of proper waveform* A normal right and left atrial pressure tracing demonstrates an increase in pressure corresponding to atrial contraction (A wave) followed by a second increase secondary to ventricular contraction (Figure 9). Catheters placed in the large thoracic veins and the occluded pulmonary artery should also demonstrate this picture, although commonly with some damping compared to atrial placement. CVP and PAOP should not be flat lines. With loss of atrial

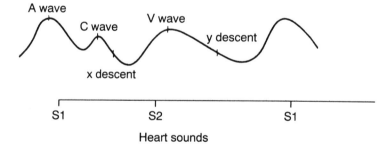

**Figure 9** Schematic representation of atrial waves seen with the pulmonary artery occlusion tracings. The A wave is due to atrial contractions, the V wave represents the pressure generated by venous filling, while the atrial-ventricular valve is closed. The C wave is due to sudden motion of the atrial-ventricular valve ring toward the atrium at the onset of ventricular systole. The x descent follows the A wave and reflects atrial relaxation. The y descent is due to rapid emptying of the atrium following opening of the atrial-ventricular valve. Reproduced with permission from Gore JM, Zwerner PL. Hemodynamic monitoring of acute myocardial infarction. In Alepert JS, Francis GS, eds. *Modern Coronary Care*. Boston: Little, Brown, 1990

## TABLE 6  CONFOUNDING VARIABLES IN VENOUS PRESSURE MONITORING

*Central venous pressure*
Improper position
Inadequate waveform
Changing right ventricular compliance
   afterload
   ischemia
   tension pneumothorax
   PEEP
   tamponade
Increased intrathoracic pressure
   PEEP
   tension pneumothorax
   increased abdominal pressure

*Pulmonary capillary wedge pressure*
Improper placement
   right ventricle
   too peripheral
   lung Zones I and II
Inadequate waveform
Changes in left ventricular compliance
   afterload
   ischemia
   ventricular filling
   tamponade
   hypovolemia
   PEEP
Increased thoracic pressure
   PEEP
   tension pneumothorax
   increased abdominal pressure

PEEP, positive end-expiratory pressure; in lung zone I ventilation (V) > perfusion (P); in lung zone II, V = P

contraction (atrial fibrillation, junctional rhythm), only the C wave will be recognized.

If a flat line is monitored the catheter may not be providing proper information. This is most likely to occur with overinflation of the pulmonary artery catheter balloon ('overwedging'), which usually results in a falsely high number (Figure 10). Confirmation that the balloon-inflated pulmonary artery catheter tip is in proper position can be obtained by aspirating blood from the occluded catheter and obtaining a blood gas. The $Po_2$, $Pco_2$ and pH of the aspirated blood are compared with those variables in an arterial blood sample. If the aspirated blood $Po_2-Pao_2$ difference is $\geq 19$ mmHg; if the $Paco_2$ – the aspirated blood $Pco_2$ is $\geq 11$ mmHg; if the aspirated blood pH – the pH of arterial blood is $\geq 0.08$, and if the aspirated blood saturation >95%, the PAOP is most likely accurate.

*Disregard for the unphysiological relationship between monitored variables*
As stated under 'Ventricular physiology', in patients with normal or good ventricular function (ejection fraction $\geq 50\%$) CVP, LAP and PAOP are similar (within 2 mmHg), if not equal. Patients with discrepancies between right and left atrial pressures should have evidence of previous or acute right or left ventricular dysfunction. Otherwise, the mechanics of the monitoring system (e.g. transducer levels, calibration, line placement) should be checked.

When pulmonary artery pressure is monitored the mean pulmonary artery pressure (PAP) should be at least 8 mmHg greater than the PAOP.

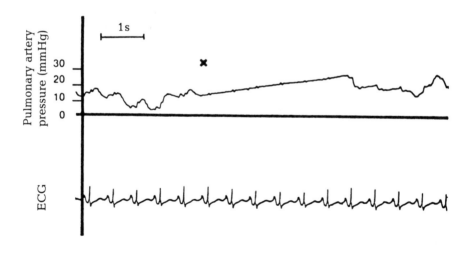

**Figure 10** A representation of the effect of overinflation of the pulmonary artery catheter balloon (X) on the pressure tracing. Characteristically the pressure increases. Reproduced with permission from Quinn K, Quebbeman EJ. Pulmonary artery pressure monitoring in the surgical intensive care unit. *Arch Surgery* 1981;116:872–6

When the PAOP is 8–10 mmHg lower than the PAP, the pulmonary artery diastolic pressure (PAD) will equal the PAOP. As mentioned previously, disease processes increase pulmonary vascular resistance, elevating PAP and PAD more than PAOP. It is unphysiological, therefore, to record a PAP of 25 mmHg and a PAOP of 22 mmHg. Most often this occurs because of poor recognition of the proper PAOP waveform and 'overwedging' the balloon catheter. However, a PAP of 30 mmHg with a PAD of 20 mmHg and a PAOP of 12 mmHg can represent evidence of increased pulmonary vascular resistance without an increase in left ventricular filling pressure. Using the PAD as a measure of ventricular filling pressure may be inaccurate in the many disease states which increase pulmonary vascular resistance.

*Diminished ventricular compliance* As described in 'Ventricular physiology', ventricular filling pressures are used as an indirect measure of ventricular volumes. The relationship between pressure and volume (compliance) is changed by a variety of mechanisms (Table 6). When compliance is diminished (increased afterload, ischemia, increased ventricular volume, pericardial tamponade) little preload (end-diastolic volume) may result in a normal or elevated pressure. Under these circumstances an elevated pressure may not indicate overstretched myocardium (a mechanism of heart failure) and measures used to reduce volume (diuretics) may aggravate hypoperfusion. Therapy should be provided to improve compliance which frequently results in better perfusion at lower pressures (i.e. afterload reduction with vasodilator therapy).

*Increased intrathoracic pressure* Intrathoracic pressure may increase because of increased pressures required for ventilation (especially with PEEP), tension pneumothorax or increased abdominal pressure. Whatever the cause, hemodynamic monitoring devices placed in the thorax will be affected by the extraluminal increase in pressure and record a pressure which represents the sum of intraluminal and extraluminal forces. The transmural pressure (intraluminal pressure–extraluminal pressure) is recognized as a more physiological measure of atrial and ventricular filling pressures. Formulae have been devised to estimate the extraluminal pressure, but recently a simple device (the saline-filled balloon-equipped nasogastric tube) (Figure 11) has been used clinically. Using this tool with increased intrathoracic pressure (application of PEEP), the increase in venous pressures was equalled by the increase in intrathoracic pressure (Figures 12 and 13). The use of such a device can greatly assist the clinical

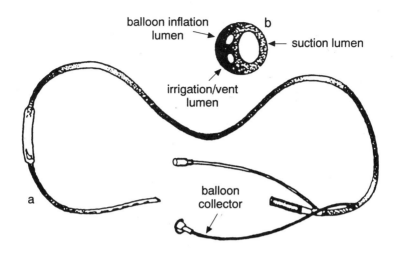

**Figure 11** Diagram of the balloon-equipped nasogastric tube (a), illustrating in cross-section (b) the lumens for suction, irrigation and balloon inflation. Reproduced with permission from Rajacich N, *et al.* Esophageal pressure monitoring: a practical adjuvant to hemodynamic monitoring with positive end-expiratory pressure. *Heart Lung J* 1988;17:483–8

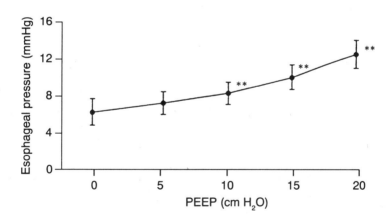

**Figure 12** The increase in esophageal pressure as positive end-expiratory pressure (PEEP) is increased. *$p < 0.05$ from baseline; **$p < 0.01$ from baseline. Reproduced with permission from Rajacich N, *et al.* Esophageal pressure monitoring: a practical adjuvant to hemodynamic monitoring with positive end-expiratory pressure. *Heart Lung J* 1988;17:483–8

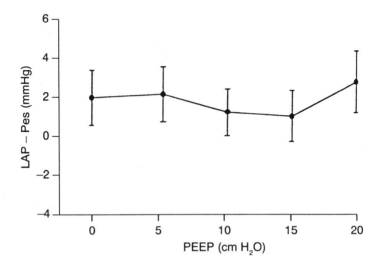

**Figure 13** The subtraction of esophageal pressure (Pes) from left atrial pressure (LAP) as positive end-expiratory pressure (PEEP) is increased demonstrates that the transmural pressure (LAP – Pes) did not change with increasing PEEP. Reproduced with permission from Rajacich N, *et al.* Esophageal pressure monitoring: a practical adjuvant to hemodynamic monitoring with positive end-expiratory pressure. *Heart Lung J* 1988;17:483–8

interpretation of venous pressure monitoring in the presence of increased intrathoracic pressure.

In addition to extraluminal effects, PEEP may produce intraluminal alterations in hemodynamic monitoring. For PAOP to equal LAP, a continuous column of fluid between the pulmonary artery segment occluded by the balloon and the left atrium is required. Because the pulmonary artery catheter is flow directed, the pulmonary artery catheter tip often locates in an area of lung which is well perfused and the continuous column achieved. The lung has been divided into the following three zones dependent on the relationship of ventilation (V) to perfusion (P): Zone I V > P, Zone II V = P, and Zone III V < P. Most often pulmonary artery catheters locate in Zone III. Increased ventilation pressures and diminished cardiac output increase the proportion of Zones I + II to Zone III. Several studies have measured a false elevation in PAOP when PEEP is applied. However, with the pulmonary artery catheter tip in Zone III, little discrepancy can be demonstrated.

*Cardiac output measurement*
The factors which can result in faulty thermodilution cardiac output measurements include temperature of injectate, technique of injection, location of proximal port and low cardiac output. The most common reasons for unsatisfactory cardiac output measurement (variability of greater than 10% in measurements taken within 5 min) is inadequate cooling of the injectate and inconsistency in the speed of injection. A fast injection results in a lower cardiac output (less dilution volume) than a slow injection. If the proximal injection port is near a venous dilator device used for percutaneous insertion, the flow of the injectate may be partially obstructed, resulting in large variations. With cardiac outputs less than 3.5 l/min, and especially less than 2.5 l/min, the thermodilution cardiac output may overestimate simultaneously obtained Fick cardiac output by 35%. (Fick method cardiac output is determined by measuring oxygen consumption and dividing this by the arterial mixed venous oxygen content difference.)

*Urine output*
Urine output may be influenced by physiological and non-physiological variables independent from renal perfusion and glomerular filtration. Osmotic substances such as glucose (commonly excreted in critical illness), vascular contrast agents and mannitol can be the reason for a well-maintained urine output despite poor renal perfusion. Since excellent renal perfusion and the resultant urine output should not result in concentrated urine, a high urine specific gravity (> 1.020) should raise the suspicion of increased osmolality as the cause of a urine output > 0.5 ml/kg/h in a critically ill patient. Similarly, a diuretic can result in increased urine output despite poor renal perfusion. This is beneficial when CHF is the etiology of poor perfusion, but can be detrimental when hypovolemia is the cause.

## Complications

*Arterial lines*
The complications of arterial line insertion include ischemia, infection, pseudoaneurysm and bleeding. Most serious is ischemia to all or part of the hand following radial artery catheterization. Before performing radial artery catheterization adequacy of collateral circulation should be assessed with a properly performed Allen test.

*Venous lines*
The complications of central venous and pulmonary artery catheters include pneumothorax, line infection, hemothorax, tamponade, pleural effusion and central venous thrombosis. Complications associated specifically with pulmonary artery lines include arrythmias, endocarditis, pulmonary infarct. Rupture of a pulmonary artery is a risk primarily in patients with pulmonary hypertension, mitral valve disease, old age, anticoagulation and hypothermia. Certainly the most immediately life-threatening complications are right ventricular arrhythmias and pulmonary hemorrhage. Arrhythmias can usually be controlled by administration of lidocaine or removal of the catheter from the right ventricle. Pulmonary hemorrhage is secondary to rupture of a pulmonary artery or branch from balloon inflation and is seen most often in the at-risk patients mentioned above. Hemoptysis, even of small quantities, may herald this potentially fatal complication. Suspicion of injury may be confirmed by radiographic demonstration of an infiltrate distal to the catheter tip. If hemoptysis is severe the patient should be placed in the lateral decubitus position which places the injured lung down, and preparations should be made for the possibility of emergency pulmonary lobectomy or pneumonectomy. Recently, transpulmonary artery catheter occlusion of the ruptured vessel has been used with success. With this potentially fatal complication in mind, the staff inflating the balloon should use gentle, slow pressure. To diminish inflation in small branches the catheter tip should be positioned in the proximal right or left pulmonary artery.

## Indications for hemodynamic monitoring

*Arterial lines*
The indications for intraoperative and postoperative arterial line insertion include arterial pressure monitoring, arterial blood gas monitoring and access to frequent blood tests. Many anesthesiologists consider constant blood pressure and frequent arterial blood gas determinations essential to proper intraoperative management of patients undergoing major procedures. Certainly, intensive care management of critically ill surgical patients is simplified by arterial access. However, the potential for serious complications must be recognized and arterial line insertion should not be simply a matter of convenience.

*Venous lines*
The indications for the placement of central venous lines include hemodynamic monitoring (Goldman Class I, II), venous access for fluid

administration, total parenteral nutrition and administration of cardiovascular drugs. Indications for the placement of pulmonary artery catheters are hemodynamic monitoring (Goldman Class III, IV) and administration of cardiovascular drugs. Considering hemodynamic monitoring, pulmonary artery catheters should be placed when measurement of PAOP, cardiac output, and/or mixed venous blood gases is/are essential for proper hemodynamic diagnosis and therapy. As previously mentioned, patients with ventricular ejection fractions > 50% are expected to demonstrate CVP = LAP = PAOP. Therefore, in patients with good cardiac function and no history of heart disease, CVP should be an adequate measure of atrial pressures. More difficult to assess is the usefulness of pulmonary artery catheters in patients with significant heart disease. Goldman's classification of cardiac risk index of cardiac complication risk is shown in Tables 7 and 8. This and similar classifications relate to the risk of a coronary event (i.e. myocardial infarction) in patients with known heart disease as well as other life-threatening cardiac complications. The use of pulmonary artery catheters and rigorous hemodynamic management for patients considered at high risk of a postoperative coronary event has been effective in reducing perioperative infarction. In addition, patients in Goldman's Class IV are more likely to demonstrate unequal atrial pressures and require cardiovascular drug manipulations during any major operation or illness. Pulmonary artery catheter placement in this group may greatly help to distinguish etiologies of poor perfusion and response to therapy, although the effect of pulmonary artery catheterization on the eventual outcome in these patients is controversial. The potential hemodynamic benefit of pulmonary artery catheter use in Class III patients is more difficult to assess, but seems warranted in patients suffering severe insults (severe inflammation and hypoperfusion, multiple trauma) or with pre-existing disease likely to produce major fluid shifts (chronic renal failure requiring dialysis). Each case should be treated individually with recognition that certain patients may benefit because of already known impairment of the circulation as well as the risk of severe impairment which can result from new disease or surgical intervention.

## CARDIOVASCULAR DRUGS

### Inotropic agents
Myocardial contraction depends on the action during systole of increased intracellular calcium on the contractile proteins actin and myosin. Cyclic AMP, which alters intracellular calcium flux, can increase calcium concentration during systole and increase the inotropic state. Most inotropic

### TABLE 7    GOLDMAN'S INDEX OF CARDIAC COMPLICATION RISK

| Clinical factor | Points |
|---|---|
| S3 gallop or JVD on preoperative examination | 11 |
| Myocardial infarction within 6 months | 10 |
| Premature ventricular beats, more than 5/min documented anytime (patients with known heart disease) | 7 |
| Rhythm other than sinus or premature atrial contractions on last preoperative ECG | 7 |
| Age >70 years | 5 |
| Emergency operation | 4 |
| Intrathoracic, intraperitoneal or aortic site of surgery | 3 |
| Important valvular aortic stenosis | 3 |
| Poor general medical condition | 3 |

JVD, jugular venous distention; ECG, electrocardiogram

### TABLE 8    GOLDMAN'S HEMODYNAMIC CLASSIFICATION

| Class | Points |
|---|---|
| I | 0–5 |
| II | 6–12 |
| III | 13–25 |
| IV | ≥ 26 |

agents either increase intracellular calcium (action of digitalis), or increase cAMP by stimulation ($\beta$-adrenergic agonists – dopamine and dobutamine) or phosphodiesterase inhibition. In general, positive inotropic agents increase cardiac contractility and produce an upward and leftward shift of the cardiac function curve (Figure 4). For the treatment of CHF or cardiogenic shock, reduction in afterload will often result in additional improvement in cardiac function. While vasodilator drugs are commonly used to reduce afterload and preload, several of the positive inotropic drugs have beneficial actions on the vasculature. Table 9 lists the relative hemodynamic actions of the commonly used inotropic agents. Of particular importance is the elevation in preload documented with the use of dopamine, even in renal doses. The mechanism for this phenomenon is unclear, but argues that dopamine is not preferable in patients with high-normal or elevated atrial pressures but may be more useful in hypovolemic states.

**Vasodilator therapy**
Vasodilator therapy may improve cardiac function by reducing afterload and/or preload. The combination of a positive inotropic drug and a vaso-dilator may further augment cardiac function (Figure 5). The relative hemodynamic effects of commonly used vasodilators are listed in Table 10.

**Diuretics**
Diuretics are used to reduce preload and improve cardiac output by moving preload from the downward side of the cardiac function curve to the up side (Figure 2). The major circulatory benefit of diuretic therapy in CHF is the improvement in cardiac output which improves oxygen delivery. The disappearance of lung water which follows lowering pulmonary capillary pressure is of secondary importance.

**TABLE 9   HEMODYNAMIC EFFECTS OF POSITIVE INOTROPIC AGENTS**

| Drug | Cardiac output | Preload | Heart rate | Systemic vascular resistance |
|------|----------------|---------|------------|------------------------------|
| Digitalis | +INC | +DEC | +DEC | ± |
| Dopamine | ++INC | +INC | ++INC | +INC |
| Dobutamine | ++INC | ++DEC | +INC | +DEC |
| Amrinone | ++INC | ++DEC | ± | +DEC |
| Milrinone | ++INC | ++DEC | ± | +DEC |

INC, increase; DEC, decrease

**TABLE 10   HEMODYNAMIC EFFECTS OF VASODILATORS**

| Drug | Preload | Afterload |
|------|---------|-----------|
| Nitroglycerin | ++DEC | +DEC |
| Nitroprusside | +DEC | ++DEC |
| Arfonad | ± | ++DEC |
| Phentolamine | ± | ++DEC |

DEC, decrease

## HYPOPERFUSION STATES

### The pathophysiology of hypoperfusion

Hypoperfusion may be defined as a decreased total body or regional blood flow sufficient to result in cellular malfunction and/or death. Hypoperfusion is the primary mechanism responsible for inadequate oxygen delivery and the immediate effects of hypoperfusion on cell viability are secondary to interruption of oxidative metabolism. However, as described in more detail below, the pathophysiological response to hypoperfusion and subsequent resuscitation can result in cellular and organ function alterations which may or may not reflect disruptions in oxidative metabolism and may or may not improve homeostasis.

### The neurohumoral response to hypoperfusion

Total body hypoperfusion is usually manifest as a reduction in cardiac output. The most frequently studied models of total body hypoperfusion cause a reduction in cardiac output from loss of volume (hypovolemic hypoperfusion) or loss of cardiac function (cardiogenic hypoperfusion). Either of these two etiologies may result in the neurohumoral response listed in Table 11. The readily apparent clinical effects of this neurohumoral response are tachycardia (epinephrine, norepinephrine, dopamine), vasoconstriction (norepinephrine, arginine vasopressin (AVP), angiotensin), diaphoresis (norepinephrine), oliguria with sodium and water conservation (adrenocorticotropic hormone (ACTH), cortisol, aldosterone, AVP), and hyperglycemia (epinephrine, glucagon, cortisol, deficient insulin). This activation of the neuroendocrine system may preserve blood flow to vital organs (heart, lungs, brain) while diminishing flow to less vital organs (kidneys, gastrointestinal tract), and serves to preserve or increase intravascular volume by limiting urine output. This response is more homeostatic under conditions of hypovolemic hypoperfusion compared to cardiogenic hypoperfusion where tachycardia, vasoconstriction, and sodium and water retention may aggravate rather than diminish hypoperfusion (see discussion below on cardiogenic states).

### Effects of hypoperfusion on inflammation

The most clearly documented association of hypoperfusion with inflammation is the effect of ischemia followed by reperfusion. Clinically this is most obvious in cases of isolated limb ischemia (compartment syndrome) and in some cases of localized intestinal ischemia. However, severe systemic hypoperfusion may result in a similar response in many tissues, particularly the gastrointestinal tract.

## TABLE 11   NEUROHUMORAL RESPONSE TO HYPOPERFUSION

*Increase*
Epinephrine
Norepinephrine
Dopamine
Glucagon
Renin
Angiotensin
Arginine vasopressin
Adrenocorticotropic hormone
Cortisol
Aldosterone
Growth hormone

*Decrease/deficient*
Insulin
Thyroxine
Triiodothyronine
Luteinizing hormone
Testosterone
Estrogen
Follicle-stimulating hormone

The mechanism responsible for ischemia reperfusion injury appears to require both local and systemic factors. A complex interaction of oxygen free radicals, thromboxane, leukotrienes, phospholipase $A_2$ and leukocytes participates in both regional and total body alterations in capillary permeability and organ function. Anatomical and physiological damage to the intestine, limb, kidney, liver and lung may follow reperfusion even when a specific organ (i.e. lung) was not initially hypoperfused. Since polymorphonuclear cells are potent producers of oxygen free radicals, these cells are central to this pathophysiology.

The potential for severe inflammation to develop during rather than following hypoperfusion is less well documented and more controversial. Some clinical and experimental studies have demonstrated an increase in inflammatory mediators and cellular activity during hemorrhagic hypoperfusion, while other studies have failed to demonstrate this increase. Curiously, CHF, which usually results in mild to moderate hypoperfusion compared to severe hemorrhage, is associated with increased blood levels of tumor necrosis factor (TNF).

In clinical hypoperfusion, particularly with trauma, it is difficult to separate tissue injury secondary only to hypoperfusion from damage from other mechanisms, such as a direct blow. Whatever the cause, hypoperfusion and inflammation commonly occur together. This combination is particularly prone to result in organ malfunction and/or death.

### Clinical diagnosis of hypoperfusion

The fundamentals of resuscitation demand attention to the airway (A), breathing (B) and the circulation (C). The presence or absence of an adequate airway is not usually difficult to ascertain. Clinical examination, chest X-rays and arterial blood gases are often sufficient to determine whether breathing is adequate to support tissue oxygenation and carbon dioxide elimination. However, recognition of an adequate or inadequate circulation often is more difficult to discern based on clinical examination and simple tests. Despite these limitations, the first step in clinical evaluation of the circulation is to examine the patient. Usually an abnormality noted on physical examination (e.g. hypotension, tachycardia, pale and/or cool extremities, altered mental status, decreased urine output) is evidence of a poor circulation and should initiate further study and therapy. Unfortunately, clinical and experimental studies suggest that significant circulation deficits (within the macrocirculation, the microcirculation, or both) may be present with little or no obvious clinical alterations. Thus, several additional tools have been advocated to assess the circulation:

(1)  Evidence of metabolic acidosis:
   (a)  Increased lactic acid;
   (b)  Increased base deficit.

(2)  Evaluation of systemic oxygen delivery and consumption:
   (a)  Augmentation of cardiac output;
   (b)  Achievement of oxygen delivery and consumption end points.

(3)  Measurement of gastric mucosal pH (pHi).

(4)  Decreased ionized calcium.

As is emphasized below, the relationship between hypoperfusion and inflammation makes the information gathered with each one of these additional modalities subject to differing interpretations.

*Evidence of a metabolic acidosis*
The long understood effects of anaerobic metabolism on the Kreb's cycle and the glycolytic pathway have resulted in the assumption that elevated

plasma or serum lactic acid is a specific indication of anaerobic metabolism secondary to inadequate oxygen supply to either the entire body (e.g. hemorrhagic hypoperfusion) or regions of the body (e.g. embolism to the superior mesenteric artery). In critical illness, however, anaerobic metabolism is not the only influence on lactate production. For instance, during severe inflammation lactate levels may increase secondary to effects on cellular metabolism (e.g. increased glucose metabolism, decreased pyruvate metabolism, the effects of nitric oxide) which do not require anaerobic conditions.

Persistent metabolic acidosis and elevated lactic acid are associated with poor outcomes in surgical critical illness. Recognition of a metabolic acidosis, therefore, should serve as a stimulus to search for a reversible process and thus possibly affect outcome. When metabolic acidosis is recognized along with an elevated lactic acid, does this mean the patient suffers solely from lack of oxygen delivery or does a component of severe inflammation also contribute to the degree of illness and potential for a poor outcome? The astute clinician should consider and address both possibilities.

*Evaluation of systemic oxygen delivery and consumption*
Difficulties with using clinical examination alone to assess the circulation have resulted in the use of more invasive methods, namely central venous and pulmonary artery catheterization. Measurements such as central venous oxygen saturation, mixed venous oxygen saturation, cardiac index, oxygen delivery and oxygen consumption have all been advocated.

The concept of supply-dependent oxygen consumption is crucial to the logic applied to the measurement of oxygen delivery and consumption in critical illness. First, under normal circumstances oxygen delivery ($Do_2$) is about four-times greater than oxygen consumption ($Vo_2$). Therefore, oxygen consumption does not decrease until $Do_2$ is reduced to about 25–30% of normal. At this point $Vo_2$ is dependent on $Do_2$ and will demonstrate a relatively linear relationship with $Do_2$. Under such circumstances tissue oxygenation falls and cells suffer during an anaerobic state.

In critical illness, particularly after resuscitation from hypoperfusion and with severe inflammation, $Vo_2$ increases. Characteristically $Do_2$ also increases. Many authors argue that the $Vo_2/Do_2$-dependency curve shifts up and to the right, increasing the magnitude of delivery-dependent $Vo_2$ and accentuating the possibility of tissues suffering from inadequate oxygen delivery. Using this logic adequate resuscitation of the circulation demands that $Do_2$ be increased until $Vo_2$ no longer increases (often achieved when the values listed in Table 12 are realized). Other authors have documented difficulties in achieving supply independent oxygen consumption. Some studies have demonstrated excellent tissue oxygen levels during severe inflammation which argue against inadequate oxygen delivery as a primary process. Despite such differences in published information, several important generalizations (listed below) can be gleaned from the large amount of data gathered in these reports. Patients who increase cardiac index, oxygen delivery and consumption in response to usual methods of resuscitation of the circulation (i.e infusion of fluids and red cells) tend to survive, especially when the increase in these para-meters approaches or meets values which are high compared to the values in non-stressed humans (Table 12). Thus, these patients become hyperdynamic with minimal intervention. Patients who do not achieve a hyperdynamic state (particularly no increase in oxygen consumption) during critical illness, with or without the infusion of inotropic agents, are more likely to succumb.

Much more controversial is whether active intervention with inotropic agents, which then do achieve a hyperdynamic state, actually affects patient outcome. Concerns have been raised that the inotropic agents them-selves can cause the measured increase in oxygen consumption which is frequently observed. If this is so, the patient's cells would not exhibit a pre-existing oxygen debt but rather a physiological response to the drug infusion. Therefore, at present it is unclear that resuscitative measures beyond the infusion of fluids and red cells to maintain intravascular volume will directly affect outcome. One thing is clear: the physician should never be satisfied with a clearly hypodynamic state (lower than normal cardiac index, oxygen delivery and oxygen consumption).

*Measurement of gastric mucosal pH*
The splanchnic circulation characteristically vasoconstricts in response to global reductions in cardiac output as well as severe inflammatory states

TABLE 12   NON-STRESSED VS. THE 'IDEAL' HYPERDYNAMIC
STATE

| Parameter | Non-stressed | Ideal |
|---|---|---|
| Cardiac index | 2.5–3.5 l/min m$^2$ | >4.5 l/min m$^2$ |
| Oxygen delivery | 400 ml/min m$^2$ | >600 ml/min m$^2$ |
| Oxygen consumption | 130 ml/min m$^2$ | >170 ml/min m$^2$ |

even when global perfusion remains intact. Despite a generous arterial circulation, the stomach mucosa is not protected from such insults, with stress gastritis the most obvious clinical correlate. Several studies have demonstrated that stomach mucosal metabolism can be assessed by indirect measurement of mucosal pH (pHi) using a device called the gastric tonometer, which uses an intragastric balloon permeable to carbon dioxide to sample the region.

These studies have demonstrated that a low stomach mucosal pH (pHi ≤ 7.32) either at the time of admission to an intensive care unit, or developing thereafter, is associated with increased risk of multiple organ failure and death. Usually a low pHi is considered indicative of inadequate oxygen delivery to all tissues, although a direct correlation between pHi and measures of total body hemodynamics and oxygen metabolism has not been regularly documented. Therefore, a low pHi may be an indirect measure of both the effect of severe inflammation upon the regional circulation of the upper intestinal tract as well as a measure of total body hypoperfusion.

Measurement of pHi may be a sensitive early warning that a tissue is suffering from disease and serve as a stimulus to determine if the disease is an inadequate global circulation, severe inflammation, or both. In one study therapeutic intervention to augment the circulation when a low pHi was recognized improved survival.

*Decreased ionized calcium*
Ionized calcium decreases with hemorrhagic hypoperfusion, during resuscitation for cardiac arrest, and during severe inflammation. Mortality is higher in patients who arrive in a critical care setting with low ionized calcium. The etiology of this phenomenon is debated, but does not appear to be secondary to inadequate parathyroid hormone (PTH) secretion or extracellular sequestration. Several studies have suggested that intracellular migration of calcium is the etiology and reflective of alterations in cellular membrane function during critical illness. Therefore, decreased ionized calcium without a clear etiology (such as elevated phosphate or decreased magnesium) may indicate ongoing hypoperfusion and/or inflammation.

**Decreased venous return – etiologies, diagnosis and treatment**
The physiology of venous return is described in detail in the cardiovascular section of this Chapter. The formula for venous return is as follows:

$$VR = \frac{(MSP - CVP)}{(RV + RA/19)}$$

where VR is venous return, MSP is mean systemic pressure, CVP is central venous pressure, RV is venous resistance and RA is arterial resistance.

*Hypovolemia*
Hypovolemia is the most common etiology of decreased venous return secondary to decreased MSP. Common etiologies of hypovolemia are hemorrhage, severe inflammation/infection, burns, trauma, excess diuresis, vomiting, bowel obstruction, pancreatitis, inadequate oral intake and peritonitis. Hypovolemia is the most common etiology of hypotension. Severe hypoperfusion secondary to hypovolemia, hypovolemic shock, has been studied most frequently in experimental and clinical hemorrhage. Hemorrhagic shock not only diminishes venous return, but also may produce additional cardiovascular alterations, such as:

(1) Increased systemic vascular resistance;

(2) Decreased ventricular contractility;

(3) Decreased ventricular compliance;

(4) Increased atrial contractility;

(5) Transcapillary refill of water to restore plasma volume;

(6) Intravascular protein replenishment from preformed extravascular protein.

Cellular effects (other than lactic acidosis from anaerobic glycolysis) which have been described include diminished transmembrane potential difference, increased intracellular sodium and decreased intracellular ATP, as well as increased cellular calcium. As mentioned above, ischemia-induced systemic inflammation has also been described.

The metabolic and/or toxic phenomena associated with hypovolemic shock, even without severe inflammation, result in loss of plasma and interstitial volume beyond that which can be accounted for by the primary disease process (i.e. hemorrhage, vomiting), with migration of interstitial fluid into cells and increased capillary permeability implicated as mechanisms.

*Physical examination in hypovolemic hypoperfusion*  The hypovolemic patient will exhibit vital signs and physical examination evidence of hypoperfusion roughly in proportion to the degree of hypovolemia. A 10% loss of plasma volume (560 ml, about the amount donated for transfusion) produces little, if any disturbance. A 20% loss may result in tachycardia and orthostatic hypotension. A 30% loss may produce hypotension while supine. However, a patient may be normotensive when supine even with greater loss of blood volume.

Agitation, tachypnea and peripheral vasoconstriction commonly accompany all significant degrees of hypovolemia. Warm extremities may be seen in inflammation despite hypovolemia and may also be present following spinal cord injury and anaphylaxis. Neck veins will not be distended unless hypovolemia is accompanied by an extracardiac increase in pressure (tension pneumothorax, pericardial tamponade, severe effort during expiration, increased abdominal pressure). An S3 gallop will not be present. An etiology of hypovolemia may also be apparent (open wound with hemorrhage, distended abdomen, femur and pelvic fractures). Agitation, tachypnea and peripheral vasoconstriction are common with any etiology of hypoperfusion. Hypotension, however, is most commonly secondary to hypovolemia. Hypotension from disruption of intrinsic cardiac function (cardiogenic shock) is much less common. CHF, a distinct clinical entity from cardiogenic shock, frequently results in increased blood pressure.

*Treatment of hypovolemia*   The circulatory, metabolic and toxic effects of severe hypovolemic hypoperfusion (also called hypovolemic shock) are best treated by rapid restoration of intravascular volume, thereby increasing MSP, venous return and oxygen delivery. In general, two types of fluid, crystalloid (isotonic – Ringer's lactate and 0.9% saline, and hypertonic saline) and colloid (red blood cells, fresh frozen plasma, albumin, processed human protein, low molecular weight dextran and hydroxyethyl starch), have been used for volume replacement. Red blood cells are very effective when needed. Once hemorrhage is arrested, administration of red cells results in increased cardiac output, increased oxygen carrying capacity, as well as little, if any, leakage of red cells into the interstitium even in the face of increased capillary permeability. Potential advantages and disadvantages of resuscitation fluids are provided in Table 13.

Fresh frozen plasma should not be used primarily as a colloid. Fresh frozen plasma should only be used when hypovolemia is accompanied by bleeding and deficiency in intrinsic or extrinsic coagulation partial thromboplastin time (PTT) > 1.5 x control, prothrombin activity (PTA) < 50%). In general, red blood cells are used to replace lost red cells and are administered until the serum hemoglobin approaches 10 g/ 100 ml. When

## TABLE 13   POTENTIAL ADVANTAGES AND DISADVANTAGES OF RESUSCITATION FLUIDS

*Crystalloid*
Advantages
   inexpensive
   readily available
   replenishes extracellular fluid (ECF)
   freely mobile across capillaries
   no increase in lung water
Disadvantages
   rapid equilibration with interstitial fluid
   lowers serum oncotic pressure
   no oxygen carrying capacity
   increase in systemically perfused interstitial fluid

*Colloid solutions (other than red blood cells)*
Advantages
   less water administered (more resuscitation per ml)
   less sodium administered
   less decrease in oncotic pressure
   acid buffer (fresh frozen plasma)
   decreased superoxide radical damage (hydroxethyl starch)
Disadvantages
   expensive (albumin, fresh frozen plasma)
   transmissible disease (fresh frozen plasma)
   increased interstitial oncotic pressure
   depressed myocardial function (albumin)
   depressed immunologic function (albumin)
   delayed resolution of interstitial edema
   coagulopathy (low molecular weight dextran)

restoration of cardiac output is difficult or does not appear adequate to meet oxygen demand, increasing hemoglobin to 13–14 g/ 100 ml may be indicated. This is most likely to be useful in patients with a cardiogenic etiology of hypoperfusion rather than simple hypovolemia. However, documentation supporting that oxygen consumption will increase with such an elevation in hemoglobin is sparse.

Much more controversial than the appropriate use of fresh frozen plasma and red blood cells are the advantages and disadvantages of the various crystalloid and colloid solutions previously listed. In general, most investigators agree that colloid administration results in less sodium administration compared to crystalloid solutions and less water administration compared to isotonic crystalloid solutions. In addition, plasma oncotic pressure is higher following colloids. Still debated is whether increased total body sodium and water gain is detrimental to organ function following resuscitation of the circulation.

Because pulmonary function is so vital, the association of pulmonary edema with increased total body sodium and water following shock resuscitation implies that either too much fluid had been administered (i.e. CHF has developed), or possibly that lowered serum oncotic pressure can produce increased lung water. The adoption of pulmonary artery catheter monitoring documented that most cases of pulmonary dysfunction during or after hypovolemic shock were not secondary to elevated pulmonary capillary hydrostatic pressure. Common clinical experience with diseases which reduce plasma albumin (cirrhosis and nephrosis) argues that patients will develop peripheral edema and not pulmonary edema with low plasma oncotic pressure. While still advocated by some investigators, most agree that pulmonary edema in hypovolemic humans is not secondary to low oncotic pressure, but rather to increased pulmonary capillary permeability. As discussed in the section on the acute respiratory distress syndrome (Chapter 4; The pulmonary system; Lung Dysfunction), the relationship between lung water accumulation and lung malfunction is complex. Etiologies of non-cardiogenic pulmonary edema may produce severe pulmonary dysfunction with little increase in extravascular lung water. The argument that zealous use of crystalloid solution results in lung malfunction has little physiological basis in animals and humans with non-cardiogenic pulmonary edema.

Peripheral edema does occur with decreased plasma oncotic pressure. Tissues supplied by the systemic circulation are commonly subjected to capillary pressures which would produce hydrostatic pulmonary edema (about 25 mmHg). Therefore, the migration of fluid across peripheral capillaries may be normally greater per unit area than in the lung and result in greater lymph flow. Another possibility is that peripheral capillaries are less permeable. Whatever the case, it appears that relatively small changes in hydrostatic and/or oncotic pressure can result in peripheral edema, implying that under normal conditions the peripheral lymphatics or other protective mechanisms are working close to maximum capacity.

Do peripheral tissues suffer because of edema? Arguments can be made that the skin (decubitus ulcers, venous stasis ulcers, aggravation of burn injury), the gastrointestinal tract (decreased absorption), thorax (pleural effusion), etc. may function poorly with increased interstitial fluid. Edema may also lower the $Po_2$ in injured tissue. However, once the underlying disease process is corrected, many edematous, hypoalbuminemic patients spontaneously excrete the interstitial fluid without recognized adverse sequelae.

Reversal of hypoperfusion is the main goal of the therapy of hypovolemic shock. Frequently crystalloid-aggravated peripheral edema formation is accepted to achieve this goal and avoid the potential harmful effects of colloids. However, more concentrated crystalloid solutions have been employed which regularly demonstrate that hemodynamic resuscitation is dependent upon the amount of sodium administered, not the amount of water. Evidence suggests that increased interstitial osmolality draws intracellular water into the interstitium, accelerates plasma refill and, subsequently, restores plasma volume and hemodynamics with little, if any, increase in peripheral edema. Serum osmolality up to 360 mosmol has been reported in man without apparent adverse effect. Other potential benefits and problems associated with concentrated sodium solutions are:

(1)  Advantages:
    (a)  Less water administration;
    (b)  Rapid resuscitation;
    (c)  Improved cardiac contractility;
    (d)  Increased urine output;
    (e)  Vasodilatation.

(2)  Disadvantages:
    (a)  Increased serum osmolality;
    (b)  Metabolic acidosis when chloride equals sodium;
    (c)  Metabolic alkalosis when chloride is less than sodium and another anion is used (acetate, lactate).

Thus, concentrated sodium solutions may be the ideal compromise, allowing effective reversal of hypovolemia with much less water and no colloid administration.

When a hypovolemic patient is receiving large volumes of crystalloid or colloid and is not responding well to therapy (most often seen in severe inflammation), dopamine administration is a logical adjunct since dopamine increases left ventricular filling pressures as it increases cardiac output. This may occur at the expense of increasing myocardial oxygen demands. Once adequate vascular volume is attained, usually the dopamine can be discontinued.

*Pericardial tamponade*

The prime mechanism for decreased venous return with pericardial tamponade is an extracavitary increase in CVP. The etiologies of tamponade in surgery are most commonly chest trauma (penetrating and blunt) and bleeding after cardiac surgery. Physical examination usually reveals evidence of hypoperfusion along with distended neck veins, muffled heart sounds and an increased paradoxical pulse (>15 mmHg). The ECG may show low voltage, the CVP will often be elevated and a chest X-ray may show an enlarging heart. With severe hypovolemia the CVP may be normal despite tamponade and may become elevated only after fluid resuscitation.

It is important to distinguish this etiology of hypoperfusion from CHF or cardiogenic shock since reducing fluid intake and administering a diuretic would reduce venous return further in tamponade. CHF usually results in a normal or elevated blood pressure. Severe tamponade results in hypotension. Therefore, tamponade simulates cardiogenic shock more than CHF. Since cardiogenic shock requires a major insult to myocardial function (see below), hypotension with an elevated CVP should increase suspicion of tamponade or a tension pneumothorax unless obvious evidence of severe myocardial malfunction is obtained.

While removal of the fluid surrounding the heart (pericardiocentesis) is the most effective therapy, venous return will also improve by increasing MSP with intravenous fluid.

*Tension pneumothorax*

Tension pneumothorax reduces venous return by producing an extracavitary increase in CVP and by increasing the venous resistance in the chest. Tension pneumothorax may occur spontaneously from rupture of a bleb, or more commonly following penetrating or blunt trauma. Physical examination reveals evidence of decreased perfusion along with decreased breath sounds over the affected thorax, tracheal deviation away from the affected thorax and distended neck veins.

Treatment consists of an emergency (within seconds to minutes) release of the tension (e.g. placing a 14-gauge needle into the chest, placing a finger in a large penetrating injury), followed by closed thoracostomy. Once again administration of intravenous fluid to raise MSP is also beneficial and neck vein distension may not be evident with severe hypovolemia.

*Increased abdominal pressure*

Increased abdominal pressure (>20 mmHg) diminishes venous return by increasing intrathoracic pressure, producing an extracavitary increase in

CVP, and increasing venous resistance in abdominal veins. Increased abdominal pressure may be particularly detrimental to renal blood flow. Abdominal pressure may be increased by a variety of mechanisms including bowel obstruction, tension pneumoperitoneum, massive bleeding, diagnostic laparoscopy, pneumatic anti-shock garment and ascites. It is most easily measured by using a bladder catheter (50–100 ml fluid inserted into the bladder via the fluid sampling port on a Foley catheter, the catheter is clamped distal to the sampling port, and pressure is measured by connecting the needle in the sampling port to standard hemodynamic monitoring tubing, using the pubis as the zero pressure level).

Physical examination will most often reveal evidence of hypoperfusion along with a tensely distended abdomen and possibly distended neck veins. The most effective treatment is to provide relief of the pressure. However, aggressive fluid management to increase MSP may be the only option selected in some cases where, for instance, exploration of the abdomen is considered prohibitively risky. When hemodynamics and respiratory function (i.e. high peak inspiratory pressures required on the ventilator) are severely impaired by increased abdominal pressure, then opening the abdomen and closing with a prosthesis or leaving the abdomen packed open may be the best alternative.

*Increased thoracic pressure*

*Positive end-expiratory pressure*   PEEP, as well as any ventilator therapy which increases mean airway pressure, also diminishes venous return by increasing CVP from an extracavitory force and increasing venous resistance in the thorax. While several other mechanisms have been argued for decreased cardiac output with increased mean airway pressure, the primary mechanism is decreased venous return. Similar to increased abdominal pressure, if the airway pressure cannot be diminished, then the primary therapy is to administer fluids to increase MSP.

*Hemodynamic monitoring with increased thoracic and abdominal pressure*
Increased abdominal and thoracic pressure will increase pressures measured in the superior vena cava, right atrium and pulmonary artery. This increase is secondary to extraluminal pressure and does not represent an increase in the pressure distending the heart. The clinician may have difficulty recognizing the magnitude of this extraluminal increase and be hesitant to administer fluid to patients with high hemodynamic pressures. Aggressive fluid administration may appear contraindicated when CVP and/or PAOP are measured as normal or elevated. However,

when this elevation is from an extracardiac increase in pressure, administration of fluid is often beneficial.

As mentioned previously, a balloon-equipped nasogastric tube has been used for estimating both the effects of increased abdominal pressure and PEEP on intracavitary hemodynamic pressures measured within the thorax (Figures 11–13). This device has been used to measure the increase in intrathoracic pressure following such interventions as pneumatic anti-shock garment or PEEP application in humans. Under these circumstances the increase in intrathoracic pressure was equal to the increase in CVP and PAOP measured simultaneously. Therefore, when elevated esophageal pressure is measured with this device, this evaluation should be subtracted from measured CVP or PAOP to estimate the transmural or intracavitary pressure(s). Knowledge that an elevated CVP or PAOP is secondary to extraluminal rather than intraluminal pressure should alleviate any anxiety about administering fluid to a patient with increased abdominal or thoracic pressure.

## Congestive heart failure

CHF is a common condition which most frequently is secondary to the etiologies in Table 14. Although difficulties with both contraction (systolic function) and relaxation (diastolic function) may coexist, an estimated 40% of patients have normal systolic function at the time of CHF. Therefore, the concept of diastolic dysfunction has gained prevalence and has implications related to therapy. Note that excessive administration of intravenous

## TABLE 14   COMMON ETIOLOGIES OF CONGESTIVE HEART FAILURE

*Systolic failure (loss of myocytes, failure to contract)*
Acute ischemia
Acute cardiomyopathy

*Diastolic failure (hypertrophy of myocytes, failure to relax)*
Hypertension
Valvular heart disease
Restrictive cardiomyopathy
Mitral stenosis
Constrictive pericarditis
Postinfarction hypertrophy

fluid is not included in the etiologies listed in Table 14. Patients without significant heart disease will sequester little intravenous fluid unless other pathophysiological conditions are present (e.g. severe inflammation). During severe inflammation fluid sequestration and weight gain are not indicative of an excess in intravascular volume. In fact, intravascular volume may be decreased despite a significant increase in total body salt and water. Only patients with underlying heart disease or unrelenting anuric renal failure will develop CHF secondary to aggressive intravenous fluid therapy. In other words, the disease is in the patient, not in the fluid.

Ventricular physiology concepts are more relevant than venous return physiology for the understanding and management of CHF. Classically, CHF is described as a fall in cardiac output secondary to overstretching one or both ventricles (markedly increased preload) and decompensation of the Starling mechanism. Decreased ventricular compliance and decreased filling with hypertrophy rather than overstretching may be responsible for the clinical physiology of CHF (salt and water sequestration, elevated ventricular filling pressures, increased extravascular lung water) without overstretching. In addition, other cardiac diseases (i.e. mitral stenosis, mitral regurgitation, left atrial myxoma) may produce a clinical picture similar to ventricular failure but with normal or increased ventricular function.

Whatever the etiology, most often the clinical presentation of CHF is secondary to increased pulmonary hydrostatic pressure along with decreased ventricular outflow via the pulmonary artery and/or the aorta. The increase in hydrostatic pressure results in increased lung water and symptoms of respiratory distress, along with mild to moderate hypoxia. This combined with a mild to moderate reduction in cardiac output decreases oxygen delivery, stimulates the sympatho-adrenal system and results in tachycardia and vasoconstriction which maintains or, more frequently, elevates mean arterial pressure. Decreased cardiac output also results in AVP release as well as renal hypoperfusion, stimulation of renin, angiotensin production and subsequent aldosterone secretion.

The neurohumoral responses to decreased cardiac output serve to further increase preload (renal conservation of sodium and water) and increase afterload (elevated mean arterial pressure), both of which may aggravate poor ventricular function and/or pulmonary water accumulation.

*Physical examination*
The clinician must remember that this disease is called congestive heart failure. Physical examination should be directed at assessing heart func-

tion. Too often clinicians infer the status of cardiac function on the basis of lung status, the amount of peripheral edema, calculated fluid balance, or the response to diuretics. Using such information CHF may be over-diagnosed in 30–40% of critically ill patients. The physical examination parameters which assess cardiac function include heart rate, rhythm, blood pressure, jugular venous pressure (JVP), S3 gallop and murmurs. Of these, the S3 gallop is the most specific, but unfortunately not the most sensitive, evidence for ventricular failure. As stated above, blood pressure is well maintained or elevated. In fact, hypotension on a cardiac basis is delegated to a distinct clinical entity: cardiogenic shock (see below). Therefore, a hypotensive patient either has cardiogenic shock or a more common cause of hypotension (hypovolemia, vasodilatation).

Clinical evidence of increased lung water (tachypnea, rales, broncho-spasm) may be present with any etiology of pulmonary edema (cardio-genic and non-cardiogenic) or may be simulated by other disease, such as atelectasis, pneumonia, COPD or asthma. Diagnostic and therapeutic decision-making based primarily on lung status can be misleading and dangerous.

*Laboratory aids*

Laboratory aids in the diagnosis of CHF include chest X-ray, measured CVP, PAOP, LAP, cardiac catheterization, echocardiogram and heart scanning. The chest X-ray may be misleading as an assessment of both the amount of water accumulated in the lungs and the etiology of water accumulation (see Chapter 4; The Pulmonary system, pulmonary fluid). With normal lungs subjected to increased hydrostatic pressure, a relatively predictable sequence of radiographic changes are noted (Table 15). If a particular hydrostatic pressure is present for more than 24 h, the chest X-ray

**TABLE 15   RADIOGRAPHIC CHANGES WITH INCREASED HYDROSTATIC PRESSURE IN NORMAL LUNGS**

| Hydrostatic pressure (mmHg) | X-ray |
|---|---|
| <15–18 | normal |
| 18–22 | cephalization |
| 20–27 | perihilar haze |
| 25–30 | rosettes |
| >30 | dense alveolar infiltrates |

should show corresponding changes. If not, another etiology of the chest X-ray findings should be considered.

Most often patients with normal hearts and patients with chronic ventricular malfunction will exhibit a CVP which is within a few mmHg of the PAOP, making CVP measurement a useful laboratory test for CHF. When acute or chronic disease is present which would be expected to produce significant discrepancy between left and right ventricular or atrial function (acute myocardial infarction (MI), mitral stenosis, mitral regurgitation) CVP may be unreliable.

PAOP, not pulmonary artery diastolic pressure, is a reliable measure of left atrial pressure. Since pulmonary vascular resistance is increased by many diseases, PAOP may be low or normal despite increased mean and diastolic pulmonary artery pressure. In fact, when a pulmonary artery catheter does not provide a good wedge pressure tracing, an elevated pulmonary artery diastolic pressure with a normal CVP should not be presumed to be secondary to increased left atrial pressure. Instead a potential etiology of increased pulmonary vascular resistance should be considered.

Pulmonary artery catheter measurements of an elevated (>18 mmHg) right and/or left atrial pressures with a low cardiac index, but without hypotension, is the most specific, readily available method to make a diagnosis of CHF in the critical care setting. Cardiac catheterization, echocardiograms and heart scanning techniques are not commonly used to make the diagnosis of CHF, but rather to determine an etiology.

*Treatment*

Just as the use of lung-related information may be misapplied to make a diagnosis of CHF, using the lung as the primary measure of therapy is also misdirected. Once arterial oxygen saturation is 90% or greater (usually at a $Po_2$ of $\geq$ 60 mmHg), little benefit in oxygen delivery is realized by further therapy directed at the lungs. The primary goal in treating CHF is to improve heart function, cardiac output, and, thereby, oxygen delivery. Commonly employed treatment options for CHF are:

(1) Reversal of underlying disease by:
    (a)   Treatment of hypertension;
    (b)   Coronary artery bypass;
    (c)   Valve replacement;
    (d)   Treatment of myopathy.
(2) Reduction of preload by:
    (a)   Decreased water intake;
    (b)   Diuretics;

(c)   Venous dilatation:
    (i)   nitroglycerin;
    (ii)   calcium channel blockers;
    (iii)   narcotics.

(3)   Reduction of afterload using:
    (a)   Nitroprusside;
    (b)   Antihypertensives;
    (c)   Diuretics;
    (d)   Narcotics.

(4)   Increase in contractility using:
    (a) Intravenous inotropes.

(5)   Increase in arterial oxygen using:
    (a) Supplemental $O_2$;
    (b) Mechanical ventilation.

Using this logic diuretics are not employed primarily to treat pulmonary edema, but to reduce preload in the overstretched heart and improve cardiac output. Since hemodynamics are the focus of treatment, hemodynamic variables (pulse, blood pressure, appearance or disappearance of an S3, skin color and temperature) as well as mental status and spontaneous urine output are more valuable determinants of cardiac response to therapy than the physical examination of the lungs, chest X-ray and arterial $Po_2$.

If reducing preload with a diuretic does not improve perfusion, then the common occurrence of well-maintained or elevated mean arterial pressure makes arterial and venous dilatation (reduced afterload and preload) the next logical step. Since increased wall tension and afterload will increase myocardial oxygen consumption, an increase in cardiac output from diuresis and vasodilatation should not increase, and might decrease, myocardial oxygen demand.

If the above therapies prove insufficient, then inotropic therapy is commonly used. Under such circumstances pulmonary artery catheter monitoring is especially useful to document that less oxygen costly therapy is inadequate, and to measure the response to drug manipulation. The end points of therapy include the following: (1) good clinical perfusion status (normal blood pressure, pulse, mental status, temperature and color of extremities, spontaneous urine output), (2) good cardiac index ($> 2.5$ l/min/$M^2$), (3) no metabolic acidosis, (4) normal lactic acid level, and (5) normal mixed venous $Po_2$ or oxygen saturation (30–35 mmHg and 65–75%, respectively).

The inotropic agents of choice for CHF are dobutamine and amrinone, both of which increase cardiac output while decreasing left ventricular filling pressures. Dopamine is not as useful because filling pressure tends to increase as cardiac output improves. Importantly, dopamine may exert this effect even in the renal dose range.

**Cardiogenic shock**
Cardiogenic shock, or hypotension on a cardiac basis, requires severe disruption of cardiac function (cardiac index <2.2 l/M$^2$) from etiologies such as:

(1)  Acute ischemia:
   (a)  Ventricular wall infarct;
   (b)  Papillary muscle infarct;
   (c)  Ventricular septal defect (VSD) rupture.

(2)  Acute valvular disease mitral: tricuspid, aortic regurgitation.

(3)  Arrythmias:
   (a)  Rapid supraventricular;
   (b)  Bradycardia;
   (c)  Ventricular tachycardia.

(4)  Other:
   (a)  End-stage cardiomyopathy;
   (b)  Severe myocardial contusion;
   (c)  Severe myocarditis;
   (d)  Severe left ventricular outflow obstruction;
   (e)  Severe left ventricular inflow obstruction.

Hypoperfusion of this magnitude, especially when secondary to myocardial infarction, is associated with high mortality.

In general, the etiologies of cardiogenic shock are not subtle, and do not gradually cause alterations in cardiac function. As mentioned, hypotension is more often secondary to hypovolemia than severe impairment of cardiac function. When a clinician makes a decision not to administer fluid to a hypotensive patient, that clinician is actually making a diagnosis of cardiogenic shock for that patient. Cardiogenic shock is the only circulatory deficit that can be worsened by the administration of fluid. Since cardiogenic shock is secondary to marked, usually obvious cardiac disease, the clinician should be able to document the occurrence of such a major insult to cardiac function. Without such documentation and the associated recognition of a disease which requires aggressive monitoring and management in a critical care setting, the clinician should consider hypotensive patients to be hypovolemic and not in cardiogenic shock.

*Physical examination*
Physical examination will reveal hypotension, tachycardia, tachypnea, peripheral vasoconstriction, distended neck veins, agitation and confusion. An S3 gallop may be apparent, and when valvular dysfunction is present associated murmurs may be auscultated.

*Laboratory aids*
Cardiogenic shock is associated with chest X-ray evidence of pulmonary edema, metabolic acidosis (lactic acidosis), increased blood urea nitrogen and creatinine, elevated CVP and PAOP. Frequently, a cardiogram will reveal evidence of acute ischemia or infarct and/or arrhythmias. An echocardiogram can provide information about ventricular wall motion and valve function.

*Treatment*
Treatment is as always based on the etiology. Arrhythmias are generally the most readily treated etiology of severe cardiac impairment. When the etiology is not an arrhythmia, the same sequence of interventions used to increase cardiac output in CHF may be used for cardiogenic shock. However, hypotension (often <90 mmHg systolic) makes the use of vasodilators alone less attractive. Therefore, a combination of inotropic support and vasodilatation is frequently employed. Mechanical support of the heart using the intra-aortic balloon pump increases cardiac output while reducing preload and afterload (Figure 14). An intra-aortic balloon pump may be more successful than high-dose dobutamine in supporting patients at the time of severe cardiac impairment. Intra-aortic balloon pump use may be adequate to support a patient until cardiac function improves or may be required until a surgical solution (e.g. replacement of the aortic valve or coronary revascularization) can be accomplished.

The complications of intra-aortic balloon pump use are lower extremity ischemia, thrombocytopenia, infection, aortic dissection and free perforation. The most frequent is lower extremity ischemia, usually on the side where the balloon pump was inserted.

## Special considerations

*Postoperative hypertension*
Postoperative hypertension and resultant increased afterload may reduce

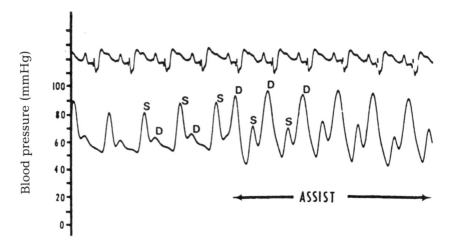

**Figure 14** The effects of intra-aortic balloon pumping on systolic (S) and diastolic (D) pressure. Systolic pressure is reduced, decreasing left ventricular afterload. Diastolic pressure is increased which increases coronary perfusion pressure. However, ventricular end-diastolic pressure is reduced, indicating a reduction in preload. Reproduced with permission from Bregman D. Management of patients undergoing intra-aortic balloon pumping. *Heart Lung* 1974;3:916–27

cardiac output without producing CHF. Etiologies of postoperative hypertension are preoperative hypertension, aortic/carotid manipulation, hypothermia, hypovolemia, vasopressor administration, delirium, CHF and pain. In patients with no previous history of hypertension, hypothermia, especially when combined with hypovolemia, can result in hypertension, presumably because of two vasoconstrictive stimuli. Restricting fluid or administration of a diuretic as treatment of this hypertension can be dangerous and aggravate hypotension when temperature returns to normal. Similarly, vasodilator therapy (nitroprusside, nicardipine, trimetaphan) must be used cautiously and may precipitate hypotension if hypovolemia is present. It is necessary to administer fluids (preferably warmed) while combating hypothermia to treat this hypertension by alleviating both stimuli to vasoconstrict.

Hypertension after cardiac or major vascular surgery is common and may be secondary to neurohumoral stimulation with the release of catecholamines or activation of the renin–angiotensin axis. Treatment with vasodilators and/or angiotensin-converting enzyme inhibitor therapy is usually effective.

Delirium is common, especially in older patients. While sedative therapy may be necessary to reduce agitation and the associated hypertension, the clinician should simultaneously search for an etiology of the delirium and not simply invoke the catch-all diagnosis of intensive care unit psychosis.

Pain by itself is not a frequent cause of hypertension, and analgesic medications may help more by sedative effect rather than true analgesia.

*Postoperative open heart hypoperfusion*
Postoperative open heart patients may suffer decreased cardiac output secondary to:

(1)   Hypovolemia;

(2)   Tamponade;

(3)   Increased afterload:
    (a)   Drugs,
    (b)   Hypothermia,
    (c)   Hypovolemia;

(4)   Congestive heart failure;

(5)   Cardiogenic shock;

(6)   Severe inflammation:
    (a)   Post-pump syndrome,
    (b)   Pancreatitis,
    (c)   Ischemic intestine.

Fortunately, these patients are usually well monitored and careful evaluation of hemodynamic variables will allow for logical therapy. As mentioned above, the combination of hypovolemia and hypothermia commonly results in hypertension despite a low cardiac output. In addition, decreased left ventricular compliance from increased afterload may result in a normal or elevated LAP or PAOP suggesting a normo- or hypervolemic state.

Keeping these concepts in mind, the management of postoperative cardiopulmonary bypass patients will generally be the same as described in previous sections. However, unique to this patient population is the risk of tamponade from mediastinal bleeding which is too rapid to be evacuated by the mediastinal chest tubes or has clotted off the chest tubes. Tamponade must be considered whenever rising filling pressures are associated with decreasing cardiac output. Since hypovolemia aggravates the fall in cardiac output with tamponade, incorrectly diagnosing CHF or cardiogenic shock followed by therapeutic decreased fluid administration and/or diuretics can be gravely detrimental. Fortunately, tamponade is usually preceded by increased mediastinal chest tube drainage and fluid resuscitation is underway when tamponade becomes more apparent. When properly diagnosed, tamponade commonly requires rapid return to the operating room to control hemorrhage.

More difficult to manage is the occasional patient who develops evidence of severe systemic inflammation following cardiopulmonary bypass. These patients with underlying heart disease may manifest a wide spectrum of cardiac alterations related to severe inflammation. The etiology and management schemes for inflammation-induced cardiac malfunction are discussed in Chapter 3; Inflammation, pathological systemic inflammation. Again, the astute clinician must be alert to the possibility that an impaired circulation may be secondary to severe inflammation.

*Postoperative major vascular surgery hypoperfusion*
Common etiologies of postoperative major vascular surgery hypoperfusion of the whole body are hypovolemia, hypothermia, hypertension, CHF and cardiogenic shock. The manifestations of total body hypoperfusion, the etiologies and the management are similar to those described above. The recognition of regional hypoperfusion (extremities, large intestine, small intestine, brain and kidneys) may be simple (obvious lower extremity ischemia) or difficult (diagnosis of intestinal ischemia). Particularly life threatening is large and small bowel ischemia and/or infarction. Clinical clues suggesting this condition are:

(1)    Surgery on abdominal or thoracic aorta;

(2)    Blood or melena per rectum;

(3)    Diarrhea;

(4)    Large fluid sequestration;

(5)    Abdominal tenderness;

(6)    Lactic acidosis;

(7)    Low mucosal pHi (sigmoid tonometer).

Physicians who regularly attend these patients may recognize subtleties of postoperative fluid requirements and abdominal findings. Inexperienced clinicians may have difficulty using this information as warning signs.

However, patients usually do not have a bowel movement during the first 24 h after major abdominal surgery and such an event, especially accompanied with blood, should lead to further study. With regional ischemia lactic acidosis will be persistent despite evidence of good total body oxygen delivery. The sigmoid tonometer, which measures the mucosal pH of the sigmoid colon, may be another tool to alert the clinician that ischemic intestine is present. The large bowel can be viewed by sigmoidoscopy or colonoscopy, but may also require reoperation for adequate evaluation. Evaluation of the small bowel is difficult and often requires reoperation for proper assessment. Ischemic and especially infarcted intestine are most often more life threatening than further surgery *per se.*

*Cardiac trauma*
Cardiac trauma may also result in hypoperfusion secondary to cardiac contusion, cardiac tamponade, blunt chamber rupture, penetrating wound, valvular disruption, or tension pneumopericardium, and present with a clinical picture which can range from no hemodynamic insult to sudden death. The diagnosis of cardiac contusion is very difficult to ascertain. In general, patients who are most severely injured are most likely to exhibit evidence of cardiac malfunction. Whether or not a majority of these patients actually have an anatomic alteration in myocardium compared to physiological malfunction is controversial. All tests considered specific for contusion (e.g. cardiac enzymes, echocardiograms, radiological imaging) may be misleading. The only test known to be truly specific is myocardial biopsy.

The necessity of aggressive cardiac monitoring for the patient suspected of having a cardiac contusion had been questioned. In essence, most severely injured patients (those at risk for cardiac malfunction) are likely to be observed in a critical care environment where alterations in cardiac function (e.g. arrhythmias, conduction disturbance, CHF, cardiogenic shock) will be recognized and managed as with any patient without a contusion.

Cardiac tamponade usually is secondary to blunt or penetrating chamber injury which will require operative repair. Chamber injury may also result in exsanguination if open to the pleural space. Acute valvular insufficiency may result in CHF or, more likely, cardiogenic shock and may require valve replacement. Tension pneumopericardium, usually associated with pneumothorax, may respond to chest tube placement on the affected pleural space or require more direct therapy (pericardial needle or chest tube insertion).

# 3

# INFLAMMATION

## Physiology

### Wound healing

The process of wound healing, the response to tissue damage, is sufficiently akin to the physiology of inflammation, whatever the inciting stimulus, to be considered simultaneously. Disorders of wound healing are often associated with factors that result in too little or too much inflammation. Overwhelming infection and organ malfunction may similarly result from an inadequate or excessive inflammatory response. Therefore, the description that follows is applicable to both.

The initial response to tissue damage by trauma is bleeding and coagulation. This is less likely but not impossible with tissue damage from such insults as ischemia and infection. Platelet activation results in the release of important chemoattractants (i.e. platelet derived growth factor (PDGF), transforming growth factor-$\beta$ (TGF-$\beta$). Damaged blood vessels initially vasoconstrict, but this is soon followed by vasodilatation and increased capillary permeability secondary to the action of agents like prostaglandin $E_2$, prostacyclin, histamine, serotonin and kinins. When blood flow is present this vascular response results in the accumulation of protein-rich edema fluid (exudate). White cells adhere to these damaged and leaky vessels.

Attracted by chemoattractants like PDGF, polymorphonuclear cells (PMNs) are the first white cells to migrate to the inflammatory site (within minutes if the circulation is good). PMNs serve to phagocytize dead tissue and foreign objects. Removal of bacteria may be assisted by opsonins and preformed antibodies. PMNs produce proteases and intracellular oxygen radicals which are critical for beneficial PMN activity. Besides proteases and oxygen radicals, PMNs can also release interleukin (IL)-1. IL-8 is a potent PMN attractant produced by many cell types after incubation with IL-1 and tumor necrosis factor (TNF). The PMNs last only for hours.

Lymphocytes are the next cells to migrate into the wound. The role of the lymphocyte is less well understood, but depletion of T cells results in impaired wound healing. Next (within hours) tissue macrophages and circulating monocytes are attracted by such substances as PDGF, TGF-$\beta$ and IL-1, migrate into the injured area and last for days to weeks. Wounds can heal without PMNs but not without macrophages which regulate most of the continuing stages of inflammation and wound healing through such mediators as IL-1, TNF, PDGF, TGF-$\beta$, TGF-$\alpha$ and fibroblast growth factor (FGF). As described in detail below, the cytokine response of macrophages appears profoundly to influence both local and systemic manifestations of inflammation.

Next, fibroblast migration and angiogenesis begin. Fibroblasts are influenced by IL-1, TNF, PDGF, TGF-$\beta$, TGF-$\alpha$, insulin-like growth factor (IGF) and epidermal growth factor (EGF). Angiogenesis is influenced by TNF, TGF-$\beta$, TGF-$\alpha$ and EGF. The combined process of fibroblast proliferation and capillary budding produce a wound that is granular in appearance (granulation tissue), very vascular and quite friable. Certain fibroblasts, myofibroblasts, have smooth muscle contractile elements which contract and diminish the area of a wound. In general, wound contraction continues until the lining cells from each edge of a wound meet (epithelialization for the skin). Therefore, little contraction will follow wounds that are closed primarily – that is, with the lining edges apposed. Much contraction may occur in secondary healing, especially when wound edges remain widely separated for long periods.

Fibroblasts make collagen, usually accelerating at 5 days after tissue damage. Before this, fibrin is the only substance besides sutures holding a wound together. Collagen synthesis is also influenced by IL-1, TNF, PDGF, TGF-$\beta$ and EGF. Since the macrophage is an important source of these factors, mechanisms that increase (glucan administration) and decrease (the combined effect of hypoxia and endotoxin) macrophage function may result in increased or decreased wound strength, respectively. A summary of cellular activity in wound healing is provided in Tables 1 and 2.

**Mediators and mechanisms of cellular activation**
Following tissue injury and/or infection many endogenous cells and cell products contribute in a complex manner to both the local and systemic

**TABLE 1   NORMAL WOUND HEALING/NORMAL INFLAMMATION**

| Events | Cells responsible |
|---|---|
| Coagulation | platelets |
| Early inflammation | polymorphonuclear cells (first few hours) |
| Later inflammation | monocytes (days), macrophages |
| Collagen and mucopolysaccharide | fibroblasts (maximum deposition 7–10 days) |
| Capillary budding | endothelial cells (maximum 7–10 days) |
| Wound contraction | myofibroblasts |
| Collagen remodeling | fewer fibroblasts and capillaries |

### TABLE 2  FUNCTIONS OF WOUND HEALING CELLS

| Cell | Function |
| --- | --- |
| Platelets | coagulation, release PDGF, IL-1 |
| Polymorphonuclear cells | phagocytosis, especially microbes, release IL-1, IL-8 |
| Macrophage | phagocytosis, stimulate fibroblast migration and growth, stimulate endothelial cell migration and growth, release FGF, PDGF, IL-1, TNF, TGF-$\beta$, TGF-$\alpha$ |
| Fibroblast | collagen deposition, wound contraction, wound remodeling |
| Endothelial cells | capillary budding |

PDGF, platelet derived growth factor; IL, interleukin; FGF, fibroblast growth factor; TNF, tumor necrosis factor; TGF, transforming growth factor

manifestations that accompany the disease process. The importance of endogenous cell activity is well illustrated by the accruing evidence that the adverse effects of endotoxin are primarily a result of endogenous cell activation rather than a direct toxic effect of the endotoxin molecule *per se*. As with all aspects of the inflammatory response, both beneficial (e.g. wound healing, control of infection) and detrimental (remote organ injury) effects of these cellular products have been described. The purpose of this section is to provide an overview of mediator activity as it relates to inflammation and then as it relates to systemic metabolic effects. Later the relationship of mediators to inflammatory alterations in the circulation will be presented. The effects of mediator action on other individual organ functions will be presented in the specific organ-related sections.

### Cytokines

Cytokines are small protein molecules produced by many cells participating in the inflammatory response to injury and infection. Several cytokines promote inflammation (pro-inflammatory), others inhibit inflammation (anti-inflammatory). TNF and IL-1, -2, -6 and -8 are considered pro-inflammatory. Table 3 lists these mediators, the origin of the cells and the primary effects on inflammation. IL-4 and IL-10 are anti-inflammatory.

### Arachidonic acid/phospholipids

Arachidonic acid (AA) in man is derived from ingested linoleic acid or as a constituent of meat. AA then becomes a component of the phospholipids

**TABLE 3  CYTOKINES (adapted from Fong Y, Lowry SF. Cytokines and the cellular response to injury and infection. In *Care of The Surgical Patient*. New York: Scientific American Inc, 1996)**

| Cytokine | Source | Inflammatory functions |
|---|---|---|
| TNF | blood monocytes | release of PMNs from bone marrow, PMN margination |
| | tissue macrophages | PMN activation, PMN migration |
| | mast cells | monocyte activation |
| | lymphocytes | lymphocyte activation |
| | endothelial cells | |
| | glial cells | |
| IL-1 | blood monocytes | release of PMNs from bone marrow, PMN migration |
| | tissue macrophages | monocyte activation, lymphocyte activation |
| | endothelial cells | |
| | lymphocytes | |
| IL-2 | T cells | T-cell proliferation, lymphokine synthesis |
| IL-6 | blood monocytes | B-cell proliferation, |
| | tissue macrophages | acute phase protein production |
| | endothelial cells | |
| | T cells | |
| IL-8 | many cells | selective PMN attraction |

TNF, tumor necrosis factor; PMN, polymorphonuclear cells; IL, interleukin

of cell membranes or other complex lipids. Once released from membrane phospholipids by the enzyme phospholipase $A_2$, AA is metabolized by two enzymatic mechanisms, cyclooxygenase and lipoxygenase. The sequential action of cyclooxygenase results in the prostaglandins listed in Table 4. The presence of cyclooxygenase and these various prostaglandins varies from tissue to tissue. For instance, the lung and spleen have all components, platelets make mostly thromboxane $A_2$, and blood vessel endothelium mostly prostacyclin (prostaglandin $I_2$). Lipoxygenase activity results in the products listed in Table 4. Lipoxygenase has been found only in the lung, platelets and white cells. 12-Hydroxyarachidonic acid (HETE) has been found to be chemotactic for PMNs and alveolar macrophages.

### TABLE 4   ARACHIDONIC ACID METABOLISM

*Cyclooxygenase*
Cyclooxygenase products
   prostaglandins G and H
   prostaglandin E, prostaglandin F, prostaglandin D
Thromboxane synthetase
   makes prostaglandin $H_2$ into thromboxane $A_2$
     which breaks down rapidly to thromboxane $B_2$
Prostacyclin synthetase
   makes prostaglandin $H_2$ into prostaglandin $I_2$ (prostacyclin) which is
   metabolized to 6-keto-prostaglandin $F_1$

*Lipoxygenase*
Lipoxygenase activity
   12-hydroperoxyarachidonic acid (HPETE)
   12-hydroxyarachidonic acid (HETE)
   5-hydroperoxyeicosatetraneoic acid (5-HPETE)
Derivatives of 5-HPETE
   leukotriene $A_4$
   leukotriene $B_4$
   leukotriene $C_4$
   leukotriene $D_4$
   leukotriene $E_4$

Leukotrienes $C_4$, $D_4$ and $E_4$ make up the substance identified previously as slow-reacting substance of anaphylaxis (SRS-A).

The lung is a major site of metabolism of AA derivatives. Many are inactivated with one passage. Other tissues that metabolize AA derivatives are spleen, kidney, adipose tissue, intestine, liver and testicle. AA derivatives exhibit several physiological effects which promote inflammation (Table 5).

Phospholipase $A_2$ also results in the release of platelet-activating factor (PAF) which promotes platelet aggregation, leukocyte activation, microvascular permeability and the metabolism of AA. Phospholipase $A_2$ has been found to be elevated in the serum of critically ill surgical patients.

*Nitric oxide*
Nitric oxide (NO) is synthesized from L-arginine by NO synthetase (NOS) which is present in endothelial cells as a constitutive enzyme (ecNOS)

**TABLE 5   EFFECTS OF ARACHIDONIC ACID DERIVATIVES THAT PROMOTE INFLAMMATION**

*Vasodilatation*
Prostaglandin Es
Prostaglandin As
Prostaglandin $I_2$ (not inactivated by the lungs)

*Platelet aggregation/stimulation*
Thromboxane $A_2$

*Leukocyte chemotaxis, aggregation, enzyme release, superoxide radical production*
Leukotriene $B_4$
Thromboxane $A_2$

and in macrophages, fibroblasts, glial cells and cardiac myocytes as an inducible enzyme (iNOS). The constitutive enzyme results in the continuous release of NO which promotes an active state of vascular dilatation as well as inhibition of platelet and PMN adhesion to endothelial cells. The inducible form responds to pro-inflammatory cytokines (TNF, IL-1) and endotoxin, and results in larger amounts of NO production, as compared to ecNOS. In these concentrations NO can be toxic against fungal, bacterial, protozoal and tumor cells. When exposed to high levels of NO endogenous cells may also suffer from the inhibition of cellular respiration and increased lactate production.

*Superoxide radicals*
The development of aerobic metabolism with cytochrome oxidase allows cells to produce substantial energy from the oxidation of glucose and metabolic intermediaries. The acquisition of this function was accompanied by the production of potentially harmful oxygen metabolites (the superoxide radical, hydrogen peroxide and the hydroxy radical) from about 1 to 2% of the oxygen metabolized. Enzyme systems (e.g. superoxide dismutases, catalases, peroxidases) have evolved which metabolize these products to harmless molecules. During the respiratory burst that accompanies phagocytosis PMN leukocytes produce superoxide, presumably to help destroy ingested organisms but also for chemotaxis.

Oxygen radicals have many adverse effects including degradation of hyaluronic acid and collagen, lipid peroxidation and damage to cell membranes and organelles. Such damage may initiate cell injury directly.

The ischemia-reperfusion model of oxygen radical injury also results in a pro-inflammatory PMN recruitment, which may amplify the original insult.

*Serotonin*
Serotonin (5-hydroxytryptamine, 5-HT) is primarily (90%) located in the gastrointestinal enterochromaffin cells. Otherwise, 5-HT is found in platelets and the central nervous system (CNS). Platelets do not synthesize 5-HT but acquire it as they pass through the intestinal circulation. 5-HT is metabolized primarily by the liver, and, when in the systemic circulation, also by the lung. The physiological effects of 5-HT are:

(1) Cardiovascular
      (a) Peripheral arterial vasodilatation,
      (b) Pulmonary arterial vasoconstriction (mild),
      (c) Venous constriction (marked),
      (d) Mild inotropic and chronotropic effect;

(2) Pulmonary
      (a) Increased minute volume,
      (b) Bronchoconstriction (mild);

(3) Blood components
      (a) Platelet aggregation,
      (b) Platelet release of thromboxane $A_2$.

*Histamine*
The actions of histamine are dependent primarily on the nature and location of the type of histamine receptor ($H_1$ or $H_2$) on a given tissue. Bronchoconstriction and gut wall contraction are mediated by the $H_1$ receptor, gastric secretion by $H_2$ receptors and vascular dilatation by receptors of both types. The various physiological responses related to inflammation are listed below.

(1) Vascular response
      (a) Arteriolar dilatation ($H_1 + H_2$),
      (b) Increased postcapillary venular permeability ($H_1$),
      (c) Venous constriction;

(2) White blood cells ($H_2$)
      (a) Prevents release of lysozymes by PMNs,
      (b) Inhibits release of antibody from B cells,
      (c) Inhibits release of lymphokines from T cells.

Histamine is located primarily in skin, intestinal mucosa and lungs. The site of histamine storage is the mast cell in tissues and the basophil cell in the blood. The allergic release of histamine from mast cells and basophils requires an antigen–IgE complex, or complement anaphylatoxins (C3a, C5a). Histamine can also be released by injury to the mast cells, most often noted in the skin (e.g. burn or scratch). Elevated plasma histamine concentrations have been noted following endotoxin administration and trauma.

*Kinins*
The kinins are blood-borne molecules which are enzymatically activated during inflammation. The most potent kinins are bradykinin and kallidin. The inflammatory effects of bradykinin and kallidin include vasodilatation of small resistance vessels and increased venular permeability.

*Endothelial molecules*
Rather than an innocent spectator subjected passively to the mechanisms of disease generated either locally or from a distance, the vascular endothelium is an active participant in inflammatory processes. Several molecules can be generated in endothelial cells which directly affect vascular tone and permeability as well as the course of inflammation.

Endothelial cell generation of NO increases vasodilatation during both physiological and pathophysiological states. Endothelin-1, a vasoconstrictor, is generated during disease. Endothelial cells stimulated with endotoxin, TNF and IL-1 generate an adhesion molecule (E-selectin) which promotes the adherence of PMNs, monocytes and T cells to vascular endothelium. E-selectin has been measured in the circulation of patients with systemic inflammation, especially when organ malfunction is present. Intercellular adhesion molecules (ICAM-1) and vascular cell adhesion molecules (VCAM-1) also may be related to inflammatory states.

The active participation of endothelial cells in inflammation may explain, in part, the clinical experience of severe inflammation developing in patients suffering severe depression of circulating inflammatory cell numbers and/or function (bone marrow transplantation patients, organ transplant patients).

## Metabolic and hormonal response to inflammation
The metabolic and hormonal response during severe inflammation is in many ways a continuation and exaggeration of the ebb and flow phases following injury (Table 6). Classically the ebb phase, as described by

**TABLE 6 SUMMARY OF METABOLIC CHANGES AFTER SEVERE INJURY OR INFLAMMATION IN HUMANS (after Stoner HB.** Metabolism after trauma and in sepsis.*Circul Shock* 1986;19:75–87)

| | | Severe inflammation | |
| --- | --- | --- | --- |
| Substance | Trauma | Ebb | Flow |
| Epinephrine | INC | N | INC |
| Norepinephrine | INC | N | INC |
| Cortisol | INC | N | INC |
| Insulin | DEC | INC | VAR |
| Glucose | INC | VAR | VAR |
| Fatty acids | DEC | VAR | DEC |
| Albumin | VAR | DEC | DEC |
| Acute reactants | VAR | INC | INC |
| Urine nitrogen | VAR | INC | INC |
| Resting energy expenditure | VAR | INC | INC |
| Glucose oxidation | DEC | INC | DEC |
| Fat oxidation | INC | INC | INC |

N, normal; INC, increased; DEC, decreased; VAR, variable

Cuthbertson (Stoner, 1986), is witnessed early after injury and during a stage commonly associated with hypoperfusion. The flow phase then follows after resuscitation of the circulation with a hyperdynamic circulation and accentuation of hypermetabolism. Hypermetabolism is characteristic of the flow phase with increased resting energy expenditure, glucose and fat oxidation. This is usually maximum at 3–4 days after injury and diminishes gradually in association with resolution of ileus, spontaneous diuresis of 'third space' and normothermia, as the inflammatory response to injury subsides. When inflammation continues, most commonly secondary to infection, the flow phase transforms into continuing hypermetabolism which will eventually result in progressive organ failure and death, sometimes despite eradication of the initial inflammatory focus.

*Carbohydrate*
Glucose is commonly elevated in the ebb phase following trauma, is frequently elevated in the flow phase, and with continuing or worsening inflammation. The combination of increased epinephrine, cortisol, glucagon, lactate and release of gluconeogenic amino acids from muscle (especially alanine) results in elevated glucose, often despite elevated insulin. As inflammation progresses glucose intolerance increases, with gluconeo-

genesis accelerated by the mass action of lactate and alanine. Glucose uptake is accelerated, particularly at major inflammatory foci such as a large wound. Therefore, elevated glucose production may provide an important energy substrate for inflammatory cells.

Elevated lactate may result from decreased oxygen delivery, but with resuscitation of the circulation inflammation is usually associated with increased oxygen delivery and consumption (see below). Other possible causes of elevated lactate are increased production by inflammatory cells or decreased processing of pyruvate through the Kreb's cycle because of enzyme abnormalities rather than lack of oxygen. For instance, active macrophages have been shown to increase glucose utilization, elevate lactate production, and proportionally increase pyruvate, a phenomenon seen in inflammation.

*Fat*
Use of fat is increased in inflammation. Some studies demonstrate fat as the major energy supply, while others demonstrate the major supply as carbohydrate. Insulin resistance is also seen at the adipocyte where lipolysis continues, despite elevated insulin.

*Protein*
The loss of protein (negative nitrogen balance) witnessed during the flow phase following injury continues at an accelerated rate in severe inflammation and appears to correlate well with organ failure. Since protein is essential for enzymes and coagulation protein synthesis, immunocompetence and diaphragm function, the relationship of progressive protein loss to increased morbidity and mortality is readily understandable.

The greatest protein breakdown occurs in skeletal muscle, the intestine and connective tissue with flux of the resultant amino acids (particularly alanine and glutamine) to the liver where protein synthesis, especially of acute phase reactants, is increased but does not equal breakdown. Amino acids are oxidized as an energy source, especially in skeletal muscle. Increased serum alanine promotes hepatic gluconeogenesis rather than protein synthesis. Glutamine, which is important for kidney and intestinal mucosal cell metabolism, may be decreased in plasma despite the release from muscle.

Increased breakdown also results in ureagenesis, ammonia and uric acid production, as well as increased creatinine release. When unchecked or not ameliorated with therapy, severe protein malnutrition can develop rapidly with progressive liver dysfunction a common terminal event.

## Mediators of the metabolic and hormonal response

The stimulation and inhibition of cellular activity which results in the metabolic and hormonal response to severe injury and inflammation can be divided into four potential pathways: the CNS, endocrine (interactions via the circulation), paracrine (cell-to-cell interactions) and autocrine (cell self-stimulation). All the mediators listed in Table 7 contribute to the observed metabolic alterations described above. No single pathway appears to be sufficient to explain the magnitude of changes measured in animals and humans.

The positive and negative feedback possibilities within this array of biological products are staggering. Further investigation to enhance the understanding of these complex interactions will be useful in the pursuit of knowledge. It is unlikely that this pursuit will result in a simple method of therapeutic intervention that will maintain the beneficial effects of this metabolic response (e.g. wound healing, acute phase reactant synthesis) while dramatically inhibiting the detrimental effects (muscle wasting). Instead, support of the patient to ameliorate the adverse metabolic effects while the primary inflammatory disease is addressed will likely remain the mainstay of management.

## NORMAL IMMUNOLOGY

### Local defense mechanisms

The components of local defense mechanisms are mechanical barriers to penetration (skin and mucous membranes) and barrier cell function (macrophages, surface propulsion, secretory immunoglobulins and normal flora). Tight epithelial cell junctions, surface chemicals, macrophages and surface propulsion such as occur with cilia in the tracheobronchial tree, IgA secretion and normal flora all serve to prevent pathogens from invading across epithelial structures. Many insults, such as antibiotics, immunological suppression and especially trauma, may interrupt these barrier functions and allow pathogens to enter deeper tissues.

### Polymorphonuclear leukocytes

Once the barrier is broken, the initial response to any insult (trauma, infection, chemical irritation) is PMN cell migration. Once released from the bone marrow PMNs remain in the circulation for 6–10 h. One third of the intravascular PMN population circulate, while two thirds marginate or roll along near the vessel wall. The migration of PMNs (chemotaxis) from the circulation to inflamed tissues is stimulated by substances called chemotactic factors (Table 8). Complement-derived products, especially

**TABLE 7    MEDIATORS OF METABOLISM FOLLOWING SEVERE INJURY AND/OR INFLAMMATION**

| | |
|---|---|
| *Central nervous system* | Cytokines |
| Hypothalamus | IL-1 |
| ACTH | TNF |
| AVP | IL-6 |
| growth hormone | Phospholipase A$_2$ |
| TSH | |
| Sympathetic nervous system | *Paracrine* |
| norepinephrine | Cytokines |
| Endorphins | IL-1 |
| | TNF |
| *Endocrine* | IL-6 |
| Adrenal cortex | Prostaglandins |
| cortisol | Superoxide radicals |
| aldosterone | *Autocrine* |
| Adrenal medulla | Cytokines |
| epinephrine | IL-1 |
| Pancreas | TNF |
| insulin | IL-6 |
| glucagon | Prostaglandins |
| Thyroid | Superoxide radicals |
| T3 | Nitric oxide |
| T4 | |

ACTH, adrenocorticotropic hormone; AVP, argenine vasopressin; TSH, thyroid-stimulating hormone; IL, interleukin; TNF, tumor necrosis factor

C5a, appear to be most important (see below for a discussion of the complement system).

Once the PMNs migrate, ingestion of organisms and dead tissue occurs, which, for microbes, is enhanced greatly by humoral factors called opsonins. Opsonins bind to the surface of microbes, interact with receptors on the phagocyte and improve ingestion. There are three types of opsonins: IgG antibodies, complement and fibronectin. Once ingested, the PMN uses a variety of mechanisms to kill microbes. Oxygen-dependent killing mechanisms include the use of hydrogen peroxide, myeloperoxidase, superoxide anion, hydroxy radicals and singlet oxygen. Oxygen-independent killing mechanisms include the use of acid, lactoferrin, lysozyme and granule cationic proteins.

## TABLE 8   CHEMOTACTIC SUBSTANCES

*Clotting of blood*
Kallikrein
Plasminogen activator
Fibrinopeptides

*Injured tissues*
Collagen fragments
Tissues factors

*Complement*
C3a
C5a
C567

*Bacteria*
Bacterial peptides

*Lymphocytes*
Lymphokines

### Monocytes and macrophages

Monocytes are intravascular cells of which approximately two thirds circulate and the remainder are adherent to vascular endothelium. When monocytes migrate into tissues they differentiate into macrophages, which have different properties depending upon the tissue. For instance, alveolar macrophages are not phagocytic, Kupffer cells in the liver are highly phagocytic, and wound macrophages attract fibroblasts to the wound. Macrophages that reside in tissues, especially the liver and spleen, make up the bulk of the reticuloendothelial (RE) defense system. The immunological functions of macrophages are listed in Table 9. RE system phagocytosis of non-bacterial particulate matter is enhanced by opsonization with $\alpha$-2 surface binding protein (fibronectin). Macrophages not only perform phagocytic functions, but also process antigens which results in both T- (cellular immunity) and B- (humoral immunity) cell activation.

### Lymphocytes and cell-mediated immunity

T (thymus-derived) lymphocytes are responsible for the cellular immunological response as exemplified by delayed hypersensitivity. As mentioned above, macrophages must first process antigens for T cells to

## TABLE 9   MACROPHAGE FUNCTIONS

*Ingestion of unwanted materials*
Microbes
Necrotic tissue
Organic and inorganic foreign bodies

*Ingestion of intracellular pathogens*
Pneumocystis
Mycobacterium
Salmonella
Listeria
Cryptococcus
Toxoplasma

*Immunological processing*
Phagocytosis of antigen
Interleukin-1 release
  T-cell differentiation
  T-cell secretion of lymphokines
    $\gamma$-interferon results in macrophage becoming highly phagocytic
    interleukin-2 results in B-cell activation

*Delayed hypersensitivity*

respond. There are primarily two types of T cells – the T-helper cell (Th, CD4) and the T-effector cell (Te). Th cells are needed for the development of cell-mediated immunity and also through IL-2 assist B-cell activation. Te cells are most capable of producing cytotoxic damage. While Te cells may directly produce cytotoxic damage, secretions of the Te cell (lymphokines) may be of greater importance for the elimination of antigens.

Another T-cell subpopulation, T suppressor (Ts, CD8) cells, inhibit both helper and effector cell function. Natural killer (NK) cells are large, granular lymphocytes which can destroy non-self cells without prior immunological processing and may be particularly important as a defense against malignant cell propagation.

### Lymphocytes and humoral immunity
Lymphocytes which produce immunoglobulins are called bursa-derived or B cells. As mentioned above, Th-cell activation is most often required for

B-cell response to an antigen. The major immunoglobulins and their primary functions are shown in Table 10.

**Complement**

Complement is a non-specific humoral defense mechanism which is composed of several protein components and can be activated by various substances. Complement serves to amplify opsonization and lysis. Beginning with the top of the complement 'cascade' each complement protein is first activated and then, subsequently, cleaves the next protein in a manner similar to the coagulation sequence. Also, like coagulation, the cascade may be activated by two routes, the 'classic' and the 'alternate' pathways (Figure 1), which lead to the same final products. The end result is vasodilatation, chemotaxis and opsonization. The biological effects of complement fragments released during the cascade are listed in Table 11.

The classic pathway is initiated by the interaction of C1, the first complement component, with IgM or IgG complexed with an antigen. IgA and IgE do not bind C1. The alternate pathway is activated by endotoxin, polysaccharides, zymosan and pyogenic cocci. Properdin is a protein analogous to C1 which is activated by the substances that activate the alternate pathway and leads to a sequence which eventually activates C3. One product of C3 activation, C3b, has a central role: it amplifies the cascade, activates C5 and is the most potent opsonin.

**Gastrointestinal mucosal barrier**

Severe inflammation is the primary etiology of death in surgical patients. Critically ill surgical patients often suffer bacteremias or fungemias, with aerobic organisms commonly found in the gastrointestinal (GI) tract (i.e. coagulace negative staphylococcus, enterococcus, *Candida, Escherichia coli, Klebsiella*). In 35–75% of these patients, a portal of entry (e.g. wound, urinary tract, sputum, central line) cannot be identified. Similar microbial invasion of the bloodstream has been noted in granulocytopenic patients, especially those with acute leukemia. Administration of oral antibiotics

**TABLE 10   IMMUNOGLOBULINS**

| Type | Function |
|------|----------|
| IgG | opsonization, activate complement |
| IgM | primary response, complement activation |
| IgE | immediate hypersensitivity |
| IgA | mucosal immunity |

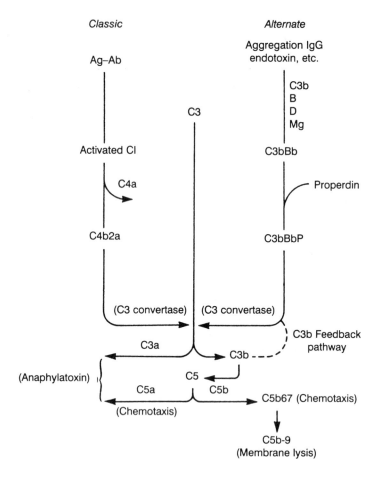

**Figure 1** A representation of the classic and alternate pathways of complement activation which can result in chemotaxis and cell lysis. Reproduced with permission from Cotan RS, Kumar V, Collins T, Robbins SL, eds. *Robbins Pathologic Basis of Disease*, 4th edn. New York: WB Saunders

effective against GI tract aerobes and fungi may diminish these septic episodes.

These studies suggest that immunocompromise from cancer, chemotherapy and critical surgical illness diminishes the 'mucosal barrier' function of the GI tract against the migration of viable intestinal organisms and/or possibly non-viable bacterial and fungal products into the

**TABLE 11   BIOLOGICAL EFFECTS OF COMPLEMENT FRAGMENTS**

| Fragment | Effect |
|---|---|
| C4a | serotonin release |
| C2b | kinin-like activity |
| C4b | immune adherence |
| C3a | anaphylatoxin, vasodilatation, chemotaxis, leukocyte mobilization |
| C3b | opsonization, immune adherence, release of platelet factor 3 |
| C5a | potent chemotaxis, ? platelet lysis |
| C567 | chemotaxis |
| C8 | initiates lysis |
| C9 | completes lysis |

mesenteric lymph nodes, liver, spleen and/or the bloodstream (collectively termed translocation). Several experimental studies have begun to elucidate the determinants of translocation (shown along with their clinical counterparts in Table 12).

Surgical patients who are subject to these insults usually have suffered hemorrhage, trauma and/or previous severe infection. In addition, these patients have received multiple antibiotics (often with activity against anaerobes), and receive total parenteral nutrition (TPN) at the time of or just preceding the translocation. Trauma and previous severe infection are known to depress immunological function (*vide infra*). Parenteral antibiotics allow growth of resistant organisms in the GI tract and often depress anaerobic bacterial concentrations. In addition, TPN may result in reduced GI tract mucosal barrier function.

The GI mucosa metabolizes the amino acid glutamine as a preferential substrate, especially during stress. Glutamine is an unessential amino acid which is unstable in solution and is not used in standard TPN. Therefore, GI mucosal energy needs may not be met as well with TPN, as compared with enteral nutrition which contains glutamine. In addition IgA, the mucosal surface antibody, may be diminished with TPN as compared with oral intake, possibly because of less antigenic stimulation. Thus, both the metabolism of the mucosal cell and the production of mucosal antibody may be suppressed by using TPN as the only nutritional source. Clinical studies that support the use of enteral nutrition over TPN to reduce infection risk will be discussed in Chapter 6; The gastrointestinal/nutritional system; Gastrointestinal dysfunction.

### TABLE 12   DETERMINANTS OF TRANSLOCATION

| Experimental factor | Clinical correlate |
|---|---|
| Aerobic organisms | *Bacteroides* rarely cultured |
| Inhibited by normal flora, especially anaerobes | follows broad-spectrum antibiotics, especially agents effective against bacteroides species |
| Promoted by anti-anaerobic antibiotics | follows broad-spectrum antibiotics, especially agents effective against bacteroides species |
| Enhanced by immunosuppression | seen in granulocytopenic patients, patients suffering from trauma and other severe inflammation |
| Enhanced with burns | seen in burn patients |
| Enhanced by malnutrition | seen in malnourished patients |
| Enhanced by parenteral feeding | TPN a major risk factor |

TPN, total parenteral nutrition

**Assessment of immunological status**

Numerous *in vitro* and *in vivo* tests have been used to assess immunological function. A listing of the various tests and the functions they assess is given in Table 13.

**Common disorders**

Disorders of immunological function have been described in a large variety of primary illnesses and as acquired phenomena accompanying trauma, infection, certain therapeutic agents and malnutrition. The conditions seen commonly in surgical patients and the associated dysfunction are listed in Table 14.

One simple clinical test is the response to recall skin antigens. The association of anergy with postoperative severe infection and death is well documented. However, the many potential etiologies of anergy make differential diagnosis difficult. For instance, a patient with cancer of the esophagus may have anergy because of the cancer, radiation therapy, chemotherapy and malnutrition. Simply addressing malnutrition may not restore adequate immunological function, whereas removing the cancer may prove more beneficial. The clinician must weigh these considerations carefully to direct therapy to improve immunocompetence.

## TABLE 13   IMMUNOLOGIC TESTS

| Cells tested | Function | Test |
|---|---|---|
| PMN | chemotaxis | test movement of PMNs from one chamber to another across a membrane (Boyden Chamber Chemotactic Index) |
| PMN | opsonization | test serum ability to allow normal PMNs to phagocytize standard test bacteria |
| PMN | phagocytosis | test PMNs ability to ingest and kill standard test microbes |
| Macrophage | chemotaxis | test macrophage movement into an injured area (Rebuck skin abrasion test) |
| Macrophage | phagocytosis | test ability to ingest facultative intracellular organisms (*Mycobacterium tuberculosis, Listeria, Salmonella*) |
| Macrophage | RE function | clearance of radio-labelled microaggregated albumin |
| T cells | numbers | T-lymphocyte count |
| T cells | proliferation | response to mitogens phytohemaglutinin, pokeweed |
| T cells | lymphokine production | assay macrophage migration inhibition factor, chemotactic factor, macrophage-activating factor |
| T cells | overall function | dinitrochlorobenzene sensitization, recall skin tests |
| B cells | overall function | serum levels of immunoglobulins, |
| Complement | overall function | serum levels of complement components |

PMN, polymorphonuclear cells; RE, reticuloendothelial system

## PATHOLOGICAL SYSTEMIC INFLAMMATION: PHYSIOLOGY

### Effects on the circulation

Severe systemic inflammation is associated with alterations in both total body and regional perfusion. Mechanisms which can reduce cardiac output during systemic inflammation are listed in Table 15.

The most common etiology of inadequate cardiac output during inflammation is decreased venous return which results from both loss of intravascular fluid and vasodilatation. Intravascular volume decreases as

### TABLE 14    SURGICAL CONDITIONS AND COMMON IMMUNOLOGICAL DYSFUNCTION

*Trauma and hemorrhagic shock*
Depressed PMN motility
Depressed lymphocyte response to mitogens
Increased suppressor T-cell activity
RE system depression
Anergy to skin recall antigens
Decreased complement
Decreased fibronectin
Depressed GI mucosal barrier

*Burns*
Depressed local cellular and humoral immunity in the burn wound
Depressed PMN chemotaxis
Depressed PMN bactericidal activity
Depressed opsonization
Increased T-suppressor cell activity
Anergy to skin recall antigens
Decreased interleukin-2
Decreased fibronectin
Depressed GI tract mucosal barrier

*Malnutrition*
Depressed PMN chemotaxis
Depressed PMN bactericidal activity
Depressed macrophage migration
Anergy to recall skin antigens
Depressed lymphocyte response to mitogens
Depressed immunoglobulin response to an antigen
Decreased complement
Depressed RE function
Depressed GI tract mucosal barrier

*Cancer*
Anergy to recall skin antigens
Decreased lymphocyte response to antigens

*Sepsis*
Anergy to recall skin antigens
Depressed opsonization
Decreased fibronectin

*(continued)*

## TABLE 14    (continued)

*Blood transfusion*
Depressed macrophage-lymphocyte stimulation
Depressed lymphocyte response to mitogens

*Steroids*
Decreased PMN chemotaxis
Decreased macrophage migration
Decreased macrophage phagocytosis
Decreased T-lymphocytes

*Chemotherapy and radiation*
Decreased delayed hypersensitivity
Decreased lymphocyte response to mitogens
Decreased humoral response
Anergy to recall skin antigens

*Antibiotics*
Depressed cellular immunity (tetracycline, chloramphenicol, clindamycin, gentamicin)
Stress on GI tract mucosal barrier especially with inhibition of anaerobic bacteria

*Anesthesia and surgery*
Depressed lymphocyte response to mitogens
Anergy to skin recall antigens
Depressed PMN phagocytosis (halothane and ether)

PMN, polymorphonuclear cells; RE, reticuloendothelial; GI, gastrointestinal

plasma exudes into the primary focus of inflammation (area of injury or infection). When systemic inflammation develops in response to the primary focus of inflammation, plasma may also exude into some or all the other tissues. Such exudation results in an increase in interstitial fluid which become protein-rich as compared with normal. In general, interstitial fluid is maintained in the extracellular space by active cellular processes, which maintain cell membrane integrity and perform such functions as sodium/potassium exchange, which keeps potassium in the cell and sodium out. Severe inflammation may interfere with active cell membrane function, decrease ion exchange capabilities and allow more interstitial water and solutes to enter cells. Depletion of interstitial fluid may be another mechanism aggravating plasma volume loss.

## TABLE 15   CIRCULATORY DISORDERS IN SEVERE INFLAMMATION – REDUCED CARDIAC OUTPUT

*Hypovolemia*
Peripheral vasodilatation
Increased capillary permeability, local or total body
Intracellular migration of fluid
Sequestration in GI tract lumen

*Myocardial depression*

*Increased pulmonary vascular resistance*
Hypoxia
Platelet emboli
Thromboxane release
Serotonin release
White cell aggregation

Ileus is common during severe inflammation, regardless of the location of the primary focus. Ileus can result in the accumulation of fluid in the lumen of the gastrointestinal tract which can be as voluminous as that sequestered during bowel obstruction. Collectively the exudation of plasma volume into inflammatory foci, the accumulation of fluid in the GI tract and the migration of fluid into cells is termed the third space, to distinguish it from normal plasma and interstitial fluid spaces. The magnitude of the third space effect is roughly proportional to the magnitude of tissue injury and/or infection present. The primary effect of third space fluid accumulation is to deplete intravascular volume and impair venous return.

Vasodilatation of systemic veins and arterioles is characteristic of severe inflammation, and several inflammatory mediators have been implicated as causative (e.g. histamine, kinins, prostacyclin, NO). Increasing the capacitance of veins decreases mean systemic (not mean arterial) pressure and may decrease venous return, especially if central venous pressure (see below and Chapter 2, The circulation, cardiovascular physiology; Venous return) does not decrease proportionally because of increased pulmonary vascular resistance.

Severe inflammation may directly depress the function of previously normal myocardial cells. Less severe inflammation may result in augmented malfunction of previously abnormal cardiac tissue. Therefore, cardiac output may be impaired in a fashion which results in a physiology consistent with an excess of intravascular volume rather than a deficit. Recognition of cardiogenic states of hypoperfusion during inflammation is important for proper therapeutic intervention (see below).

Severe inflammation is associated with increased pulmonary vascular resistance. This increase in right ventricular afterload may result in dilatation of the right ventricle, decreased right ventricular ejection, and impaired filling of the left ventricle. Right atrial pressure may increase and impair venous return.

### Effects of the circulation on severe inflammation

Both regional and global deficits in the circulation can aggravate inflammation. Interruption of a region of the circulation to a tissue will result in partial to complete necrosis of the previously perfused region. Tissue necrosis will result in inflammation at the site of tissue injury and the magnitude of cellular injury will usually determine if the resultant inflammatory response remains local or becomes systemic. In other words, the more tissue death, the more inflammation, the more likely a systemic inflammatory response will occur. The relationship between the amount of tissue damage and the degree of systemic inflammation is best illustrated by the physiology following burn injury of varying depths and quantities of skin.

Ischemia-reperfusion can result in both local and systemic inflammatory responses, likewise dependent on the amount of tissue that becomes ischemic (i.e. calf muscles from an embolism to the popliteal artery vs. total body ischemia from profound hemorrhagic shock) and then reperfused.

Global and regional hypoperfusion is an etiology of disruption of the gastrointestinal mucosal barrier which can allow inflammatory stimulants to migrate from the intestinal lumen into the portal circulation, potentially stimulating Kupffer cells, or the general circulation, stimulating inflammatory cells elsewhere.

### Effects on cell metabolism

The effects of severe inflammation on metabolism have been studied in many cell systems, with liver, inflammatory cell and skeletal muscle models used most frequently. Two broad categories of cellular metabolic alterations have been most frequently described: alterations in cell membrane function and alterations in intracellular energy metabolism.

*Alterations in cell membrane function*
Decreased cell membrane function is characterized by such abnormalities as altered electrical gradients, increased permeability and increased intracellular calcium. These all suggest that cell membranes may lose important barrier functions, which can result in potentially toxic accumulations of intracellular substances which then markedly disrupt cellular function or cause cell death.

*Alterations in intracellular energy metabolism*
Documentations of changes in muscle and liver cell utilization of glucose and amino acids as well as the increase in lactic acid production are numerous and alluded to in the Mediator and mechanisms of cellular activation section of this Chapter. Whether these alterations are adaptive and needed for cell survival or maladaptive and toxic is controversial. This reflects the difficulty in discerning when inflammation and the consequences of inflammation are a benefit (what is referred to in this treatise as physiological inflammation) or a detriment (referred to as pathological inflammation).

## PATHOLOGICAL SYSTEMIC INFLAMMATION: DIAGNOSIS AND TREATMENT

### Clinical diagnosis of severe systemic inflammation
The clinical manifestations of severe systemic inflammation include:

(1) Vital signs:
    (a) Temperature elevation, hypothermia,
    (b) Tachycardia,
    (c) Tachypnea,
    (d) Hypotension with warm or cold extremities;

(2) Change in mental status;

(3) Respiratory insufficiency;

(4) Ileus;

(5) Oliguria, increased urine protein;

(6) Elevated hemoglobin, thrombocytopenia, leukocytosis, leukopenia;

(7) Increased serum glucose, decreased ionized calcium.

These manifestations are as potentially varied as the many organs that may manifest malfunction. Most patients will demonstrate hemodynamic alterations, but sometimes abnormal lung, CNS, hematologic and/or other organ states represent the primary evidence of inflammation rather than hemodynamic changes. Therefore, a high index of suspicion of the patient at risk augmented by evidence gathered during physical examination and with selected laboratory tests will support the diagnosis of significant inflammation.

### The patient at risk

The first category of risk is that a patient has recently acquired a disease (e.g. severe pancreatitis) or sustained an injury (e.g. unstable pelvic fracture with ruptured spleen) which is characterized by severe inflammation. The second category of risk is that a patient has an underlying condition (e.g. immunosuppression following liver transplantation) or recent procedure (e.g. elective colon resection for carcinoma) which makes systemic inflammation, particularly from infection, more likely. Any patient who has suffered a significant episode of hypoperfusion (e.g. cardiogenic shock following an acute myocardial infarction, upper gastrointestinal (UGI) hemorrhage sufficient to result in hypotension) is also at risk for developing systemic inflammation either at the time of the hypoperfusion or days later.

### Physical examination

*Vital signs*
Usually severe systemic inflammation is manifest as a decrease in blood pressure, increase in heart rate, increase in respiratory rate and elevated temperature. Patients with underlying cardiac disease may present with hemodynamics more consistent with congestive heart failure (elevated blood pressure and tachycardia). Hypothermia may be present in the most severe cases.

*General overview*
The patient is usually restless and may demonstrate mental status alterations ranging from delirium to coma. In fact, mental status changes may precede obvious hemodynamic and/or respiratory findings. This sometimes leads to misdirection in evaluation (computed tomography of the brain). Such alterations in CNS function are rarely focal and most consistent with a metabolic encephalopathy.

If intravascular volume is decreased the skin will be cool, possibly mottled, with vasoconstriction most often evident in both the upper and lower extremities. Capillary refill will be decreased.

*Lungs*

The lung examination may demonstrate clear lungs (even with the acute respiratory distress syndrome (ARDS) – see Chapter 4), but may also exhibit rales, rhonchi and bronchospasm. Examination findings consistent with consolidation (e.g. tubular or tubulovesicular breath sounds, egophony) may assist in locating an inflammatory process, but are clearly not peculiar to systemic inflammation. The lung examination is not sufficiently specific to make a diagnosis of systemic inflammation or other etiology of diffuse pulmonary malfunction.

*Cardiovascular examination*

Hypotension and tachycardia are usually present along with crisp heart tones. After intravascular volume restitution extremities will be warm, demonstrating good capillary refill. Hypotension with warm hands and feet usually represents the response to inflammation, although anaphylaxis and a high spinal cord injury could produce similar findings. Jugular venous pressure will be low by clinical examination. As a result of plasma exudation and the other causes of plasma volume loss, the patient usually is sequestering fluid. This can be sudden or, if the patient has been monitored in a hospital setting, the positive fluid balance and an increase in weight may have been documented for several days prior to an acute deterioration.

Myocardial depression from inflammation might result in an elevated jugular venous pressure as well as hypertension and an S3 gallop. Severe myocardial depression sufficient to result in hypotension and a clinical picture identical to cardiogenic shock is possible. However, such myocardial malfunction is much less common than are circulatory deficiencies secondary to hypovolemia. The clinician must be very careful to distinguish the fluid sequestration and positive fluid balance of severe inflammation from the same phenomena seen with cardiogenic states. Treating hypovolemia with fluid restriction and diuretics will result in further circulatory embarrassment.

Fluid sequestration implies that fluid is administered because of an inadequate circulation. Often the circulation is assessed by using urine output. Decreased urine output secondary to severe inflammation is most often secondary to inadequate cardiac output and, therefore, a marker of an inadequate circulation.

*Abdominal examination*

Abdominal distention, decreased or absent bowel sounds, and tympany may accompany any severe inflammatory process and represent the ileus which can develop with or without a primary disease or injury in the abdominal cavity.

## CNS examination

As stated above, mental status changes are common and usually non-focal, consistent with a metabolic encephalopathy.

## Laboratory studies

### Hematologic

An increase in total white blood count, particularly young PMNs, is most common, Leukopenia denotes more severe disease and usually consists mostly of immature PMNs. The platelet count usually decreases and evidence of consumption of coagulation proteins with breakdown of fibrinogen (increased prothrombin time, increased partial thromboplastin time, and increased fibrin spit products or D-dimer) also denotes more severe disease. Hemoglobin may increase as plasma exudes into inflammatory sites. Such an increase may be a very useful tool in assessing intravascular volume resuscitation, since plasma volume is likely to be inadequate until the hemoglobin has at least returned to the patient's baseline value (such an increase may also be secondary to desiccation or, more commonly, to inadequate replacement of measured or unmeasured losses).

### Lung studies

A decrease in arterial $Po_2$ and $Pco_2$ is characteristic of severe systemic inflammation as well as many other lung disease states. A chest X-ray may be clear and/or demonstrate loss of lung volume as well as evidence of pulmonary fluid accumulation, most often from a non-cardiogenic pathophysiology. The clinician should recognize that respiratory symptoms, signs and laboratory data during severe inflammation may be indistinguishable from those seen commonly with congestive heart failure (CHF), and should be alert to the dangers of the misdiagnosis and management of severe inflammation effects on the lung as CHF (see Chapter 2, The circulation; Hypoperfusion states and Chapter 4, The pulmonary system; Lung dysfunction).

### Urine studies

Oliguria is common during severe inflammation and is most often secondary to an inadequate circulation, resulting in laboratory tests consistent with a prerenal state (e.g. elevated urine specific gravity, low urine sodium, increased urine osmolality, elevated blood urea nitrogen: creatinine ratio).

Dating from at least the time of Meleney's description of synergistic bacterial gangrene, increased urine protein has been witnessed during severe inflammatory conditions. Therefore, it is possible that renal microvasculature (glomerular or otherwise) responds to the same mediators which result in increased capillary permeability elsewhere. Increased urine protein excretion may indicate that systemic inflammation is present, especially when no local renal disease (i.e. glomerulonephritis) is evident.

*Serum chemistry*
Elevated blood glucose is common during inflammation. Decreased total serum calcium has been recognized for many years to be associated with one particular severe inflammatory disease, namely pancreatitis, and the amount of decrease correlates with the severity of disease. Ionized calcium represents the calcium which is not bound to albumin and is not, therefore, influenced by albumin concentrations, which can change significantly during critical illness. Ionized calcium is also better correlated with parathyroid hormone release compared to total calcium.

Ionized calcium decreases with any disease which results in either severe hypoperfusion or inflammation (see Chapter 5, The renal system; Renal failure and selected metabolic disturbances). In addition, the magnitude in decrease correlates with the severity of disease. While not specific for inflammation, ongoing severe inflammation must be considered possible in any patient with decreased ionized calcium. In contrast, a normal ionized calcium would be unusual during severe inflammation and/or hypoperfusion. Therefore, a normal value without recent calcium administration would suggest that a severe systemic insult is not present.

Electrolyte and/or arterial blood gas information consistent with a metabolic acidosis as well as an elevated lactic acid level are often seen in severe inflammation. Like ionized calcium, these abnormalities do not distinguish severe inflammation from a decrease in either regional or global perfusion. Persistent metabolic acidosis could mean that either disease is present and should prompt further diagnostic and, possibly, therapeutic efforts.

**Treatment**

*Treat the underlying cause*
Once severe inflammation is recognized the first principle of treatment is to discover the underlying cause and initiate appropriate therapy.

Treatment of severe inflammation should include control of etiology, support of organ function, antagonism of inflammatory and metabolic mediators, and enhancement of immunological function. While infection and infection-like processes (e.g. infusion of endotoxin) are the most commonly considered etiologies of severe inflammation, reactions to drugs and/or transfusions, as well as tissue injury without infection (e.g. early severe pancreatitis) can result in severe systemic inflammation indistinguishable from that seen with the invasion of microorganisms. The management guidelines for common inflammatory conditions in surgery are presented in the individual organ-related Chapters in this manual.

While the search for the primary disease is underway and therapy is initiated, vital organ function must be supported until the primary process comes under control. Unfortunately, sometimes systemic inflammation continues despite adequate resolution of the initiating insult. In some patients inflammation appears to become self sustaining, as if a positive feedback system has developed in one or more of the organs suffering from systemic inflammation. As discussed below, novel therapies focused upon interruption of various steps in the inflammatory process are being studied to determine if this can ameliorate the adverse effects of severe inflammation and improve clinical outcomes. In addition, therapies designed to enhance immunological function may prevent subsequent inflammatory insults secondary to infection or microbiological byproducts.

*Support organ function*

Most of the details of organ support during severe inflammation are presented in the individual organ system Chapters. Since the importance of cardiovascular support is paramount in the management of severe inflammation, the management principles for that organ system are given special attention here (Table 16). The reader is referred to Chapter 2, The circulation; Hypoperfusion states for information regarding the accurate diagnosis of disorders of the circulation.

Most often the patient suffering from severe inflammation is hypovolemic and will respond to the infusion of fluid with an increase in cardiac output such that hypotension is alleviated, if not completely reversed, and the extremities change from cool to warm. Urine output and mental status usually improve. Unfortunately, pulmonary function does not usually improve dramatically with treatment of hypovolemia alone. Ionized calcium and metabolic acidosis may or may not improve from simple improvement in the circulation.

## TABLE 16   CARDIOVASCULAR SUPPORT DURING SYSTEMIC INFLAMMATION

*Accurate diagnosis of state of circulation*

*Therapy according to circulation condition*
Hypovolemia
    crystalloid (lactated Ringer's, 0.9% saline)
    dopamine
    colloid
    hypertonic saline
    red blood cells
Cardiogenic state
    dobutamine
    amrinone
    vasodilators
    intra-aortic balloon pump
Oxygen delivery endpoints
    $CI \geq 4.5$ l/min/m$^2$
    $O_2D \geq 600$ ml/min/m$^2$
    $VO_2 \geq 170$ ml/min/m$^2$
    $O_2$ consumption not delivery dependent
Use of arterial constrictors
    high cardiac index
    low systemic resistance
    suspicion of fixed stenoses

CI, cardiac index; $O_2D$, oxygen delivery; $VO_2$, oxygen consumption

This Chapter of the manual will not discuss in depth the controversies related to crystalloid vs. colloid administration (see Chapter 2, The circulation; Hypoperfusion states). The authors agree with studies that have demonstrated no substantial benefit to colloid administration, especially during inflammatory states. Red blood cell transfusion should be reserved for patients with ongoing hemorrhage or levels of hemoglobin below 10 g/100 ml who manifest abnormalities consistent with inadequate oxygen delivery. For patients with hemoglobin levels above 10 g/100 ml, simply increasing hemoglobin does not appear to significantly improve oxygen consumption. Dopamine is administered commonly during severe inflammation. Since dopamine tends to increase left ventricular end-diastolic pressure as cardiac output increases, this drug has a physiological effect similar to fluid infusion and is most useful when hypovolemia is the primary abnormality.

The diagnosis and treatment of a cardiogenic state usually requires more complicated monitoring than blood pressure, pulse, skin color, mental status, urine output and electrolyte monitoring. Insertion of a pulmonary artery catheter allows more precise measurement of cardiac filling pressures and the response to inotropic and/or vasodilator manipulations. During severe inflammation myocardial depression may be a manifestation of decreased myocardial catecholamine receptor function. Amrinone which does not require this receptor function, and which may have anti-inflammatory properties of its own, may be the inotropic agent of choice during severe inflammation.

The distinction between hypovolemic and cardiogenic hypoperfusion with the respective use of appropriate management strategies to achieve clinical endpoints such as good urine output and mental status is considered by several studies to be inadequate therapy for severely inflamed patients. These studies support the concept that the circulation is deficient until the cardiac index, oxygen delivery and oxygen consumption values listed in Table 16 have been achieved. More demanding than this list is the concept that an adequate circulation has been achieved only when oxygen consumption does not increase following continuing increases in oxygen delivery (Figure 2). In other words, oxygen consumption is no longer delivery dependent.

Difficulties with the conclusions from these studies are presented in Chapter 2, The circulation; Hypoperfusion states. In brief, concerns have been raised that these studies demonstrate the epidemiological characteristics of survivors better than the beneficial effects of a therapeutic intervention. However, any patient suffering severe inflammation who demonstrates significant malfunction from any organ can be considered to have a deficient circulation. The guidelines in Table 16 may be useful in discerning if such a deficiency is indeed present.

During hyperdynamic, elevated cardiac output, low systemic resistance states, the use of an $\alpha$-receptor stimulant (e.g. norepinephrine, neosynephrine) may be indicated, especially when certain vessels with fixed stenoses (e.g. renal, carotid, coronary arteries) are suspected to require higher mean arterial pressure for adequate perfusion. When employed, such vasoconstrictor therapy should be accompanied by documentation that global perfusion (i.e. cardiac index) does not decrease.

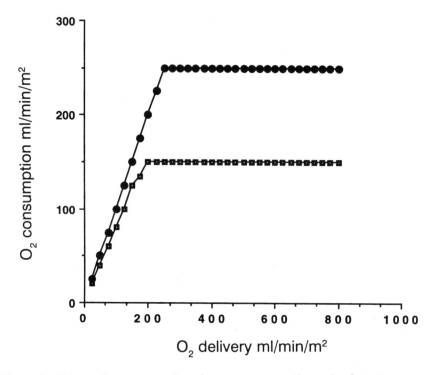

**Figure 2** Schematic representation of oxygen consumption as it relates to oxygen delivery during 'normal' or less inflammation (■—■), as compared to 'increased' or more inflammation (●—●) conditions. When oxygen consumption continues to increase as oxygen delivery increases, consumption is considered 'delivery dependent'. Once consumption has leveled off, further augmentation of oxygen delivery is not beneficial

*Antagonism of inflammatory mediators/steroid administration*
Much experimental and clinical research has evaluated the antagonism of inflammatory and metabolic mediators in severe inflammatory states (Table 17). Many such studies show promise, but none has become standard therapy.

As stated in the introduction to this Chapter, inflammation has beneficial effects (e.g. wound healing, defense against invasive organisms) which are important for survival during critical illness. Therefore, a successful outcome depends greatly on a balance between the beneficial and detrimental effects of inflammation. Therapy that

## TABLE 17   ANTAGONISM OF INFLAMMATORY AND METABOLIC MEDIATORS IN SEVERE INFLAMMATORY STATES

*Interference with endotoxin effects*
Clearing endotoxin from the circulation
   anti-endotoxin antibody
   binding toxin to membrane
   filtering toxin out
Interfering with endotoxin binding to effector cells (i.e. bactericidal/
   permeability-increasing protein)

*Interference with activation of pro-inflammatory cytokines*
Steroids
Non-steroidal anti-inflammatory agents
IL-1 converting enzyme inhibition

*Interference with the activity of increased pro-inflammatory cytokines*
Anti-TNF, Anti-IL-1 antibodies
Bind TNF and IL-1 with excess receptors
Block effector cell receptors, i.e. administration IL-1 receptor antagonist
Continuous blood filtration

*Administration of anti-inflammatory cytokines*

*Interference with superoxide activity*
Decrease production
Increase scavenging

*Interference with secondary mediators*
Cyclyooxygenase system
Nitric oxide system
Complement
Histamine, serotonin, kinin system
Coagulation system

*Interference with inflammatory cell activation by blocking activation*
   *receptors (i.e. inhibition of leukocyte integrin and selectin)*

IL, interleukin; TNF, tumor necrosis factor

aggressively suppresses inflammation (i.e. pharmacological doses of anti-inflammatory steroids) may result in short-term benefits, such as hemodynamic and pulmonary function improvement, but the loss of the beneficial effects of inflammation may result in death secondary to recurrent infection or wound breakdown. With all treatments designed to limit severe inflammation, this balance between detrimental and beneficial effects for both the short term (hours to days) and long term (days to weeks) must be evaluated. The use of steroids for severe inflammation is particularly illustrative of the difficulties with this balancing process.

Alterations in adrenocortical function following severe hemorrhage and inflammation have been recognized for many years. For most patients an elevated blood cortisol level is considered part of the normal response to a severe stress which requires admission to an intensive care unit. However, some stressed patients may exhibit depressed adrenocortical function, exemplified best by cases of meningococcal bacteremia with adrenal hemorrhage, and other cases of anatomical interruption of adrenal tissue. Over the past several decades, measurement of lower than expected blood cortisol concentrations during severe inflammation, without anatomic disruption of the adrenals, has prompted speculation that severe inflammation may result in a pathophysiological suppression of adrenal function from such mechanisms as TNF and IL-1 interference with adrenal cortisol synthesis. Therefore, severe inflammation may be associated with down-regulation of an endogenous negative feedback system which would serve to check the progress of inflammation.

Administration of pharmacological doses of anti-inflammatory steroids demonstrated acute beneficial effects in experimental models of septic shock and ARDS. The short-term benefits documented in these experimental studies did not prove transferable to long-term benefits in humans. As stated above, the known adverse effects of pharmacological steroids on host defenses and wound healing may have disrupted the proper balance between the detrimental and beneficial effects of inflammation.

For all of the therapies listed in Table 11 this balance must be considered. The benefits of inflammation are primarily effected at local sites (the focus of tissue injury or infection). The detrimental effects are primarily systemic (e.g. alterations in circulation, pulmonary function). Therapies that allow local inflammation to continue while the systemic inflammation is suppressed may promote the proper inflammatory balance.

Two therapeutic concepts that appear suitable for achieving this balance are blood filtration methods, which may remove molecules causing systemic alterations, and the use of anti-inflammatory substances which can be titrated to diminish systemic inflammation while allowing the local inflammation to proceed. Continuous veno-venous hemo-filtration is a model of the former (see Chapter 5, The renal system; Renal failure and metabolic disturbances). The administration of physiological doses of hydrocortisone may be a simple model of the latter.

When severe inflammation is associated with less than expected blood cortisol concentrations (i.e. <15 µg/dl), several studies have reported improved hemodynamic and pulmonary function when low-dose (150–300 mg/day) hydrocortisone is administered. Such a dose, which is little more than the reported endogenous release of cortisol during stress, would not be expected to severely limit local inflammation, as compared with pharmacological doses of methylprednisolone (2 g). Thus far, no long-term outcome studies have been reported using this dosage in patients with 'suppressed' cortisol concentrations. Further study is necessary to determine if morbidity and/or mortality can be affected by such a relatively simple intervention.

## Immunological enhancement

Unchecked severe inflammation may be secondary to deficient host defenses present either before the inflammatory insult or developing as a result of the inflammatory response. All aspects of host defenses (epithelial barriers, white cell function, cellular immunity, humoral immunity) can be decreased following severe tissue injury and hypoperfusion, as well as less acute alterations secondary to such processes as malnutrition and malignancy.

Persistent deficits in host defense are associated with increased infection and mortality risk in critically ill surgical patients. Strategies for improving host defenses are several but center on the principles of good surgical intervention.

(1)  Maintenance of an excellent circulation;

(2)  Surgery for drainage and debridement;

(3)  Nutritional support – preferably enteral vs. TPN;

(4)  Proper use of antibiotics;

(5)  Administration of immunoenhancement agents:
    (a)  Glucan,
    (b)  IL-2,
    (c)  Immunoglobulins.

### TABLE 18    DISORDERS OF WOUND HEALING

*Inadequate hemostasis*
Inadequate operative control
Thrombocytopenia
Platelet disorders
Anticoagulant treatment
Coagulopathy

*Diminished inflammatory response*
Inadequate blood supply
   inadequate debridement of devitalized tissue
   large and small arterial disease
      atherosclerosis
      diabetes
      radiation
   low cardiac output
   vasoconstriction
   tissues normally with little blood supply – subcutaneous fat
PMN dysfunction
   pharmacological steroids
   non-steroidal anti-inflammatory agents
   chemotherapy agents
   malnutrition
   diabetes
   alcohol ingestion
   radiation
   severe trauma
   severe systemic inflammation
Macrophage dysfunction
   pharmacological steroids
   non-steroidal anti-inflammatory agents
   chemotherapy agents
   malnutrition
   remote sepsis
   diabetes
   radiation
   severe systemic inflammation

*(continued)*

## TABLE 18    (continued)

*Decreased fibroblast proliferation*
Decreased migration secondary to macrophage malfunction
Radiation
Chemotherapeutic agents
Thrombocytopenia

*Decreased endothelial proliferation*
Decreased macrophage function
Thrombocytopenia

*Disorders of collagen synthesis*
Vitamin C deficiency
Protein depletion
Tissue hypoxia

*Disorders of wound contraction*
Pharmacological steroids

PMN, polymorphonuclear cells

## WOUND HEALING DISORDERS

### Effects of hypoperfusion and systemic inflammation
Hypoperfusion can result in decreased wound healing in two ways: as a result of inadequate oxygen supply to meet the needs of essential cells, and also by initiating systemic inflammation which can also affect adversely the function of cells essential for normal wound healing. Systemic inflammation from any cause may also alter oxygen supply by decreasing total body and regional perfusion and promoting edema formation in the perfused tissues.

### Disorders of repair
Common disorders of wound healing are listed in Table 18. The central role of the macrophage is illustrated, being affected by many conditions and therapeutic agents which adversely affect wound healing. In addition, even a brief preoperative illness has been demonstrated to adversely affect wound healing. The surgeon enhances wound healing by removing

devitalized tissue, ensuring good blood supply, relieving tension between apposed tissues and treating diseases that adversely affect wound healing, i.e. drain sepsis, reverse hypoperfusion (regional or total body), minimize detrimental drug therapy, correct coagulopathies, control blood glucose and provide nutrition.

# 4

# THE PULMONARY SYSTEM

Mechanical ventilation
      Fundamentals
      Strategies to improve oxygenation and decrease the adverse
         hemodynamic effects of positive-pressure ventilation
      Strategies to reduce the risk and incidence of ventilator-
         induced lung injury
      Complications of intubation
      Weaning
Extracorporeal pulmonary support
      Extracorporeal membrane oxygenation
      Extracorporeal lung assistance
      Complications of extracorporeal lung support
      Support personnel

## INTRODUCTION

The lung primarily accomplishes two life-sustaining processes: the addition of oxygen to and the removal of carbon dioxide from the blood (gas exchange). Approximately 300 million alveolar-capillary units with ventilation (V) and perfusion (Q) accomplish this task. This Chapter describes the various relationships of V to Q, the mechanics of respiration, fluid movement in the lung, basic monitoring, definitions of respiratory failure and indications for ventilator support. The use of mechanical ventilation with positive pressure is so common that separation of the physiology of negative-pressure spontaneous ventilation from the physiology of positive-pressure mechanical ventilation is impractical. Therefore, features of both are often intermixed in the following discussion. Subsequent sections will expand on the use of mechanical ventilation.

## LUNG VOLUMES

Figure 1 is a graphic representation of lung volume components which are meaningful for both negative-pressure and positive-pressure respiration. Tidal volume is the most frequent volume of air moved into and out of the lungs, usually without extra effort, but can be greater (close to vital capacity) or less than 'normal' because of disease. Functional residual capacity (FRC), the amount of volume remaining in the lung after a normal expiration, is particularly relevant to upcoming discussions of respiratory failure and ventilatory management. Critical closing volume (CCV, not shown in Figure 1) is the lung volume at which small airways collapse, resulting in microatelectasis. Normally CCV is less than FRC. However, with increasing age, chronic lung disease and acute lung disease CCV may become larger than FRC resulting in significant atelectasis and an increase in physiological shunt fraction (see below).

### Dead space and alveolar ventilation

Dead space (VD) is the amount of tidal volume (usually about 30%) that does not come in contact with pulmonary blood and cannot aid gas exchange. Dead space has two components: (1) anatomic – nose, mouth, trachea, bronchi, bronchioles; and (2) physiological – areas of lung parenchyma which are well ventilated but poorly perfused (i.e. V/Q approaches infinity) (Figure 2). Alveolar ventilation (VA), the ventilation of perfused alveoli, is the difference between tidal volume (VT) and VD.

$$VA = VT - VD$$

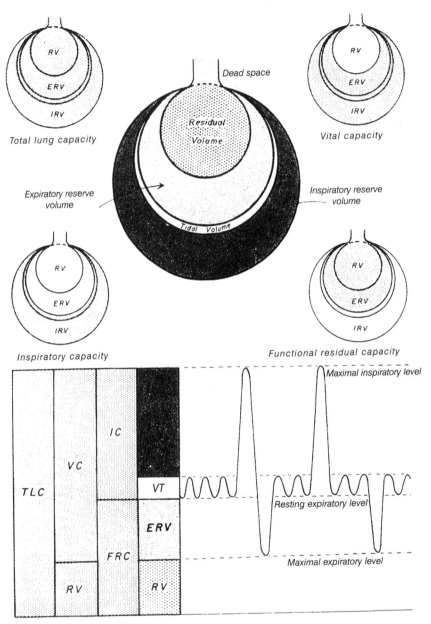

**Figure 1** A schematic and spirographic representation of static lung volumes important to pulmonary physiology. RV, residual volume; ERV, expiratory reserve volume; IRV, inspiratory reserve volume; TLC, total lung capacity; VC, vital capacity; IC, inspiratory capacity; FRC, functional residual capacity; VT, tidal volume. Reproduced with permission from Comroe JH. *Physiology of Respiration.* Chicago: Year Book Medical Publishers, 1968

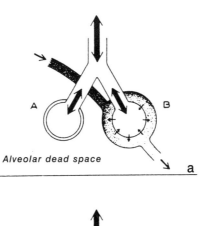

Alveolar dead space a

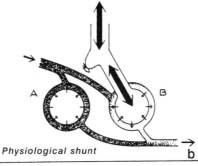

Physiological shunt b

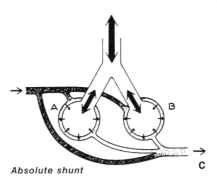

Absolute shunt c

**Figure 2** Schematic representations of (a) lung units with ventilation and no perfusion (alveolar dead space). There is uniform ventilation to A and B, with no blood flow to A. (b) Lung units with perfusion to A and B but no ventilation (physiological shunt) to A. (c) Lung units with uniform ventilation and blood flow to A and B, but venous blood bypasses alveoli (absolute shunt). Reproduced with permission from Comroe JH. *Physiology of Reproduction.* Chicago: Year Book Medical Publishers, 1968

**Determinants of arterial $P_{CO_2}$ and $P_{O_2}$**

The determinants of arterial $P_{CO_2}$ and $P_{O_2}$ ($P_{aCO_2}$, $P_{aO_2}$) are listed in Table 1. $P_{CO_2}$ is directly proportional to the ratio of dead space to tidal volume (VD/VT). As dead space ventilation approaches tidal volume, carbon dioxide cannot be eliminated (VD/VT = 1). Methods used to reduce an elevated $P_{CO_2}$ include reduction of dead space (i.e. tracheostomy to replace an endotracheal tube) or an increase in tidal volume (i.e. relief of bronchospasm). Increasing rate of respiration to lower $P_{CO_2}$ will be successful only if areas of lung are present which have a low VD/VT ratio. If the entire lung has a high VD/VT ratio, simply increasing respiratory rate will be ineffective.

The carboxyhemoglobin dissociation curve is steep and almost linear, as compared to the oxyhemoglobin dissociation curve (Figure 3). Increasing oxygen saturation reduces affinity and facilitates $CO_2$ release in the lungs; lower oxygen saturation increases affinity and augments $CO_2$ removal from the tissues. The nature of this curve allows a well-ventilated and perfused area of lung to markedly reduce $CO_2$ content and compensate significantly for lung areas not engaged in gas exchange.

Carbon dioxide is the end product of the metabolism of carbohydrate, protein and fat. Increased metabolic demands (e.g, exercise, infection) increase $O_2$ use and $CO_2$ production. The ratio of $CO_2$ production to $O_2$ use is the respiratory quotient (RQ), which is 1.0 for carbohydrate and protein and 0.7 for fat. Hypermetabolic states which use primarily carbohydrate

**TABLE 1   DETERMINANTS OF ARTERIAL $P_{CO_2}$ AND $P_{O_2}$**

$P_{CO_2}$
- Ratio of dead space to tidal volume (VD/VT)
- Anatomic dead space
- Physiological dead space
- Carboxyhemoglobin dissociation curve
- $CO_2$ production

$P_{O_2}$
- Alveolar gas equation
- $F_{iO_2}$
- $P_{CO_2}$
- Ventilation–perfusion inequality
- Shunt
- Decreased cardiac output
- Diminished diffusion capacity

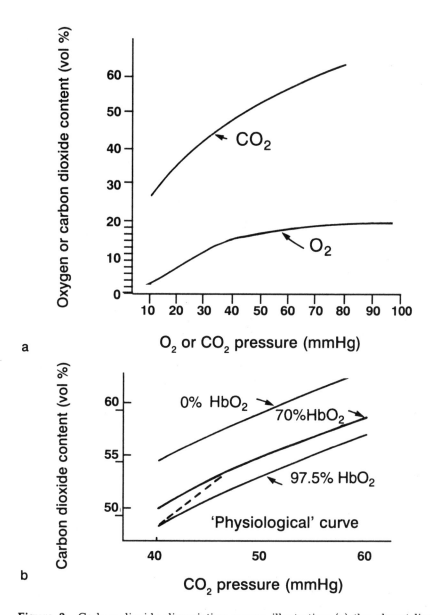

**Figure 3** Carbon dioxide dissociation curves illustrating (a) the almost linear relationship between the pressure of carbon dioxide and the content, and (b) increasing oxygen saturation reducing affinity and facilitating CO$_2$ release in the lungs. Reproduced with permission from Comroe JH. *The Physiology of Respiration*. Chicago: Year Book Medical Publishers, Inc., 1968

and protein (severe inflammation) result in more $CO_2$ production than states that use primarily fat (starvation without inflammation).

The alveolar gas equation determines alveolar $Po_2$ ($PAo_2$) and, therefore, the highest possible $Pao_2$.

$$PAo_2 = Fio_2 \ (713) - PAco_2 \left[ Fio_2 + \frac{1 - Fio_2}{R} \right]$$

Where $Fio_2$ is the fraction of oxygen in inspired air, $PAco_2$ is the mean alveolar $Pco_2$ and R is the respiratory exchange ratio.

The barometric pressure is 713 mmHg because at sea level (760 mmHg) the partial pressure of water vapor in the alveolus at 37°C (47 mmHg) must be subtracted. This difference is then multiplied by the percentage of oxygen in the inspired air ($Fio_2$). Next, the partial pressure of carbon dioxide in the alveolus must be measured and, following further calculations dependent upon $Fio_2$ and the respiratory quotient, the product is subtracted. Rising body temperature and elevated $Pco_2$ can both lower $Pao_2$, but the effect will be less as $Fio_2$ increases. The alveolar gas equation is the clearest demonstration of the interaction between oxygen being added to the blood and $CO_2$ being eliminated. Otherwise, the two processes are best thought of as separate.

Ideally, the ventilation and perfusion of alveoli are perfectly matched (V/Q = 1). Areas that are ventilated but not perfused (V/Q = infinity) are physiological dead space units; areas that are perfused but not ventilated (V/Q = 0) are physiological shunts. A shunt represents venous blood that does not come in contact with ventilated alveoli (Figure 2). Just as with dead space, there is a normal anatomic component of shunting (5–6% of cardiac output) which consists of the blood supply to the bronchioles and heart, which then drains directly into the pulmonary veins or the left ventricle, respectively. Areas of lung that simulate dead space will affect $Pao_2$ via the alveolar gas equation. Areas that simulate a shunt will diminish $Pao_2$ by the admixture of venous blood with newly oxygenated blood.

With minimal shunting, mixed venous oxygen content will have little effect on $Pao_2$. Increasing the shunt increases this influence. Under these circumstances, variables that decrease mixed venous oxygen (decreased cardiac output, increased oxygen utilization) can significantly diminish $Pao_2$ and may lead to therapy directed at improving lung function. Similarly, increasing cardiac output may make $Pao_2$ improve and lead to a false interpretation that the lung is better. Measurement of cardiac output and calculation of the shunt percentage, as well as oxygen delivery and consumption, can help sort out the influence of cardiac output and oxygen consumption on arterial oxygen concentration.

$$\frac{\dot{Q}s}{\dot{Q}_T} = \frac{[PAo_2 - Pao_2] \times 0.0031}{[Cao_2 - C\bar{v}o_2] + [PAo_2 - Pao_2] \times 0.0031}$$

Where $\dot{Q}s$ is shuntflow, $\dot{Q}_T$ is cardiac output, $Cao_2$ is arterial oxygen content and $C\bar{v}o_2$ is mixed venous oxygen content.

Oxygen content $= 1.34 \times Hgb$ (g/dl) $\times$ oxygen saturation $+ 0.0031 \times Po_2$

The average V/Q relationship of a normal lung may be close to unity, but gravity is an important determinant of the relative ratio of ventilation to perfusion in different areas of the lung. For instance, pulmonary blood flow may be nine times greater at the base compared to the apex in upright man. Ventilation, however, is greatest at the apex. The influence of gravity on V/Q distribution is particularly important when measuring vascular pressures, especially the pulmonary artery occlusion pressure (PAOP). West (1964) divided the lung into three zones which describe the ratio of intra-alveolar pressure (PAV) to pulmonary arterial (Pa) and venous (Pv) pressure: zone 1 PAV >Pa > Pv; zone 2, Pa > PAV > Pv; zone 3, Pa > Pv >PAV (Figure 4). PAOP equals pulmonary venous pressure and, therefore, measures left atrial pressure most reliably in zone 3 where the catheter tip is vertically below the left atrium. Fortunately, since the catheter is flow directed, most often the tip does locate in zone 3.

Diminished diffusion capacity is generally of little clinical significance in surgical critical care and likely to cause hypoxemia only when $Fio_2$ is low (high altitude), with thickened alveolar-capillary membranes (interstitial fibrosis), or with shortened exchange time (very high cardiac output).

## Pulmonary mechanics

The mechanics of respiration listed below are important determinants of the need for respirator support. The major components of pulmonary mechanics are:

(1) Inspiratory pressure;

(2) Expiratory pressure;

(3) Compliance/elastance;

(4) Resistance;

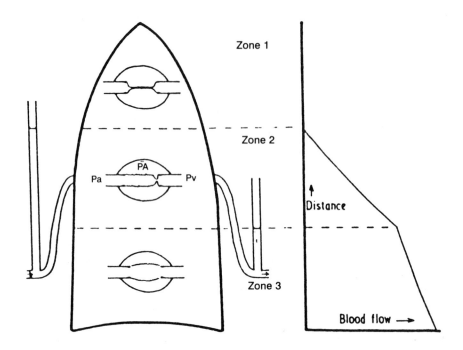

**Figure 4** Schematic illustration of the relationship between alveolar pressure (PA), pulmonary arterial pressure (Pa) and pulmonary venous pressure (Pv) in different zones of the lung. In zone 1, PA is greater than both Pa and Pv. In zone 2, Pa is greater than PA and Pv. In zone 3, Pa is greater than Pv which is greater than PA. Reproduced with permission from West JB, Dollery CT, Naimark A. Distribution of blood flow in isolated lung; relation to vascular and alveolar pressures. *J Appl Physiol* 1964;19:713–24

(5) Airway pressures;

(6) Work of breathing.

The following text provides a brief description of the fundamentals which can be applied commonly in clinical practice.

*Muscles of respiration*
The diaphragm is the major muscle of respiration. During quiet respiration, the costal and crural fibers which insert on the central tendon push the abdominal viscera down and produce negative intrathoracic

pressure. The intercostal muscles are much less important, unless diaphragmatic weakness or paralysis is present, in which case there is inward displacement of the abdominal wall during inspiration. Other muscles assisting inspiration are the scalenes and the sternocleidomastoids. Maximal contraction of inspiratory muscles can generate a negative intrapleural pressure of 60–100 mmHg.

Expiration is usually passive. Active expiration incorporates all the muscles of respiration, with the abdominal muscles most important. Pressures up to positive 119 mmHg have been documented.

*Compliance/elastance*
Expansion of the lungs can be likened to the expansion of a balloon. Comparing two balloons subjected to the same increment in transmural pressure, if balloon 1 expands to a larger volume than balloon 2, then balloon 1 has more compliance but less elastance. Compliance is the ratio of the change in pressure to the change in volume. Elastance is the opposite of compliance and represents the intrinsic elastic component which resists deformation by stress. The relationship between transmural inspiratory and expiratory pressures and lung volumes is determined by the compliance of the chest wall and lungs (total compliance).

$$\text{Compliance (C)} = \frac{\Delta V}{\Delta P}$$

$$\text{Total compliance (CT)}: \frac{1}{CT} = \frac{1}{CW} + \frac{1}{CL}$$

Where CW is chest wall compliance and CL is lung compliance. Without disease, CT is determined mostly by the elastic recoil properties of the lung (CL) and thorax (CW). With negative-pressure inspiration CT equals approximately 0.1 l/cmH$_2$O. Under conditions of mechanical ventilation in patients with normal lungs and chest walls, CT is approximately 0.05 l/cmH$_2$O. Certain diseases (e.g. circumferential thoracic burns) diminish primarily chest wall compliance, while others (e.g. pulmonary edema) diminish primarily lung compliance. Critically ill patients commonly develop alterations in both components of total compliance.

The compliance described above is measured at a given inflation volume held constant (static compliance). The relationship between volume and pressure can be plotted (pressure–volume curve, Figure 5) and the slope of this curve represents compliance. As can be seen in the figure, a normal lung exhibits a similar relationship between pressure and volume as pressure is gradually increased and then decreased. With certain

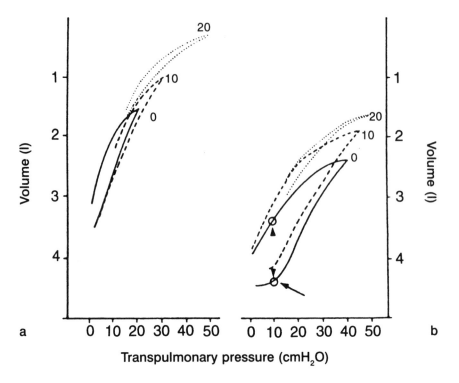

**Figure 5** Static pressure–volume curve as an indication of compliance. The slope of the curve represents compliance. (a) Shows compliance of a normal lung and (b) shows the compliance of a lung from a patient with acute respiratory distress syndrome. Both a and b show the change or lack of change in compliance with the addition of positive and expiratory pressure (PEEP). The diseased lung (b) exhibits a more normal volume pressure relationship following the application of PEEP. Reproduced with permission from Marcy TW, Marcini JJ. Inverse ratio ventilation in ARDS: rationale and implementation. *Chest* 1991;100:494–504

diseases (acute respiratory distress syndrome (ARDS) in this case) the pressure–volume curve exhibits significant hysteresis, indicating that compliance changes as lung volume units open when pressure is increased and then close as pressure is decreased. The changes in static compliance (effective compliance) with different inflation volumes can be plotted (Figure 6) to produce a characteristically sigmoidal curve. An

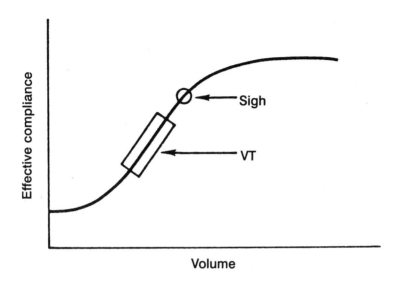

**Figure 6**   Effective compliance vs. lung volume. Compliance is greatest in the mid-volume range, where tidal volumes (VT) usually occur. The increase in volume of a sigh normally remains in the range where compliance can still increase. Reproduced with permission from Rochon RB, Mozingo DW, Weigelt JA. New modes of mechanical ventilation. *Surg Clinics N Am* 1991;71:843–57

increase in compliance is greatest in the mid-volume range (where tidal volumes usually occur) and is least at total lung capacity (top right of the curve) and low lung volumes (bottom left of the curve) near FRC or residual volume (RV).

*Resistance*
Any fluid (air is considered a fluid) moving through a tube meets resistance to flow. Because of this resistance the pressure measured at the end of the tube will be less than the pressure measured at the beginning of the tube. This difference in pressure is related to both the resistance and the flow rate of the fluid.

$$\text{Resistance (R)} = \frac{\text{pressure beginning (PB)} - \text{pressure end (PE)}}{\text{Flow rate}}$$

$$\text{Airway resistance (RAW)} = \frac{\text{PM} - \text{PALV}}{\text{Flow rate}}$$

where PM is pressure at mouth, PALV is alveolar pressure and resistance is described in units $cmH_2O/l/s$ (normal 2–3 in the spontaneously breathing adult). The pressure drop during laminar flow is calculated by:

$$PB - PE = K1 \times L \times 1/r^4$$

where K1 is a constant related to flow rate and viscosity, L is length of tube, and r is the radius of the tube. The pressure drop during turbulent flow is calculated by:

$$PB - PE = K2 \times (\text{flow rate})^2$$

where K2 is a constant related to length and radius of tube along with viscosity and density of the gas.

Flow in tubes can be described as linear and turbulent. Variables which influence the pressure drop (and thereby resistance) across a tube during linear flow are the viscosity of the fluid, the length of the tube, and the radius of the tube. The influence of radius on resistance during laminar flow is profound. With a sufficient increase in flow rate in a tube (the critical flow rate) turbulent flow develops. With turbulent flow all of the variables which influence the pressure drop during linear flow are in effect; however, in addition, the density of the gas and the square of the flow rate are important variables.

*Airway pressures*
During negative-pressure ventilation the lung is subjected to little potential damage from pressure effects. Positive-pressure ventilation, however, results in several airway pressure alterations which may cause beneficial effects (improved oxygenation and carbon dioxide removal) and detrimental effects (decreased cardiac output and lung damage). The airway pressures that have received the most attention are as follows: peak inspiratory pressure (PIP), the pressure at end inspiration (plateau pressure, Pplat), mean airway pressure (Paw), mean alveolar pressure (Palv), transalveolar pressure (Ptrans), and positive end-expiratory pressure (PEEP).

PIP is the maximum pressure generated in the airway during gas flow (Figure 7). PIP can be influenced by compliance, airway resistance, tidal volume and the rate of flow of gas. Pplat is the pressure in the airway at the end of inspiration during a positive pressure tidal volume, but before exhalation begins. Pplat (Figure 7) is a measure of peak alveolar pressure. At the onset there is a drop from PIP as gas distributes from the upper to the lower airways. Pplat is mostly affected by compliance. Paw is calculated from the area under the pressure curve during a ventilatory cycle

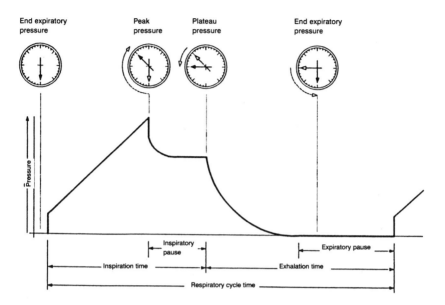

**Figure 7** Pressures of the respiratory cycle during controlled mechanical ventilation. Reproduced with permission from Depuis YG. *Ventilators: Theory and Clinical Application*, 2nd edn. St. Louis: Mosby Year Book, 1992

(inspiration and expiration). Paw is influenced by resistance to inspiratory flow, the duration of inspiration compared to expiration (I : E ratio), compliance and end-expiratory pressure.

Palv is the mean pressure in the alveolus during the entire respiratory cycle. Palv is influenced by most of the variables which influence Paw except that resistance to expiratory flow is more important than inspiratory flow resistance. Palv is closely approximated by Paw in many clinical circumstances, especially when inspiratory and expiratory resistance are nearly equal. However, when expiratory resistance is higher than inspiratory resistance, Paw will underestimate Palv, especially when minute ventilation is high. That is, when air meets more resistance leaving the alveolus than when air is brought to the alveolus, alveolar pressure will increase in proportion to the amount of air brought to the alveolus each minute. In patients with lung disease, especially pulmonary edema, Palv is directly related to opening alveoli, shunt reduction and improved oxygenation.

Palv also has a direct influence upon pleural pressure (Ppl) which is influenced by the compliance of the lung (CL) and the chest wall (CW), as described by the following formula:

$$\Delta Ppl = \Delta Palv \times \left( \frac{CL}{CL + CW} \right)$$

Therefore, as Palv increases, Ppl will increase to a greater extent when CL is high and when CW is low (for example, a patient with bullous emphysema who has an increase in CL may notice a significant increase in Ppl following a circumferential chest wall burn which would decrease chest wall compliance). Ppl is inversely related to alterations in venous return. That is, an increase in Ppl will result in a decrease in venous return. Therefore, an increase in Palv in compliant lungs will have a more significant effect on Ppl and venous return than an increase in Palv in non-compliant lungs. On the other hand, non-compliant lungs will develop more of an increase in transpulmonary pressure (Ptrans) as Palv increases.

Ptrans is the pressure difference between the alveolus and the pleural space, as described by the following formula:

$$Ptrans = Palv - Ppl$$

As discussed in the mechanical ventilation section of this Chapter, Ptrans is an important determinant of the risk of ventilator-induced lung injury. Increasing Palv in the compliant lung appears to relatively increase the risk of hemodynamic compromise compared to ventilator-induced lung injury, whereas increasing Palv in the non-compliant lung appears to relatively increase the risk of ventilatory-induced lung injury compared to hemodynamic compromise. However, high Palv may result in both adverse effects regardless of lung compliance.

PEEP is pressure present in the airway at the end of expiration. Pressure at the end of expiration contributes to Paw and Palv. PEEP is often applied to the ventilator circuit as part of ventilator management (external PEEP). In addition, disease states that result in a failure to return to passive FRC before the onset of the next inspiration (high expiratory resistance – dynamic hyperinflation), and ventilator settings that result in a similar phenomenon (increased I : E ratio) can result in increased alveolar pressure at the end of expiration (auto-PEEP). For patients on a ventilator auto-PEEP may be present whenever the flow tracing shows flow at the end of exhalation. Total PEEP is the sum of externally applied PEEP and auto-PEEP. Measurement of end-expiratory occlusion pressure (the airway pressure at end-expiration with the expiratory port occluded) provides total PEEP. The difference between this and externally applied PEEP is auto-PEEP. Auto-PEEP can increase Paw and Palv in the same fashion as external PEEP and, therefore, has the same potential to influence hemodynamics and transalveolar pressure.

### Work of breathing

The work of breathing is performed to overcome airway resistance and the recoil of the lungs and chest wall. Work of breathing determinants are:

(1) Airway resistance;

(2) Lung and chest wall compliance;

(3) Oxygen consumption and production;

(4) V/Q coordination;

(5) Minute ventilation.

Change in volume multiplied by the pressure difference forcing the change in volume equals work. The work of breathing increases as the volume inflated increases because compliance is less at higher volumes.

The work performed to stretch the lungs and chest wall becomes potential energy for expiratory work. Since the airway narrows during expiration, resistance increases, but normally not enough to inhibit expiration. With increasing resistance (i.e. bronchospasm) more work must be performed during expiration to raise the intrathoracic pressure above atmospheric, which in turn compresses the airway.

A common physiological response to the increased work of breathing is tachypnea, often with a reduction in tidal volume. However, increasing respiratory rate with small volumes is an ineffective method of increasing ventilation in the presence of increased airway resistance (more work per unit time). Increasing rate with small tidal volumes is more effective in the presence of diminished compliance. Tachypnea often accompanies increased oxygen consumption and especially increased carbon dioxide production. Each may require increased minute ventilation (both rate and tidal volume) and, therefore, more work per unit time. V/Q mismatch, which results in either increased physiological dead space or poorly ventilated non-compliant areas, will increase respiratory rate and work. Hyperventilation and increased work may also result from such conditions as metabolic acidosis, anxiety, systemic inflammation and thyrotoxicosis.

The work of breathing may be measured in mechanical units or by oxygen consumed by the respiratory apparatus. Normally, the respiratory muscles consume less than 5% of total body oxygen. With increasing work, respiratory muscle oxygen demand increases.

The etiologies of the symptom dyspnea are many, and the potential interactions of these various etiologies are complex. However, when considering respiratory muscle oxygen demand, dyspnea may be considered the 'angina' of the respiratory muscles, indicating inadequate oxygen supply for the demand. Any disease that increases the work of breathing will increase oxygen demand and potentially produce dyspnea. In addition, any disease which reduces oxygen supply to the muscles (i.e. hypovolemic, cardiogenic hypoperfusion) may produce dyspnea. Using this approach therapy for dyspnea may be directed to both reducing the work of breathing (e.g. decreasing airway resistance, improving compliance, reversing acidosis, treating systemic inflammation) and increasing the oxygen supply to the muscles (e.g reversing hypovolemic hypoperfusion). Despite such efforts respiratory muscles may fatigue, resulting in worsening pulmonary function and the need for mechanical ventilation (see section on Mechanical ventilation).

**Pulmonary fluid**
The physiology of the movement of intravascular fluid and protein into and out of the pulmonary interstitium has been well studied and is described by Starling's equation.

$$Jv = LpA\,[(Pc - Pt) - \sigma\,(\pi c - \pi t)]$$

Where Lp is hydraulic conductance or the speed at which fluid can pass through the microvascular exchange barrier, A is the surface area available for exchange, $\sigma$ is the reflection coefficient, or the relative permeability of the microvascular membrane to plasma proteins, Pc is microvascular hydrostatic pressure, Pt is tissue hydrostatic pressure, $\pi c$ is plasma colloid oncotic pressure, and $\pi t$ is tissue oncotic pressure. In the lung, as in other organs, the migration of fluid and protein, especially albumin, into the interstitial space at the high pressure end of capillaries is partially returned to the circulation as the hydrostatic pressure falls, but also returns to the circulation via the lymphatics. Interstitial and subsequent alveolar edema does not occur until the lymphatics are overwhelmed. Pulmonary lymphatics may be capable of removing six to eight times the usual amount of interstitial fluid before edema develops.

Starling's equation and the physiology of lymphatic drainage allow for several etiologies of pulmonary edema:

(1) Increased pulmonary microvascular pressure;

(2) Increased capillary permeability;

(3) Obstructed lymphatics;

(4) Decreased oncotic pressure.

One representation of the 'true' hydrostatic pressure in the pulmonary capillary is called pulmonary microvascular pressure (Pc), which is determined by both mean PA pressure (PAP) and PAOP, as well as arterial and venous resistance.

$$Pc = \frac{PAP \times Rv + PAOP \times Ra}{Ra + Rv}$$

Where PAOP is pulmonary artery occlusion pressure, Ra is pulmonary arterial resistance, and Rv is pulmonary venous resistance. The most common etiology of an increase in Pc is left heart failure. When Pc is elevated secondary to heart failure a good correlation between radiographic indices of increased lung water, measurement of extravascular lung water (EVLW) and hydrostatic pressure has been documented (Table 2). With other etiologies of pulmonary edema (i.e. ARDS), the correlation of hydrostatic pressure and radiographic findings (especially using portable technique) with EVLW is poor. Other potential etiologies of increased microvascular pressure include increased pulmonary venous resistance and increased PA pressure secondary to pulmonary arteriolar constriction, which has been seen with a variety of pulmonary insults. Common etiologies of pulmonary arteriolar constriction include:

(1) Hypoxia;

(2) Hypercapnia;

(3) Bronchospasm;

## TABLE 2   RADIOGRAPHIC CORRELATION WITH HYDROSTATIC PRESSURE INCREASE IN NORMAL LUNGS

| PAOP (mmHg) | Radiographic finding |
| --- | --- |
| <16–18 | normal |
| 18–22 | cephalization |
| 22–25 | perihilar haze |
| 25–30 | periacinal rosette |
| ≥ 30 | dense alveolar infiltrates |

(4) Pulmonary edema (any etiology);

(5) Severe inflammation;

(6) Pulmonary embolism.

Increased capillary permeability (permeability pulmonary edema) is an important mechanism for the increase in lung water in ARDS. Many etiologies of increased permeability which accompany the several disease states associated with ARDS have been described. Both experimental and clinical studies have documented the increased migration of plasma proteins into the interstitium and alveoli. In addition, pathological examination has documented increased 'pores' in pulmonary endothelial cells or the junctions between cells. This information supports increased capillary permeability as the etiology of pulmonary edema in ARDS, but not necessarily the etiology of poor oxygenation (see Lung dysfunction section).

The most common diseases obstructing lymphatics are malignancies that either invade the mediastinal lymphatics (lymphoma, metastatic lung cancer) or spread in the interstitium of the lung (breast cancer, leukemia). This form of pulmonary edema is usually unresponsive to common treatment (treatment of the circulation and/or inflammation) but may improve if the malignancy is treated.

The concept that reduced oncotic pressure may result in pulmonary edema has been controversial for at least 30 years. Prior to intense investigation, the clinical entities of hepatic cirrhosis and nephrotic syndrome have often been associated with low serum albumin, peripheral edema and little, if any, pulmonary edema. Therefore, these well-described entities provide some information that simply lowering serum albumin does not result in florid pulmonary edema in humans. Guyton & Lindsey (1959) demonstrated that dogs would produce increased lung water with decreased oncotic pressure at normal hydrostatic pressure. Results of human studies in patients with and without pulmonary disease have been conflicting, but generally support the evidence that cirrhotic and nephrotic patients have illustrated – that a significant reduction in colloid oncotic pressure with normal hydrostatic pressures does not result in a significant increase in EVLW.

## PULMONARY MONITORING

### History and physical examination
Pulmonary monitoring begins with history and physical examination. History should provide information regarding severity of dyspnea, cough,

sputum production, smoking, bronchospasm, previous lung infections and previous thoracic surgery. Physical examination observation is the first, and often only, maneuver required for the diagnosis of mild, moderate or severe respiratory distress. Skin color (cyanosis), mental status (anxiety, agitation), respiratory rate, depth, symmetry and pattern of respiratory muscle use provide clues relevant to the work of breathing and gross gas exchange inadequacies (e.g. lack of motion of hemithorax, marked tachypnea, shallow respiration, flail chest). Auscultation helps determine the presence or absence of air movement, and can provide evidence of increased lung water, consolidation and bronchospasm. Percussion helps delineate the presence of excess air (tympany) or excess fluid (dullness). However, observation alone is often adequate to diagnose respiratory distress worthy of mechanical support.

## Pulmonary mechanics

Pulmonary mechanics measurement is useful both before and after surgery and for assessing the need for respiratory support with mechanical ventilation. Since the bulk of chronic lung disease is secondary to smoke-induced obstruction of airways, chronic obstructive pulmonary disease (COPD), preoperative pulmonary risk for both non-thoracic and pulmonary resective surgery is correlated with indices of expiratory function, such as spirometric measurement of the amount of air forcibly expired after a maximal inspiration (amount expired in one second (FEV1)), total amount expired (forced vital capacity (FVC)), mid-expiratory flow rate (MEFR) and the maximum ventilation in one minute (MVV) (Table 3). Problems with inspiration usually represent upper airway difficulties which are readily apparent on physical examination (stridor) and are rarely chronic. Neuromuscular disease is usually chronic and risk is commonly measured by the maximum force generated during inspiration (maximum inspiratory force (MIF)) and vital capacity (Table 3).

Postoperatively, MIF and vital capacity (VC) are useful mechanical indices of a patient's ability to begin spontaneous respiration. MIF less than 25 cmH$_2$O and VC less than 15 ml/kg body weight represent poor mechanical indices.

## Blood gases

Arterial and mixed venous blood gases have been discussed previously (Chapter 2, The circulation; hemodynamic monitoring). Patients with preoperative evidence of poor ventilation ($Pa_{CO_2} > 45$ mmHg) are more likely to have postoperative respiratory dysfunction. As described in

**TABLE 3   PULMONARY FUNCTION AND PULMONARY RISK**

| Function | Measurement | Risk |
|---|---|---|
| *Risk with COPD* | | |
| FEV1 | >2 l | normal |
| FEV1 | 1–2 l | slight |
| FEV1 | 0.5–2 l | moderate |
| FEV1 | <0.5 l | severe |
| FEV1/FVC | <40% | moderate |
| FEV1/FVC | <25% | severe |
| *Risk with pulmonary resections* | | |
| FEV1 | <2 l | moderate |
| MVV | <50% predicted | moderate |
| MEFR | <20% predicted | moderate |
| *Risk with neuromuscular disease* | | |
| VC | >50% predicted | normal |
| VC | <25% predicted | severe |
| MIF | >25 cmH$_2$O | mild |
| MIF | 15–25 cmH$_2$O | moderate |
| MIF | <15 cmH$_2$O | severe |

COPD, chronic obstructive pulmonary disease; FEV1, amount of air forcibly expired in 1 s; FVC, forced vital capacity; MVV, maximum ventilation in 1 min; MEFR, midexpiratory flow rate; VC, vital capacity; MIF, maximum inspiratory force

Chapter 2, continuous monitoring of mixed venous saturation as well as peripheral oxygen $Po_2$ and saturation are sensitive to alterations in perfusion and cannot be used reliably as the only monitor of pulmonary function.

**Respiratory failure**
Diminished lung function is common after surgery and trauma (Table 4). Respiratory failure may accompany any one of these etiologies. The definition of respiratory failure is varied, and can be as broad as the need for ventilator support for longer than 48 h, and as specific as requiring many mechanical, oxygenation and ventilation indicators. Mechanical indicators of respiratory failure are respiratory rate > 35 breaths/min, vital capacity < 15 ml/kg and inspiratory force < 25 cmH$_2$O. Oxygenation indicators of respiratory failure are $Po_2/Fio_2$ < 250 mmHg A–a difference in O$_2$

## TABLE 4   ETIOLOGIES OF DIMINISHED LUNG FUNCTION

*Atelectasis*
Secretions
Hypoventilation

*Hypoventilation*
Anesthesia
Narcotics
Supine position
Splinting – thoracic > upper abdominal > lower abdominal
Chest wall trauma
Obesity

*Lung injury*
Contusion
Acute respiratory distress syndrome
Aspiration
Smoke inhalation

*Lung infection*
Aspiration pneumonia
Nosocomial pneumonia

> 350 mmHg and a shunt fraction >10%. Ventilation indicators of respiratory failure are VD/VT > 0.6 and $P_{CO_2}$ > 60 mmHg. As mentioned under History and physical examination, observation of the patient's mental status and the rate and depth of respiration will often be adequate to determine who needs respiratory assistance. Allowing a patient to suffer markedly increased work of breathing because blood gases are 'OK' places too much emphasis on gas exchange and too little on the mechanics of respiration. Such patients commonly tire and deteriorate suddenly. Unless the etiology of respiratory failure can be reversed rapidly (i.e. placement of a chest tube for a pneumothorax, rapid resolution of bronchospasm), the patient should receive mechanical ventilation.

Respiratory failure can be thought of as secondary to primarily mechanical difficulties (mechanical failure) or secondary to gas exchange difficulties within the parenchyma (alveolar failure) (Table 5). Ventilator support may be required to assist primarily with one or both of these deficits.

### TABLE 5    ETIOLOGIES OF RESPIRATORY FAILURE

*Mechanical failure (PaCO$_2$)*
COPD
Respiratory muscle paralysis or weakness
Flail chest
Large airway obstruction
Bronchospasm
Depression of respiratory center
Decrease energy supply to respiratory muscles

*Alveolar failure (Pao$_2$)*
Pulmonary edema – any etiology
Pneumonia
Atelectasis
Pneumothorax
Lung contusion
Pulmonary embolism

COPD, chronic obstructive pulmonary disease

**Indications for mechanical ventilation**
The indications for mechanical ventilation are respiratory failure, anesthesia, paralysis and therapeutic hyperventilation. General anesthesia and therapeutic paralysis are common but are often short-term reasons for mechanical ventilation. Respiratory failure is the most common reason for long-term support. Indications for intubation are to establish an airway, respiratory toilet and administer mechanical ventilation.

**DRUG THERAPY**

Most often drug therapy that improves lung physiology does not treat a chronic underlying lung disease. Instead, this therapy treats an acute disease which has further diminished lung function, such as pneumonia or congestive heart failure. The most common chronic lung disease requiring therapy in surgical patients is COPD. Pharmacology for this disease is limited primarily to bronchodilators, which not only diminish airway resistance but also improve diaphragm function. Corticosteroids are effective but have the disadvantage of potentially decreasing host defenses and wound healing, especially when used in pharmacological doses (100 mg methylprednisolone every 8 h). Since surgical patients are subject to severe infection and wounds, corticosteroids are usually avoided except as necessary to replace suppressed adrenal function under stress (approximately 150 mg hydrocortisone per day). Curiously such physiological therapy may be sufficient to avoid severe bronchospasm in COPD patients.

## LUNG DYSFUNCTION

### The effects of hypoperfusion on the lung
The main effect of hypoperfusion either to the entire lung or to regions of the lung is an increase in physiological dead space. During systemic hypoperfusion, little alteration in oxygenation occurs. Once hypoperfusion has been reversed, the effects of the initiating insult (hemorrhage, severe inflammation) will be manifest, depending on the degree of resultant systemic inflammation.

### The effects of systemic inflammation on the lung
Decreased lung function is a characteristic phenomenon of severe systemic inflammation. A marked increase in both physiological shunting, physiological dead space and a variable increase in EVLW often result in the institution of mechanical ventilation for the condition most often designated as the acute respiratory distress syndrome or ARDS. Therefore, rather than limit ARDS to clinical circumstances where an increase in EVLW is obvious, ARDS will be considered present whenever significant alterations in physiological shunt and dead space occur in the setting of systemic inflammation. This definition of ARDS is different from many and does not include such local diseases of the lung as aspiration, smoke inhalation, viral and other pneumonia, and bilateral pulmonary contusions. The purpose of this distinction is to emphasize the concept that an inflammatory insult distant from the lung proper is responsible for the witnessed alterations in lung physiology. This has important implications when diagnosis and therapy are considered (see below).

Pathophysiological studies demonstrate that severe systemic inflammation results in alterations in blood flow through the microvasculature of the lung (e.g. microembolism, platelet trapping, plugging by white cells), as well as increased capillary permeability and active inflammation at the alveolar–capillary interface.

Cells and endogenous substances that have been associated with the lung alterations in ARDS are:

(1) Polymorphonuclear leukocytes;

(2) Platelets;

(3) Alveolar macrophages;

(4) Histamine;

(5) Serotonin;

(6) Thromboxane;

(7) Tumor necrosis factor;

(8) Superoxide molecules;

(9) Activated complement;

(10) Leukotrienes.

As implied by the above definition of ARDS, clinical ARDS can occur with any disease distant from the lung proper which results in significant systemic inflammation such as:

(1) Severe infection;

(2) Severe trauma;

(3) Major burns;

(4) Ischemia/reperfusion;

(5) Severe bone injury;

(6) Severe pancreatitis.

The importance of EVLW accumulation for both the pathophysiology and the management of ARDS is controversial. First, since ARDS does not represent pulmonary edema secondary to congestive heart failure, attributing the EVLW of ARDS simply to overzealous fluid administration is erroneous. In ARDS EVLW does increase as pulmonary capillary pressure increases. However, as mentioned previously, the oxygenation alterations in ARDS are not explained solely by EVLW and, therefore, therapy that might increase EVLW in ARDS cannot be considered a primary reason for oxygenation deficits. Second, decreased oncotic pressure cannot explain either the magnitude of EVLW in ARDS or the oxygenation deficit. While decreased oncotic pressure may aggravate pulmonary edema when hydrostatic pressure is elevated, this has not been demonstrated when hydrostatic pressure is normal in humans. Third, since EVLW is not correlated with oxygenation deficits, therapy directed primarily at reducing lung water will not likely improve oxygenation. As described below, any therapy for ARDS resulting in a decreased cardiac output may not only be ineffective but may aggravate the inflammatory state which resulted in ARDS and, therefore, may worsen arterial hypoxemia by both mechanisms.

Since oxygenation alterations are not simply secondary to increased EVLW, other features of ARDS appear to be equally important as potential causes of the increased physiological shunt. These features include focal atelectasis, patchy alveolar consolidation, decreased compliance and decreased FRC.

The primary management principles of ARDS are:

(1) Make the proper diagnosis;

(2) Support oxygenation and ventilation;

(3) Maintain or improve cardiac output;

(4) Diagnose the underlying cause;

(5) Treat the underlying cause;

(6) Anti-inflammatory therapy;

(7) Prophylaxis.

Making the proper diagnosis of ARDS can be difficult, especially since several other diseases can produce acute respiratory distress and abnormalities on both the chest radiograph and in arterial blood gases.

### Differential diagnosis of ARDS

It is necessary to differentiate ARDS from the following:

(1) Congestive heart failure;

(2) Pulmonary embolism;

(3) Massive aspiration;

(4) Bilateral pneumonia;

(5) Smoke inhalation;

(6) Bilateral pulmonary contusion;

(7) Major atelectasis.

First and foremost is differentiating ARDS from congestive heart failure (CHF). Unfortunately, many clinicians understand only one mechanism for developing increased lung water, namely CHF. Because of this, disease states responsible for ARDS are often treated initially as CHF. Since therapy such as depletion of intravascular volume may reduce cardiac output when ARDS is present, this can be particularly detrimental to the patient suffering from ARDS (see below). Therefore, careful clinical and laboratory assessment is essential to distinguish ARDS from CHF (see Chapter 2, The circulation; Hypoperfusion states). Because ARDS usually results from systemic inflammation, the patient with ARDS will often exhibit clinical symptoms, signs and laboratory data consistent with inflammation such as: hypotension, tachycardia, warm extremities, elevated white blood count, decreased platelet count and metabolic acidosis (see Chapter 3, Inflammation).

A chest X-ray is rarely sufficient to differentiate etiologies of bilateral diffuse interstitial and alveolar infiltrates. One feature of ARDS – non-homogenous alterations in lung parenchyma – can be useful for diagnostic purposes. CHF usually results in homogenous interstitial and alveolar infiltrates, and a chest computed tomography scan rather than a standard chest X-ray can usually distinguish non-homogenous alveolar disease from homogenous disease. However, diseases resulting in patchy disruption of pulmonary vasculature (i.e. COPD) may result in non-homogenous alveolar patterns even in CHF.

Early in ARDS the chest X-ray may look clear and appear more consistent with pulmonary embolism. A lung scan may be necessary to distinguish this possibility; more rarely a pulmonary angiogram is necessary.

Aspiration sufficient to produce severe pulmonary malfunction and bilateral infiltrates is usually massive and would be witnessed by someone (e.g. family member, emergency medical transport personnel, hospital personnel). Following massive aspiration upper intestinal contents will likely be seen in the upper airway at the time of intubation.

Distinguishing ARDS from bilateral pneumonia can be particularly perplexing. This is especially the case when the patient has had ARDS for some time and secondary infection is possible. ARDS should be readily distinguished from smoke inhalation and pulmonary contusion by knowledge of the patient's history. Large segments or lobes of atelectasis should be distinguishable from ARDS by differences noted on the standard chest X-ray.

Support of oxygenation and ventilation are discussed below in the Mechanical ventilation section. Any therapy used to support the lung should not result in decreased cardiac output. The reasons for this are as follows: (1) inadequate tissue perfusion will aggravate any inflammatory state through the variety of mechanisms described in Chapter 3, Inflammation, and (2) when a significant increase in physiological shunt is present a decrease in cardiac output will likely result in a decrease in mixed venous oxygen saturation. The admixture of this blood through the shunt physiology in the lung will aggravate arterial oxygenation difficulties. An increase in cardiac output with a resultant increase in mixed venous oxygen saturation may result in an improvement in arterial oxygen levels, even though the lungs themselves have not improved. If this happens, the magnitude of lung support, like the concentration of inspired oxygen or PEEP levels, may be decreased while maintaining satisfactory arterial oxygen saturation. The guiding dictum is: 'do not sacrifice the heart for the lungs'

Increased pulmonary vascular resistance (PVR) is characteristic of the lung response to injury and the resultant right heart malfunction may be a primary determinant of an inadequate circulation. Under such circumstances methods directed at reducing PVR may allow a lung treatment to improve the circulation. Initial attempts at using such agents as nitroprusside and prostaglandin $E_1$ to dilate the pulmonary vasculature demonstrated that the primary effect was augmentation of the cardiac output from the systemic effects of the drug rather than the effect on the pulmonary vasculature. Inhaled nitric oxide may result in exactly the desired effect: a reduction of PVR and an improvement in pulmonary function.

While the circulation and pulmonary function are supported or improved, the primary management principle for ARDS is to locate and treat the underlying inflammatory disease responsible for ARDS. Sometimes the disease is understood (e.g. ARDS with severe pancreatitis) and under therapy; sometimes the disease is not known (e.g. ARDS day 6 after elective colon resection) and an etiology of severe inflammation must be sought. ARDS is not treated by respirator and circulatory adjustments. The patient is kept alive by these interventions until the true cause is identified and managed appropriately.

Rarely, a patient may develop ARDS without any discernible etiology. Since the lungs contain inflammatory cells, it is possible that an initiating inflammatory insult will stimulate diffuse pulmonary inflammation, which then continues unabated when the initial inflammatory focus is treated. Sometimes diffuse pulmonary infection appears to continue the inflammation. Sometimes no unequivocal inflammatory focus is found, even at postmortem. Such cases of ongoing severe ARDS may cause death with or without multisystem organ involvement.

Anti-inflammatory therapy early in ARDS has been studied in experimental and clinical trials. Use of pharmacological doses of steroids has not proved beneficial. Other strategies, such as the use of non-steroidal anti-inflammatory agents, antihistamines, antiserotonin agents, inhibitors of PMN adherence in the lung, inhibition of thromboxane production and continuous filtration of the blood, have been advocated and continue under investigation.

Inflammation in all tissues results eventually in fibrosis. Prolonged ARDS (for weeks) may result in significant fibrosis and may impair mostly mechanical (decreased compliance) aspects of breathing, which may make weaning from the ventilator difficult and/or cause long-term pulmonary disability. Steroids have been reintroduced into the management of later, fibrosing ARDS, and initial reports demonstrate therapeutic benefits.

Prophylaxis against ARDS may be best considered as a strategy serving to limit systemic inflammation. With the understanding of the importance of thromboxane in the pathophysiology of ARDS, two studies have demonstrated that ketoconazole, an imidazole antifungal agent which inhibits thromboxane synthesis, is effective in preventing ARDS in patients at risk.

**Chest trauma**
Chest trauma may result in any or all of the following conditions: rib fractures, flail chest, pulmonary contusion, pneumothorax, tension pneumothorax, hemothorax, ruptured thoracic aorta and penetrating thoracic visceral injury. Respiratory failure most commonly is secondary to multiple rib fractures (mechanical failure) and/or pulmonary contusions (alveolar failure). Flail chest is defined as instability of the chest wall, which allows paradoxical movement of a chest wall segment (inward movement during inspiration). This usually requires at least three ribs broken in two places. The most common mechanism for flail chest is a blow to the lateral thoracic cage, which produces anterior and posterior stress. The association of lung contusion with flail chest results from the close apposition of the lung to the force of injury. Single lateral-rib fractures are most often secondary to anterior and/or posterior blows, which cause the lateral stress on the ribs and usually little parenchymal insult.

With rib fractures the patient may be tachypneic, splinting the affected area and exhibit marked tenderness and/or bony crepitus at the injury site. With flail chest similar tachypnea, splinting and tenderness will be noted along with paradoxical chest wall movement. Physical examination will also be altered by concomitant processes such as pneumothorax and hemothorax.

Mechanical ventilation is employed only when either or both mechanical lung and alveolar lung function are inadequate. The simple presence of a flail chest does not mandate mechanical ventilation. In fact, more often contusion-induced inadequate alveolar function is a greater problem than mechanical instability. Frequently, simple mechanical failure can be ameliorated by adequate pain relief (e.g. rib blocks, epidural anesthesia). Mechanical stabilization of the thorax is rarely indicated.

Pneumothorax and tension pneumothorax may be secondary to iatrogenic injury. Tension pneumothorax can cause a life-threatening reduction in venous return. Simple pneumothorax will produce tachypnea, decreased breath sounds, tympany and a shift of the trachea towards the affected side. Tension pneumothorax will be similar but also may cause hypotension, distended neck veins and tracheal deviation away from the disease. Both are usually treated by closed thoracostomy. Hemothorax may be present with or without a pneumothorax. The initial treatment requires placement of a chest tube, usually in the fifth or sixth interspace in the mid-axillary line.

Penetrating thoracic trauma may require diagnostic evaluation in the intensive care unit (ICU), especially for the possibility of missed injury. This is accomplished with the use of radiographic or echocardiographic studies to evaluate the heart, great vessels and the esophagus.

Severe blunt thoracic injury, especially secondary to deceleration, is associated with thoracic aorta rupture. This diagnosis may not have been entertained until the patient arrives in the ICU. Clinical clues to aortic injury include mechanism of injury, a wide mediastinum, first rib fracture(s), an apical cap, nasogastric tube deviation and hypertension. Of these the mechanism of injury should most alert the clinician that the thoracic aorta requires investigation, with such modalities as a chest CT transesophageal echocardiography or angiography. Other vascular injuries, particularly subclavian, may also produce many of the signs listed and when suspected should be evaluated angiographically.

## Pneumonia, lung abscess and empyema

*Pneumonia*
Pneumonia is a frequent etiology of respiratory failure or prolongation of respiratory failure in ICU patients. ICU pneumonia mortality averages about 50%. Risk factors that promote parenchymal lung infection in the ICU include:

(1) Colonization of oropharynx;

(2) Intubation of trachea;

(3) Depressed immunocompetence;

(4) Previous antibiotic exposure;

(5) Increased stomach flora;

(6) Aspiration;

(7) Pulmonary contusion;

(8) Pulmonary edema (any etiology).

Critically ill patients may have their oropharynx colonized with nosocomial organisms in 24 h. Intubation of the trachea bypasses a normal barrier to the migration of organisms and may reduce ciliary propulsion of organisms cephalad. Critical illness globally diminishes immunocompetence, which enhances the progression of colonization to invasion. Previous antibiotic use often suppresses endogenous flora increasing the concentration of resistant organisms from the environment (*Serratia, Pseudomonas, Enterobacter, Hemophilus influenza*) and endogenous flora (*Escherichia coli, Klebsiella*). Intubation of the trachea with endotracheal or tracheostomy tube balloon inflation does not protect fully against aspiration of small amounts of either oropharyngeal or gastric contents.

The role of stress ulcer prophylaxis with control of acid production in the stomach in the development of ICU pneumonia is controversial. Presumably control of acid allows for more rapid growth of potential pathogens in the upper gastrointestinal tract as compared with no prophylaxis or the use of sucralfate which, in some reports, does not alter stomach acid concentrations. While many reports support the use of sucralfate, several investigators have found no benefit. Possibly more important than this controversy is discerning which patients are at risk for stress ulceration/gastritis and limiting prophylaxis to that group (see Chapter 6, The gastrointestinal/nutritional system; Gastrointestinal dysfunction).

Arising commonly in the milieu of other etiologies of surgical sepsis, the diagnostic and therapeutic challenges in ICU pneumonia can be large. Proposed diagnostic criteria include:

(1) Elevated temperature;

(2) Elevated white blood cell count;

(3) Consolidation on physical examination;

(4) Positive sputum culture;

(5) Many polymorphonuclear cells on Gram stain of sputum;

(6) Consistent infiltrate on CXR.

These are especially useful when no previous pulmonary insult has predated the suspicion of pneumonia. Diagnosis of pneumonia can be especially difficult when the lungs have previously suffered a non-infectious insult (e.g. aspiration, pulmonary contusion, ARDS, cardiogenic pulmonary edema) which causes infiltrates and promotes subsequent bacterial invasion. Under these circumstances the use of expectorated or suctioned sputum, fever and elevation of white blood cell count, and even a chest x-ray may not be sufficiently specific to allow the confirmation of pneumonia. Microscopic evaluation and culture of tracheobronchial secretions in ventilated patients is insufficiently sensitive and/or specific to either make a diagnosis of pneumonia or to decide which pathogens to treat. However, a positive blood culture of an organism also found in the sputum, or finding an empyema with organisms found in the sputum are not sufficiently sensitive. Therefore, other techniques have been proposed to increase specificity in those patients with infiltrates, sputum cultures with pathogens, and signs of systemic inflammation:

(1) Bronchoscopic sampling for quantitative culture, no protected brush (sensitivity 100%, specificity 100% – one report);

(2) Bronchoscopic protected brush specimen (PBS) quantitative culture (sensitivity 38–100%, specificity 60–100%);

(3) Non-bronchoscopic protected brush specimen;

(4) Bronchoscopic bronchoalveolar lavage (BAL) quantitative culture (sensitivity 72–88%, specificity 71–100%);

(5) Directed (left or right lung) wedged suctioning without bronchoscopy – not quantitative;

(6) Non-directed endotracheal aspiration – quantitative;

(7) Lung biopsy.

In general, it is detrimental to patient outcome to either under diagnose or over diagnose pneumonia. Under diagnosis can result in progressive lung damage and possible death. Over diagnosis and subsequent treatment can result in antibiotic toxicity and superinfections with resistant organisms.

Each of the techniques mentioned has proponents and detractors. Obviously, open lung biopsy should be used only when diagnostic/therapeutic risk/benefit ratios are carefully scrutinized. BAL has the disadvantage of frequently decreasing pulmonary function, sometimes for extended periods, and therefore is not an advantage in patients with severe oxygenation or ventilation difficulty. The non-directed quantitative aspiration technique may be the most reasonable method of discerning who should and should not be treated in the ventilator-dependent patient with multiple old and/or new pulmonary infiltrates.

Once the diagnosis of pneumonia is made, treatment should be directed whenever possible at the organism(s) known to be responsible for the pneumonia. ICU pneumonia can be polymicrobial and, therefore, choosing to treat only one of several pathogens found through microbiological analysis is illogical unless some additional information (positive blood culture, pleural fluid culture) identifies a single pathogen.

Common bacterial pathogens in ICU pneumonia include *E. coli, Klebsiella, Pseudomonas, Serratia, Enterobacter* and *Staphylococcus aureus*. When a patient demonstrates signs of severe systemic inflammation broad-spectrum therapy, which includes antimicrobials effective against nosocomial *S. aureus* and the most prevalent nosocomial Gramnegative organisms, is warranted until more specific microbiological data are available, at which time more precise therapy may be provided.

Often prophylaxis is more effective than therapy. Since pneumonia organisms most often come from the oropharynx and are found in the stomach, the concept of decontamination of the stomach and oropharynx with non-absorbable and systemic antibiotics as well as antibiotic ointments has been tried with varying success to prevent both pneumonia and other infectious complications (see Chapter 6, The gastrointestinal/ nutritional system; Gastrointestinal dysfunction). The results of these studies, especially the effect of such prophylaxis on ICU mortality, generally do not support such aggressive use of antibiotics in this fashion.

As mentioned, aspiration is the primary mechanism whereby organisms gain entry to the tracheobronchial tree. This is not to say that every instance of aspiration leads to pneumonia. Aspiration of acidic gastric contents most often produces a chemical injury to dependent lung segments (basal lower lobe segments, superior segment of lower lobes, posterior segment of upper lobes). Sometimes the injury is bilateral and diffuse, producing an X-ray similar to pulmonary edema from other etiologies.

Simple acid-induced injury predisposes to infection but does not guarantee infection. The aspiration pneumonitis may progress to bacterial pneumonia or may resolve spontaneously. The natural history for the chemical injury is to begin resolving in 48–72 h. If no resolution is apparent, bacterial invasion may be presumed, and following sputum culture appropriate antibiotics begun. Antibiotics should not be started at the time of initial aspiration unless marked upper intestinal bacterial growth is known or suspected (e.g. small bowel obstruction, alkaline gastric pH). Steroids have no role in the therapy of aspiration.

Similarly, pulmonary contusion predisposes to lung infection. Pulmonary contusion also begins to diminish both physiologically and radiographically in 48–72 h postinjury. The persistence or progression of an infiltrate at this time should be suspected as evidence of pneumonia and warrants antibiotic therapy if clinical infection is apparent.

Antibiotics work well with bacterial pneumonia because the lung has excellent blood supply and the infection has a mechanism for drainage via the tracheobronchial tree. Therapy, therefore, includes chest physiotherapy, suctioning and sometimes bronchoscopy.

## Lung abscess

Lung abscess is pneumonia which has progressed to suppuration, and is often accompanied by a large communication with the tracheobronchial tree. Antibiotics, chest physiotherapy, suctioning and bronchoscopy are usually effective. Occasionally percutaneous drainage is required, which can result in a bronchopleural fistula and can make ventilation difficult.

## Empyema

Empyema must be considered in any patient who shows clinical signs of infection and evidence of a pleural effusion. Pneumonia, chest-tube trauma and esophageal injury are risk factors for empyema. In trauma patients chest tubes are often hurriedly inserted as a life-saving procedure, with less-than-ideal sterile technique, into bloody fluid. Elective chest tube placement at the time of pulmonary surgery is much less likely to be contaminated. A chest X-ray will often locate pleural fluid which can be sampled for culture. After previous pulmonary pathology and thoracic surgery, distinguishing pleural fluid from thickened pleura or locating thoracic fluid may be impossible with standard chest radiography. In this setting chest ultrasound and/or computed tomography have proved useful for locating and sampling suspicious collections. Once diagnosed as infected fluid, empyema therapy requires external drainage and sometimes decortication (removal of the surrounding fibrous capsule to allow full expansion of the lung) to eradicate the infectious focus.

## Postoperative thoracotomy management

Patients undergoing thoracotomy with or without pulmonary resection are at risk for the complications of hemorrhage, pneumothorax, decreased chest wall mechanics, pneumonia and empyema. Hemorrhage may be of a magnitude to obstruct chest tubes and risk tension pneumothorax or hemothorax. Significant hemorrhage (> 200 ml/h) may require reoperation for control. Decreased chest wall mechanics from rib resection, pain and tight dressings may inhibit weaning from mechanical ventilation. Epidural catheterization for instillation of long-acting narcotics and anesthetics has helped improve mechanical function in such patients.

Complications peculiar to pulmonary resections are:

(1) Supraventricular arrhythmias;

(2) Pulmonary edema;

(3) Bronchopleural fistula;

(4) Twisted lung segment;

(5) Mediastinal shift.

Supraventricular arrhythmias are common enough after pulmonary resection that many thoracic surgeons administer digitalis preoperatively. Postpulmonary resection pulmonary edema is most likely non-cardiogenic in origin, and may be secondary to a disturbance of pulmonary lymph drainage. The same principles used in treating ARDS apply. Severe V/Q mismatch may develop when a segment of lung is not properly positioned to maintain bronchial and vascular patency. This usually appears as a lobar or entire lung opacity which will not respond to bronchoscopy. Mediastinal shift, similar to that seen with tension pneumothorax, may follow pneumonectomy with subsequent imbalance of thoracic pressures. This can usually be remedied by instillation or withdrawal of air into/from the pneumonectomy side.

A very difficult complication is a large bronchopleural fistula which is often associated with intrathoracic infection. When present with external drainage, a bronchopleural-cutaneous fistula is present. Both predispose to recurrent parenchymal pulmonary infection and difficulty with ventilation. Much of each tidal volume may be lost via the fistula, increasing the VD/VT ratio and $P_{CO_2}$. Low-pressure high-frequency jet ventilation may be required to provide adequate gas exchange with less loss of tidal volume via the fistula. Operative closure when infection is present is usually unsuccessful but may be useful once infection is controlled.

## Pulmonary embolism

Pulmonary embolism is most commonly secondary to lower extremity deep venous thrombosis (DVT). Factors that predispose to DVT are trauma, stasis and hypercoagulable states. Trauma refers to direct trauma to a vein.

Stasis refers to diminished perfusion. Hypercoagulable states occur commonly following injury.

The incidence of DVT in elective surgical patients, especially those undergoing orthopedic procedures, has been well studied. The incidence in critically ill surgical patients is less well documented but presumed to be significant. Patients with spine fractures and paraplegia, as well as those with lower extremity injuries, are at highest risk. Other factors, such as older age, long duration of immobilization and multiple transfusions in trauma patients, also increase risk. Importantly, DVT may occur in such high-risk patients despite prophylactic measures.

The diagnosis of DVT is suggested by the physical examination findings of unilateral edema, painful calf to palpation and pain on dorsiflexion of foot. The high false-negative and false-positive rate for physical examination stresses the importance of a high index of suspicion and a willingness to obtain more objective studies. Laboratory diagnosis includes venous ultrasound duplex and venogram.

Pulmonary embolism is also often diagnosed on the basis of a high index of suspicion, although history and physical examination may be more specific than for DVT (Table 6). Again, laboratory tests are more objective and a positive lung scan (high probability) is usually enough to initiate therapy. Both high probability and normal scans are sufficiently diagnostic to require no further investigation. However, intermediate and

### TABLE 6   DIAGNOSIS OF PULMONARY EMBOLISM

*History*
Chest pain
Hemoptysis
Dyspnea

*Physical examination*
Pleural friction rub
Accentuated pulmonic second heart sound

*Laboratory*
Decreased $P_{O_2}$
Decreased $P_{CO_2}$
Clear chest X-ray, less commonly a peripheral lung density
Positive lung scan
Positive pulmonary angiogram

low probability scans should prompt further investigation, most often pulmonary angiography, particularly if the index of suspicion remains high. Pulmonary angiogram is indicated with an equivocal lung scan, when anticoagulation is otherwise contraindicated, and often to prepare the patient for further therapy (vena cava filter, emergency embolectomy). More recently transesophageal echocardiography and spiral chest computed tomography have been used to locate massive pulmonary embolism (e.g. emboli caught in the proximal pulmonary arteries).

The mechanism for reduction in $Po_2$ is unclear. Obstruction of pulmonary blood flow to the well-ventilated lung should result in an increase in dead space with little effect on $Po_2$, and possibly an increase in $Pco_2$. Instead, most often arterial blood gases reveal a decrease in both $Po_2$ and $Pco_2$. When measured, physiological dead space is commonly increased, but the stimulus to increase tidal volume and rate most often overcomes the dead space increase. This may not be the case in patients with increased physiological dead space (COPD). In these patients pulmonary embolism may be responsible for the increased $Pco_2$.

So, why does the $Po_2$ decrease? A fall in $Po_2$ implies decreased ventilation to perfused areas of lung, an increase in physiological shunt similar to that seen in ARDS. Serotonin release, probably from the thrombus, appears capable of producing the physiological abnormalities noted, illustrating that physiologic shunting can increase without an increase in lung water. Also, obstruction to pulmonary flow and increased pulmonary artery pressure may result in increased perfusion to poorly ventilated lung segments, overcoming normal autoregulation which attempts to match perfusion to ventilation. Investigators have also documented a physiology more like that described for ARDS, including an increase in extravascular lung water.

The therapy of submassive pulmonary embolism includes anticoagulation, thrombolytic agents, treating the source and prevention of future emboli. Surgical patients can usually receive anticoagulation (heparin) unless the risk of hemorrhage at the surgical site is life threatening (e.g. intracranial surgery). Pulmonary embolism physiology may be ameliorated with heparin, but mostly the physiology abates as part of the natural history of the disease and anticoagulation is used primarily to prevent further clot propagation at the initial DVT focus. Thrombolytic therapy is usually contraindicated in patients with surgical sites or wounds, because of the potential to disrupt clots resulting in uncontrolled hemorrhage and/or wound collagen digestion. However, thrombolytic therapy with urokinase infused directly into the clot has been shown to be safe within the first 14 days following surgery in one report. The use of thrombolytics during this time might be considered more appropriate for massive embolism rather than for embolism which is not immediately life threatening. When anticoagulation or thrombolytic therapy are contraindicated or ineffective (e.g. recurrent emboli on adequate anticoagulation), therapy is directed at preventing further emboli, usually by placing a filter in the inferior vena cava below the renal veins.

Massive pulmonary embolism (> 50% pulmonary artery occlusion) results in hypotension and occasionally cardiac arrest. If cardiopulmonary resuscitation successfully restores some, but not adequate, cardiac output, thrombolytic therapy should be considered first. The other option is removal of the embolus using either cardiopulmonary bypass or a percutaneous suction device. Further emboli must be prevented using an inferior vena cava filter.

DVT and embolism present particularly difficult management problems when located in thoracic veins and/or when infected. Placement of a filter is impractical in the superior vena cava, and if anticoagulation is contraindicated or ineffective, the only therapeutic option may be thoracic vein thrombectomy. Deep vein septic phlebitis and/or embolism is usually treated with anticoagulation and antibiotics. Once again, if anticoagulation is contraindicated or ineffective, thrombectomy may be required to remove the infected focus.

Prophylaxis strategies against DVT and subsequent pulmonary embolism in critically ill patients include intermittent pneumatic compression, anticoagulant therapy with low-dose unfractionated heparin, low molecular weight heparin, warfarin, and inferior vena cava filter placement. Because critical illness often comes on suddenly, it is impractical to initiate prophylaxis before DVT risk begins (as in elective surgical practice). Provision of intermittent pneumatic compression of the lower extremities, low-dose heparin or both is recommended when mechanically possible (e.g. no prohibitive trauma to the extremities) and when not contraindicated (e.g. coagulopathy from hypothermia). Otherwise, a high index of suspicion and frequent use of DVT surveillance techniques, such as venous duplex, may enable an early diagnosis and prompt therapeutic intervention with such therapies as anticoagulation and vena cava filter placement.

## MECHANICAL VENTILATION

### Fundamentals
Since respiratory failure may occur primarily from mechanical (inability to spontaneously eliminate carbon dioxide) or alveolar (inability to add

oxygen) failure, mechanical ventilation may be used to improve pulmonary function related to one or both of these mechanisms (indications for intubation of the tracheobronchial tree and mechanical ventilation are listed previously). Mechanical ventilation can improve minute ventilation and the VD/VT ratio in patients with increased work of breathing or decreased function of respiratory muscles. This results in improved $Paco_2$. Mechanical ventilation can also open collapsed alveoli, which improves functional residual capacity, decreases physiological shunting and improves $Pao_2$.

The types of readily available ventilators include:

(1) Negative pressure;

(2) Positive pressure – volume regulated;

(3) Positive pressure – pressure regulated;

(4) Positive pressure – pressure support;

(5) Positive pressure – high frequency.

Negative-pressure ventilators (iron lung) used for polio victims are impractical for critically ill patients who require much attention to the thorax. One of the most commonly used ventilators is the volume-regulated positive-pressure type, which delivers a predetermined tidal volume. As a safety precaution, the maximum pressure allowed to deliver the tidal volume is also predetermined (the 'pop off' pressure), which, when exceeded because of coughing, bronchospasm, or agitation, results in the external release of part of the tidal volume. The common ventilatory modes used with volume ventilators are:

(1) Controlled mechanical ventilation (CMV);

(2) Assist control (AC);

(3) Intermittent mandatory ventilation (IMV);

(4) Synchronous intermittent mandatory ventilation (SIMV).

With CMV the patient receives only a set tidal volume at a prescribed rate. This mode is used only when spontaneous ventilatory effort is absent (e.g. high cervical spinal cord injury, therapeutic hyperventilation) or undesirable (e.g. therapeutic paralysis). AC is in effect when every inspiratory effort sufficient to activate the respirator initiates delivery of a full tidal volume. AC uses a minimum rate which will establish CMV if the patient no longer initiates inspiration. The negative pressure required to trigger AC can be adjusted and a patient may not generate enough inspiratory effort to engage AC with every breath. These two modes of volume ventilator management require the least respiratory work, with CMV requiring less work than AC.

IMV establishes a minimum rate of positive-pressure volume ventilation which is augmented by the patient's own negative-pressure respiration. With many ventilators the patient must generate more negative pressure to open the IMV valve than would be required if the patient were simply connected to air at atmospheric pressure (T-piece). This increases the work of breathing. Some ventilators employ a pressure assist to open the IMV mechanism and reduce the work of breathing.

The presumed benefits of IMV include an easier weaning regimen, exercise of respiratory muscles and less positive pressure, resulting in less depression of cardiac function and less risk of ventilator-induced lung injury. IMV is useful for patients who are expected to wean rapidly from a ventilator since it requires little manipulation of the patient and/or the ventilator. If tolerated at a low rate, a patient is ready to discontinue ventilatory support. However, for patients with marginal mechanics or increased work of breathing, IMV unassisted ventilation may increase diaphragm oxygen requirements enough to produce dyspnea, tachypnea and agitation. Therefore, other methods of weaning may be better tolerated. The potential advantages of IMV for respiratory muscle exercise are not well documented; neither is improved cardiac function. The risk of ventilator-induced lung injury relates to several variables which may or may not be significantly reduced using IMV (see page 42).

SIMV provides a positive pressure respiration for a certain ratio of breaths initiated by the patient. If the patient wishes to breath 20 times a minute and SIMV is set to 1 : 2, the respirator will assist every other breath; if set to 1 : 3, assistance will be with every third breath.

For all these devices tidal volumes are set commonly at 5–15 ml/kg. The tidal volume selected should avoid localized alveolar overdistension. Selecting a tidal volume located on the steep portion of the P–V curve along with limiting PIP and peak alveolar pressure will diminish the risk of overdistension. Peak alveolar pressure $< 35 \, cmH_2O$ is a commonly accepted goal. The use of low tidal volumes and allowing $Pco_2$ to be elevated during mechanical ventilation (permissive hypercapnia) will be discussed later in this Chapter.

Respiratory rate is adjusted according to the mode of ventilator therapy (see below); however, for CMV generally it is set in the range of 8–12/min.

Usually increasing rate will result in a decrease in arterial $P_{CO_2}$. However, with COPD and other diseases with increased expiratory resistance the physician should consider expiratory time allotment when adjusting rate. Since expiration is delayed in these patients, inadequate expiration time may result in air trapping. This is most likely to occur during rapid respiration. Under such circumstances reducing the respirator rate may improve $CO_2$ elimination and diminish dynamic hyperinflation. When IMV or SIMV are used the rate will be set so that only a portion of the patient's breaths are provided by positive pressure. Therefore, the patient's spontaneous negative-pressure ventilation capability will greatly influence $CO_2$ elimination.

The initial $F_{IO_2}$ is set according to knowledge of the patient's acute and/or chronic respiratory status, but is often in the range of 40–50%. Arterial blood gases are then used to stimulate further respirator adjustments. The goal is to achieve an oxygen saturation of $\geq$ 90%, which is usually achieved with an arterial $P_{O_2} \geq$ 60 mmHg. The use of PEEP and other methods to improve oxygenation and potentially avoid oxygen toxicity is discussed later.

An inspiratory flow rate of 60 l/min is usually sufficient with volume-controlled ventilation. Patients with COPD may benefit by increasing flow rates to 100 l/min which may increase expiratory time and diminish gas trapping.

Pressure-regulated ventilators deliver a volume of air until a preset pressure is attained. When first introduced this method produced an unreliable regulation of tidal volume and was virtually abandoned when volume-regulated ventilators were introduced. More recently pressure-limited ventilator management has been reintroduced as pressure-support ventilation (PSV). With this method a preselected pressure is maintained as a square wave during an inspiration and ends when the patient's inspiratory flow decelerates below a certain level (e.g. 25% of peak flow). Although this method can be used without the patient initiating a breath (pressure control ventilation (PCV)), it is often used with the patient breathing spontaneously. Under these circumstances the patient controls the rate, rhythm and time of inspiration during the ventilator support. Volume is not regulated directly with this mode and may change abruptly if the patient does not initiate a breath or develops a change in lung or chest wall compliance. PSV, therefore, requires careful monitoring and a back-up rate of volume ventilation if the patient stops initiating a pressure-support breath.

Since the patient initiates each breath, PSV reduces the potential for asynchronous efforts by the patient and the ventilator, as compared to volume ventilator modes. PSV also eliminates the work required to open the IMV or SIMV valves with those methods and reduces the work of breathing. Respiratory rate may decrease and tidal volume increase with increasing levels of PSV. Clearly, with this method the PIP is controlled by the clinician and not by the tidal volume as in volume ventilation.

## Strategies to improve oxygenation and decrease the adverse hemodynamic effects of positive-pressure ventilation

### Positive end-expiratory pressure

High concentrations of inspired oxygen ($Fio_2 \geq 60$) may result in direct lung injury or aggravate microatelectasis. Ventilator adjustments that result in an arterial $Po_2 > 60$ mmHg and an arterial oxygen saturation > 90% while maintaining $Fio_2 < 60$ are usually considered beneficial. As will be discussed further, oxygen delivery to tissues depends on cardiac output and hemoglobin concentration. Therapies that allow a reduction in $Fio_2$ but which reduce cardiac output may decrease tissue oxygenation, despite improvements in arterial oxygen concentrations. Therefore, any strategy to decrease $Fio_2$ which might compromise cardiac output should be used with caution and with careful hemodynamic monitoring.

PEEP is used commonly to improve arterial oxygen concentration in patients with respiratory failure, primarily of the alveolar type. End-expiratory pressure maintains the patency of airways that would otherwise collapse as the volume of the lung decreases during expiration towards the critical closing volume, which is commonly increased and greater than FRC in acute illness. PEEP-induced increased air at end-expiration is measured as an increased FRC, which then correlates inversely with the calculated shunt fraction.

In general, PEEP is used when patients cannot achieve 90% oxygen saturation ($Po_2 \geq 60$ mmHg) at a $Fio_2$ of 0.6 or less. The most common pulmonary disease for which PEEP is effective is pulmonary edema of any etiology, or similar disease which produces bilateral decreased compliance and decreased FRC. PEEP does not prevent ARDS, nor does it significantly decrease lung water. PEEP is used to achieve adequate arterial oxygen saturation while diagnostic and/or therapeutic interventions are employed to diagnose and/or treat the underlying disease.

PEEP is usually introduced at a level of 5 cmH$_2$O and increased at 2.5–5 cmH$_2$O increments, with 20–30 cmH$_2$O considered high levels and more likely to result in complications such as decreased cardiac output, artifacts in hemodynamic monitoring, increased shunt and barotrauma. PEEP complications are more likely to develop in less diseased lungs with closer to normal compliance. Under these circumstances the pressure effects of PEEP can produce greater distension of alveoli and transmission of pressure to other intrathoracic organs.

While PEEP may improve arterial oxygen saturation, PEEP-induced cardiac impairment may reduce oxygen delivery. Proposed mechanisms for PEEP-induced decreased cardiac output are decreased venous return, myocardial depression and dilatation of the right ventricle. The primary mechanism is diminished venous return. PEEP results in an increase in Paw and Palv which is then variably transmitted to the pleural space, depending on lung compliance. An increase in pleural pressure results in an extracardiac increase in central venous pressure (CVP) as well as an increase in thoracic venous resistance, both of which inhibit venous return (see Chapter 2, The circulation; Hypoperfusion states). In addition, more direct cardiac impairment from a physiology similar to cardiac tamponade may be present. Increasing mean systemic pressure (MSP) by fluid infusion returns cardiac output close to or to baseline, pre-PEEP values. If myocardial depression or right ventricular distension were major mechanisms of decreased cardiac output, aggressive fluid infusion should aggravate rather than improve compromised cardiac status.

Since PEEP increases intrathoracic pressure to a variable degree, depending on such factors as lung and chest wall compliance, the influence of PEEP on pressures measured within the thorax has been difficult to assess. An elevation in CVP and PAOP with falling cardiac output following PEEP administration may be considered evidence of cardiac decompensation. However, if the elevation of cardiac chamber pressures were secondary to increased pleural pressure, cardiac output changes would be better attributed to decreased venous return. In the past, measurement of PEEP effects on extracardiac pressure required placement of monitors at the time of open-heart surgery or other invasive techniques. Otherwise, a maneuver such as acutely discontinuing PEEP was advocated as a method of estimating the influence of PEEP on hemodynamic monitors. The first method obviously cannot be used in non-open-heart surgery patients, and a non-invasive method is preferred. The second method presumes that cardiac status will be similar without PEEP as with PEEP, the only difference being the increase in intrathoracic pressure. Because cardiac output is affected by PEEP and PEEP changes ventricular compliance, this presumption is false. In addition, abrupt discontinuance of PEEP may result in decreased arterial oxygen saturation which may take minutes to hours to recover. Therefore, a non-invasive method which allows PEEP to continue and provides an estimate of PEEP-induced effects on hemodynamic monitors is desirable.

Such a device has been used in the following manner: a balloon-equipped nasogastric tube which is filled with saline and uses standard saline transducers provides a reasonable estimate of the contribution of increased intrathoracic pressure on cardiac chamber pressures. With this method the clinician can determine if decreasing cardiac output is secondary to factors adverse to venous return or myocardial dysfunction (see Chapter 2, The circulation; Hemodynamic monitoring).

When pulmonary disease is unilateral PEEP administration may aggravate the intrapulmonary shunt. Compliant less-diseased lung will suffer more alveolar distension, increased pulmonary vascular resistance and decreased perfusion. More perfusion will be directed to the diseased non-compliant lung, aggravating the shunt. One method advocated to avoid this problem is synchronous ventilation of each lung with different ventilators. However, most often recognition of this complication of PEEP will result in decreasing PEEP and continuing measures to maintain or increase cardiac output.

As stated in the 'Differential diagnosis of ARDS' section, ARDS does not result in a homogeneous injury to the lung. Throughout both lungs there are relatively compliant and non-compliant regions. Therefore, PEEP may cause overdistension of some lung units while having little effect on others. Such compliant regions may be particularly susceptible to lung damage from overdistension and/or high transalveolar pressures.

PEEP administration with volume ventilators results in increased PIP, Paw and Palv. Depending upon total lung and lung unit compliance, PEEP may also increase transalveolar pressure throughout the lung. Barotrauma may result (see below). Gross evidence of barotrauma (pneumothorax, pneumomediastinum, pneumoperitoneum) can usually be controlled with chest tube insertion to the most affected thorax.

*Inverse ratio ventilation*

As presented above and in the 'Differential diagnosis of ARDS' section, acute lung injury which falls under the rubric of ARDS is associated with non-homogeneous lung units which exhibit variations in compliance and sometimes resistance. As a result, the time constants (TC = resistance × compliance) in various areas will vary and the time necessary to inflate and deflate regions of lung will not be uniform. The actual functioning lung may be compliant but comprise only a fraction of normal lung volume. As stated by Marcy and Marini (1991)'...the functioning lung in ARDS is not so much stiff as it is small'.

With standard volume ventilator management the ratio of the time of inspiration to the time of expiration (I : E) is characteristically 1 : 3. With IRV inspiration time is prolonged relative to expiration, increasing the I : E ratio. This allows less compliant alveolar units more time to open and less time to collapse. An increase in mean airway pressure accompanies less peak airway pressure compared to using PEEP. In general, patients require sedation and paralysis to tolerate this mode of therapy. Ratios up to 4 : 1 have been reported in adults. Most often external PEEP can be reduced as well as $Fio_2$. Curiously $CO_2$ elimination often improves also, suggesting a decrease in physiological dead space with this mode of ventilation.

The shortened duration of expiration has the potential to allow gas trapping and auto-PEEP. The resultant increase in mean airway and mean alveolar pressure may augment oxygenation, but have implications regarding increased pleural pressure and decreased venous return. Therefore, careful attention to mean airway pressure, measurement of total PEEP and cardiac output is required when using this method.

While IRV can be applied with volume ventilators, most often PCV has been used (PCV+IRV). The indications for PCV+IRV may be either ineffective oxygenation with other methods or fear of barotrauma (see below) from high PIP.

One method of implementation is as follows (after Lain):

(1) Sedation usually with paralysis;

(2) Choose a pressure maximum for PCV (estimate at about 50% of the previously needed peak pressure);

(3) Initial I : E of 1 : 1 with the plan to increase this over several hours;

(4) Decrease extrinsic PEEP as dictated by oxygenation;

(5) Try to keep initial Paw the same as that prior to initiation of PCV+IRV, but Paw is expected to increase as I : E increases;

(6) Try to keep PIP > 20, < 40 cmH$_2$O.

*Prone position ventilation*
Another method which has been utilized to improve perfusion to ventilated areas of lung and/or improve ventilation to perfused areas of lung is changing the position of the ventilated patient from supine to prone. Most often this management has been applied in patients with ARDS. Characteristically, the $Pao_2/Fio_2$ ratio improves significantly with

little change or sometimes a decrease in $Paco_2$. Patients have been maintained in the prone position for as little as 1 and as long as 66 hours. On average, there is a noted increase in the $Pao_2/Fio_2$ ratio by 2 hours, although occasionally 24 hours have passed before improvement has been noticed. Major concerns are the possibility of endotracheal tube displacement, difficulty gaining vascular access, and the potential of peripheral nerve injuries or injuries to the eyes from excessive pressure. Clearly cautious positioning and attention to all pressure points must be employed to safely use this method. However, the promising results with early reports clearly place prone positioning as one possible strategy for improving oxygenation in severe ARDS.

## Strategies to reduce the risk and incidence of ventilator-induced lung injury

The potential lung injuries that can occur during positive-pressure ventilation are considered secondary to either an increase in pressure (barotrauma) or an increase in lung unit distention (volutrauma). The intimate association between the effects of pressure and over-distention are sufficiently difficult to separate that the more inclusive terminology of ventilator-induced lung injury will be used for this section. Such injuries include pneumothorax, pneumomediastinum, pneumoperitoneum, pneumopericardium, pulmonary interstitial emphysema, tension air cysts, gas emboli and induction of an ARDS-like pathology. The potential etiologies of ventilator-induced lung injury are high peak-inspiratory pressures ($> 40 \, cmH_2O$), high transalveolar pressures ($> 35 \, cmH_2O$), alveolar overdistension, shear forces and surfactant depletion. Patients with ARDS are at particular risk. Strategies for limiting such injuries include:

Strategies for limiting such injury include:

(1) Permissive hypercapnia;

(2) Inverse ratio ventilation;

(3) Prone ventilation;

(4) High frequency ventilation;

(5) Airway pressure release ventilation.

*Permissive hypercapnia*
Of these, the least complicated to use is permissive hypercapnia which is accomplished by reducing the tidal volume, sometimes to as low as

5 ml/kg, to decrease Pplat to < 40 cmH$_2$O or PIP < 45 cmH$_2$O. Oxygenation and hemodynamics have not been noted to change, despite $P_{CO_2}$ increases as high as 79 mmHg and arterial pH as low as 7.2. In general, this method has not been regularly used in patients with head injury and intracranial hypertension unless the effects of increasing $P_{CO_2}$ can be measured with intracranial pressure monitoring. In addition, patients with cardiac arrhythmias and renal failure with metabolic acidosis are considered less than optimal candidates.

*Inverse ratio ventilation*
The use of PCV+IRV is more commonly used to reduce the risk of ventilator-induced lung injury in patients with severe oxygenation difficulties than to treat the oxygenation difficulties *per se*. Whether these methods of ventilation can actually improve outcome needs further study. The possibility that limiting barotrauma will diminish the intrinsic inflammation in the lung and, thereby, decrease the severity of systemic inflammation is certainly intriguing as clinicians attempt to limit the deleterious effects of ongoing inflammation not only in the lung but in other tissues so commonly injured by severe systemic inflammation.

*High-frequency ventilation*
High-frequency ventilation (HFV) is a modality of respiratory support which, in general, encompasses three methods:

(1) High-frequency positive pressure ventilation (HFPPV);

(2) High-frequency jet ventilation (HFJV);

(3) High-frequency oscillation (HFO).

These methods were designed to provide adequate gas exchange at lower airway pressure, thereby reducing the risk of barotrauma and cardiac impairment.

HFPPV was the first method developed and is similar to CMV, with tidal volumes in the range of 3–6 ml/kg and rates usually 60–80/min, but sometimes up to 150/min. HFJV is the type used most in the USA. Gas under high pressure (500–3000 mmHg) is delivered through a catheter into an endotracheal tube. The jet of air captures or entrains air surrounding the jet with the tidal volume equal to the jet air plus the entrained (E) air (tidal volume = Vjet + VE). Usually Vjet and VE are close to equal (within 10%). HFO uses an oscillator which vibrates a column of air at frequencies up to 3000/min and uses small tidal volumes (1–3 ml/kg).

The movement of air into and out of the lung is dependent on two processes: convection, which results in the movement of relatively large volumes over a small surface area (air movement in the larger airways); and diffusion, which moves smaller amounts over a larger surface area (terminal airways and alveoli). Conventional ventilators rely mostly on convection to move air within the larger airways, as does HFPPV. With HFJV convection is still important, but diffusion is presumably enhanced by kinetic energy added to the system. HFO depends primarily on diffusion as oxygen is added and carbon dioxide removed from the circulation.

HFV has been used in a variety of disease states (bronchopleural fistula and ARDS) and procedures (bronchoscopy, laryngoscopy, pulmonary resection, tracheal suctioning and transtracheal ventilation). In general, HFV has been found to be most useful in the treatment of bronchopleural fistula (especially HFJV), whereby adequate gas exchange at low pressure diminishes the loss of tidal volume from the fistula. In addition, either the small size of the HFJV catheter, the lower airway pressures employed, or the ability to place the catheter directly into the trachea have been found beneficial for the procedures listed above in which HFV has been used. Claims that this therapy would improve outcomes in ARDS, diminish barotrauma and decrease hemodynamic complications have not been supported in prospective trials (see below).

*Airway pressure release ventilation*
With airway pressure release ventilation (APRV), continuous positive airway pressure (CPAP) is applied to inflate the lungs and the pressure released intermittently to allow expiration. In patients who do not make an inspiratory effort, APRV is similar to pressure-controlled inverse ratio ventilation. However, APRV can be used in patients with respiratory efforts. This method is designed to limit PIP and, thereby, presumably, ventilator-induced lung injury. Further study is required to determine if this mode has distinct advantages compared to more commonly used techniques.

## Complications of intubation
Besides the potential problems of decreased cardiac output and lung injury associated with mechanical ventilation, complications of tracheal and/or tracheostomy must be considered. Complications of such intubation include colonization of tracheobronchial tree, vocal cord injury, tracheomalacia, tracheostenosis, tracheoinominate fistula, tracheoesophageal fistula and paranasal sinusitis with nasotracheal intubation.

Colonization of the tracheobronchial tree occurs rapidly (see Pneumonia section, this Chapter). Endotracheal tubes are generally well tolerated for 3 weeks without significant vocal cord injury. Therefore, unless prolonged respirator dependency or respiratory toilet access is expected, tracheostomy is usually delayed until after 3 weeks. The currently used low-pressure cuffs are much less likely to produce the erosive complications, but attention is still required to ensure that cuff pressures are less than 20 mmHg.

The association of nasotracheal intubation and paranasal sinusitis has been well documented. This may by a cryptic source of infection in critically ill surgical patients and may only be diagnosed by sampling sinus fluid discovered by plain or computed tomography X-rays of the face.

## Weaning

Since the need for mechanical ventilation is secondary to either mechanical or alveolar failure, the criteria for weaning relate to both mechanical and alveolar function, the former being the primary reason for failure to wean. Commonly employed mechanical weaning criteria are inspiratory force $\geq$ 20 cmH$_2$O, vital capacity $\geq$ 15 ml/kg, $P$a$CO_2$ $\leq$ 50 mmHg and FEV1 $\geq$ 500 ml. Alveolar weaning criteria are $P$a$O_2$/F$IO_2$ $\geq$ 200 and shunt fraction $\leq$ 15%. Several studies have questioned the validity of many of these standard criteria. For instance, not all patients must achieve a $P$a$CO_2$ $\leq$ 50 mmHg. $P$a$CO_2$ may be allowed to remain in the 50s if the patient is known to have severe COPD and previous $CO_2$ retention. All proposed weaning criteria are guidelines and patients, especially the elderly, may wean without meeting several.

The clinical response of the patient during weaning is the best measure of the weaning process. Any patient who has a marked increase in pulse, blood pressure and respiratory rate is not tolerating weaning. Dyspnea may in part reflect an imbalance between diaphragmatic energy supply and demand. Any process that increases diaphragmatic energy demand (i.e. work of breathing) can make weaning difficult. Sometimes this may be simply the first time the diaphragm is expected to do any work after a period of rest.

Methods that have been advocated to enhance weaning are:

(1) Treatment of reversible disease e.g. ARDS, pneumonia, bronchospasm, pulmonary embolism, hypoperfusion, ischemic heart disease, remote inflammatory disease and severe metabolic acidosis;

(2) Increase diaphragm function using theophylline, upright position, ?exercise, ?nutrition, investigate possible paralysis;

(3) Tracheostomy to decrease deadspace and decrease resistance;

(4) Pressure support ventilation;

(5) Physiological PEEP.

The most important is to treat disease within or remote from the lung which may inhibit pulmonary function (e.g. pneumonia, CHF, severe inflammation, bronchospasm). Assuming the upright position improves diaphragm function in most patients. Theophylline not only reduces bronchospasm but improves diaphragm contractility. Tracheostomy will reduce physiological dead space and airway resistance, as compared to endotracheal tubes. Often patients who are having difficulty weaning have prolonged endotracheal intubation and will require a tracheostomy to protect the vocal cords.

Exercise of the diaphragm is controversial and is one of the presumed advantages of gradually decreasing IMV as a method of weaning, as compared to gradually increasing periods of time off the respirator on a T-piece. Patients with good respiratory function tolerate rapid IMV weaning well. Patients with poor respiratory function often develop dyspnea on IMV, even with IMV set at a rate close to or above a patient's positive-pressure ventilation. Apparently even a slight demand for diaphragmatic work in such patients induces dyspnea. The IMV valve may require more work than a T-piece, with short periods of time on a T-piece better tolerated. An alternative is to provide pressure assistance to help open the IMV valve. Slowly decreasing pressure support ventilation may be the best-tolerated method to gradually increase the work of breathing in anticipation of discontinuing the ventilator.

With critical illness muscle wasting is common and presumably the diaphragm suffers along with other skeletal muscle. Nutrition that reduces negative nitrogen balance would be expected to improve all muscle function. However, metabolism of carbohydrate, fat and protein results in $CO_2$ production (carbohydrate > fat), which may aggravate difficulties in $CO_2$ elimination, stimulate respiration and increase work of breathing. Providing nutrition with higher fat content and less $CO_2$ production may be less detrimental (see Chapter 6, The gastrointestinal nutritional system; nutritional therapy). Muscle wasting is also associated with the prolonged complete and/or partial paralysis induced by paralytic drugs. Recognition of partial paralysis is important and will at least provide an understanding of weaning difficulties in certain patients.

Patients suffering sufficient respiratory embarrassment to require mechanical ventilation often are subject to severe systemic inflammation, use of a neuromuscular blocking agents for ventilator management, and corticosteroids for underlying inflammatory diseases. Such patients may develop a neuromuscular disorder which has been described as critical illness polyneuropathy. In addition, a more direct injury of muscle may occur to the point of actual muscle necrosis. Precise diagnosis of these conditions may require electromyographs and/or nerve and muscle biopsies. Recognition that a patient is suffering from a defined neuromuscular disorder has important implications vis-a-vis prognosis, plans for continuing ventilator management, and interventions that may be directed at primarily improving lung function. Any patient exhibiting an unexpected degree of weakness or lack of motor response during or shortly following any severe critical illness is a candidate for careful neurological/neuromuscular evaluation.

Low levels of PEEP (3–5 cmH$_2$O) have been advocated as more 'physiological' than respiration via an endotracheal tube or tracheostomy at 0 PEEP. Presumably the larynx produces an expiratory effect similar to low levels of PEEP, and FRC measured after extubation is closer to that measured with 'physiological' PEEP than with a T-piece at atmospheric pressure alone. Proponents of this use of low-level PEEP argue that weaning is enhanced by improving FRC.

Weaning from the ventilator does not necessarily mean that a patient will tolerate extubation. Extubation requires sufficient control of the oropharynx and control of respiratory secretions to allow maintenance of a clear airway. Patients with neurological insults are the most obvious group who may not need a ventilator but still need an airway. Tracheostomy may be indicated in such patients primarily for airway and not because it improves the mechanics of respiration.

## EXTRACORPOREAL PULMONARY SUPPORT

During respiratory failure, support of pulmonary function using the ventilator management methods described in the previous sections is usually successful. However, for patients with severe lung damage, mechanical ventilation may itself aggravate injury by the mechanisms described previously. The intersection in time of recognition of a finite limit to medically enhanced *in vivo* performance of failing organs with a growing appreciation of the potential for iatrogenic insults led to increasing interest in safer and more effective means of replacing the function of the lungs similar to the use of dialysis for the replacement of renal function. Based on this concept, techniques that provide gas exchange without mechanical ventilation may provide adequate support to sustain life and allow the damaged lung to recover without inciting further injury, even from the ventilator itself (see 'Strategies to reduce the risk and incidence of ventilator-induced lung injury section).

### Extracorporeal membrane oxygenation

Extracorporeal membrane oxygenation (ECMO) in the critical care setting was the inevitable child of cardiopulmonary bypass in the operating room. In the late 1960s ECMO was introduced to the neonatal ICU and eventually applied to adults. Pediatric extracorporeal pulmonary support found a niche in babies with immature lungs and it has become a standard practice. There was less success in older patients. Oxygenation could be accomplished but patients expired from their underlying fatal diseases. Eventually ECMO for adults was abandoned. It was expensive in time and resources and it was not effective in preventing death.

In the late 1980s there was a change in focus from extracorporeal oxygenation to extracorporeal carbon dioxide removal. This change in focus, together with a better understanding of the pathophysiology of pulmonary failure in the ICU, led to a resurgence of interest in the clinical application of extracorporeal lung support. Extracorporeal pulmonary support unquestionably allows effective exchange of oxygen and carbon dioxide at minimal airway pressures. It allows prolongation of patient survival. It may permit effective treatment of the underlying cause of pulmonary failure or it may allow spontaneous recovery of the patient's native lungs.

### Extracorporeal lung assistance

Extracorporeal lung assistance (ECLA) is usually provided through a venovenous access circuit. This approach reduces the risk of air embolism by avoiding the left heart circulation. If hemodynamic support is desired, arterial access can be added. Large-bore wire coil-reinforced access catheters have proved to be the most satisfactory means of vessel cannulation. When a venovenous circuit is used the drain catheter, with multiple distal side perforations to improve flow, is placed in a femoral vein. The blood return line is placed so that it empties near the right atrium. Arterial access in adults is usually via the femoral artery. Heparin-bonded polyvinylchloride tubing is used for the extracorporeal circuit. It must be strong enough to tolerate the pressure of the extracorporeal pump. All tubing connections are factory sealed to prevent separation during use which can be both dangerous and dramatic. A servoregulated blood pump mechanically maintains flow at a constant rate. The more severe the patient's pulmonary process the greater the extracorporeal flow rate of oxygen enriched blood required to maintain oxygenation.

The key components of the ECLA circuit are the artificial lungs. Two microporous hollow-fiber membrane lungs are arranged in parallel. Each membrane lung has an integral heat exchanger and, in the present model, each lung has an individual blood pump. An air trap and bubble alarm are placed downstream of the membrane lungs to capture any air bubbles before they reach the patient. Oxygen, the sweep gas, is delivered to the membrane lungs through a standard flow meter. Blood sampling ports are located on either side of the bioartificial lungs.

### Complications of extracorporeal lung support

Bleeding is the major complication of extracorporeal pulmonary support. The extracorporeal circuit sequesters platelets and heparinization, with its associated problems, is required. In addition, there may be spontaneous bleeding caused by the flow characteristics of the external roller pump running at high flow rates. Hemolysis is a well-recognized complication in extracorporeal support. It may be due to pressure gradients, shear forces, or trauma to erythrocytes from the extracorporeal pump. Elevated levels of carbon monoxide have been observed as well.

Activation of the inflammatory cascade is another phenomenon associated with extracorporeal support. The complement component, particularly C3a, is prominent. Reductions in circulating leukocytes occur simultaneously with the initiation of extracorporeal support. A change to heparin-bonded components for the external circulation may reduce complement activation.

Some complications specific to out-of-body blood circulation lead to potentially catastrophic problems. Should the extracorporeal circuit spontaneously fracture or disconnect, there is the potential for air embolism as well as massive bleeding. Factory welding of tubing connections and constant vigilance minimize but do not eliminate these dangers. Clotting in the circuit occurs and with time failure of the extracorporeal organ is to be expected. Patients who depend on an external bioartificial lung for survival can become very unstable even during planned controlled membrane and tubing exchanges. For this reason, one external lung is replaced at a time. One practice is to have a complete standby circuit including pumps and monitors ready at all times at the bedside in case of an unplanned adventure.

**Support personnel**

Extracorporeal pulmonary support is advanced technology which requires dedicated personnel when it is in use. A pump assistant, internist and two nurses are commonly assigned to the patient. One nurse provides the usual critical care clinical services needed. The second nurse is one of a cadre of specially trained practitioners who look after the extracorporeal support system. In addition to ECLA they are also trained in continuous hemodiafiltration techniques as well as being regular, often senior members of the ICU nursing staff. A bioengineer is another integral component of the ECLA team.

Extracorporeal pulmonary support may develop into a practical life saving ICU system in the future, but at present it is a promising last effort for selected patients. It has serious complications and risks. It does not cure lung failure but it may keep patients alive long enough for other curative measures to be effective. Partial cardiopulmonary bypass using an arteriovenous circuit may be used to augment flagging cardiac performance. ECLA requires constant attention to the patient and to the ECLA system. It is labor- and resource-intensive, but it has resulted in some spectacular successes. Further extensions are being explored for its use as a bridge to transplant and as an intraoperative adjunct in liver trauma surgery to permit vascular isolation of the liver. At the time of writing, one patient has undergone repair of a traumatic rupture of the thoracic aorta on ECLA.

# 5

# THE RENAL SYSTEM

Basic physiology
       Renal circulation
       Glomerular filtration
       Tubular reabsorption
       Coupled ion transport
Monitoring of renal function
       History and physical examination
       Urine specific gravity
       Urine electrolytes
       BUN and serum creatinine
       Urinalysis
Drugs
       Diuretics
Fluid and electrolytes
       Body fluid compartments
       Basic fluid and electrolyte therapy
       Common electrolyte abnormalities
       Acid–base physiology
Renal failure and selected metabolic disturbances
       The effects of circulation on renal function
       The effects of inflammation on renal function
       Renal failure
       Hemodynamic management of renal failure
       Management of 'renal' kidney failure

## BASIC PHYSIOLOGY

The kidneys serve primarily to preserve intravascular volume, maintain normal acid–base status, and excrete products of metabolism. For surgeons, the mechanisms involved in preserving intravascular volume and acid–base status are most important, and are emphasized below. The excretion of metabolic products is of greatest concern when this process is interrupted during renal failure and receives more attention later in this Chapter; Renal failure and selected metabolic disturbances section.

### Renal circulation

The renal circulation has the following four components: outer cortex (75%), juxtamedullary cortex and outer medulla (20%), vasa recta and inner medulla, and perirenal and hilar fat (combined 5%). The high rate of outer cortical blood flow is ideal for glomerular filtration, the slow blood flow in the vasa recta helps maintain osmotic gradients in the peritubular space. During reduced renal blood flow, outer cortical perfusion is reduced and juxtamedullary cortical and outer medullary flow increases. This adjustment maintains blood flow where urinary concentration mechanisms are most active. In acute renal failure outer and juxtamedullary cortical flow are further reduced, but medullary flow can be relatively well maintained.

### Glomerular filtration

The first process in the formation of urine is glomerular capillary ultra-filtration of blood. This results in a filtrate which is low in protein and contains all solutes not bound to non-filterable proteins.

Glomerular filtration (the amount of blood filtered) is measured by determining the clearance from the plasma of a substance which is filtered but neither secreted nor absorbed by the renal tubules. Dividing the amount excreted in the urine over a given amount of time by the plasma concentration of that substance in normal adult humans results in a value of 100–125 ml/min (144–160 l/day).

### Tubular reabsorption

The 100–125 ml/min of glomerular filtrate enters the proximal renal tubule which, along with the rest of the tubular system, reabsorbs approximately 98% of the filtered water and solutes, mostly in the proximal tubule (two-thirds to seven-eighths of glomerular filtrate). Obviously, without reabsorption vascular volume loss would be rapidly lethal. Two mechanisms have been described for reabsorption in the proximal tubule: active and passive. Active absorption may exhibit characteristics of transport maxima (TM) or gradient-time (GT) limitations (Table 1). Passive absorption of water, and consequently urea, follows osmotic gradients established primarily by the active transport of sodium. Since water absorption is passive preservation of vascular volume depends primarily on sodium absorption.

TM-limited reabsorption mechanisms, such as that for glucose, demonstrate the ability to remove a substance from the tubules until a maximum concentration in tubular fluid is exceeded. A similar mechanism has been described for phosphate, sulfate and amino acids.

Sodium is the major solute reabsorbed with a GT mechanism. Sodium can be absorbed up to a maximum concentration difference between intraluminal sodium and peritubular cell sodium. The maximum concentration difference achieved also depends on the time of contact of the sodium with the tubular cell establishing the concentration difference. Therefore, the rate of glomerular filtration and proximal tubular flow has a regulatory influence on the degree of proximal tubular sodium reabsorption. Otherwise, local or systemic physiological processes have little effect on the proximal tubule.

The distal nephron (distal convoluted tubules and collecting ducts) reabsorbs much less water and fewer solutes, but is more responsive to

**TABLE 1    MECHANISMS OF TUBULAR REABSORPTION**

*Active*
Transport maxima
   glucose
   phosphate
   sulfate
   lactate
   $\beta$-hydroxybutyrate
   acetoacetate
Gradient-time limitations
   sodium
   chloride
   bicarbonate

*Passive*
Water
Urea

local or systemic physiological alterations. Using the counter-current mechanism established by the loop of Henle, the distal nephron can establish high ion and osmolar concentration gradients between tubular fluid and peritubular plasma, and respond to mineralocorticoid and arginine vasopressin (AVP; also known as antidiuretic hormone (ADH)1) secretion for enhanced sodium and water reabsorption, respectively.

**Coupled ion transport**
The reabsorption of sodium is the major active transport mechanism of the entire nephron. The variables that determine sodium reabsorption and the renal response to these physiological influences provide excellent underpinning for further discussions of the renal response in disease. The three major determinants of sodium reabsorption are glomerular filtration, aldosterone and a 'third factor', possibly atrial natriuretic factor (ANF). As mentioned, glomerular filtration rate determines the time available for sodium reabsorption in the proximal tubule. Rapid filtration rates diminish reabsorption, while slow rates enhance it.

Aldosterone augments sodium absorption in the distal tubule and is released as the end product of the renin–angiotensin–aldosterone hormonal axis. Renin is released from the juxtaglomerular cells of the kidney as a response to diminished renal perfusion, diminished sodium supply to the distal tubule, and $\beta$-adrenergic stimulation. Renin converts renin substrate (produced in the liver) into angiotensin I which is converted mostly in the lungs into angiotensin II, a potent arteriolar vasoconstrictor and a stimulus for aldosterone release from the adrenal cortex. Both renin and aldosterone levels have been shown to fluctuate markedly in normal humans during salt deprivation and salt loading, with an inverse relationship to sodium excretion under both circumstances.

However, glomerular filtration and aldosterone do not explain de Wardener's observation that despite partial renal artery occlusion of one kidney and the maintenance of constant glomerular filtration and aldosterone'levels, a large sodium infusion produces a sodium diuresis in the clamped kidney, approaching that of the unclamped kidney. Atrial extracts producing sodium diuresis in rats, ANF(s) have more recently been isolated and synthesized that can both promote natruresis and vasodilatation of large arteries. Natruresis from ANF probably results from increased glomerular filtration possibly secondary to selective constriction of glomerular efferent arterioles. In addition, ANF appears to reduce renal renin secretion and to reduce basal and stimulated release of aldosterone. ANF also may block the vasoconstrictive effects of angiotensin II. Thus,

ANF may serve as a negative feedback mechanism, possibly released with atrial distension, to offset the active renal and hormonal mechanisms for maintaining blood pressure, preserving sodium and increasing blood volume.

The transport of chloride, hydrogen ions, bicarbonate and potassium are all intimately related to sodium transport. In the proximal tubule chloride is absorbed passively and depends on active sodium absorption. To maintain electroneutrality in the tubular lumen, hydrogen ions are exchanged for sodium and result in increased intracellular bicarbonate. The secreted hydrogen ions react with bicarbonate and reduce bicarbonate concentration in the lumen. Both intracellular and intraluminal reactions of hydrogen ions and bicarbonate are facilitated by carbonic anhydrase. In the distal tubule hydrogen ion secretion continues, especially when sodium absorption is high (aldosterone secretion). To preserve anion electroneutrality, either chloride or bicarbonate must accompany sodium. During states of chloride deficiency or strong sodium reabsorption (e.g. hypoperfusion of the kidneys, loss of chloride from the stomach, elevated aldosterone or cortisol levels, diuretics) sodium–hydrogen exchange is augmented and results in increased bicarbonate absorption (or intracellular production) and excretion of hydrogen in the face of a metabolic alkalosis (paradoxical aciduria). Potassium excretion is also responsive to electroneutrality requirements and is commonly increased in states of sodium reabsorption, even in the face of hypokalemia.

## MONITORING OF RENAL FUNCTION

The common clinical parameters used to monitor renal function are rate of urine flow and blood urea nitrogen (BUN) and serum creatinine (CR), which are discussed in detail below.

### History and physical examination

The first step in evaluating the etiology of oliguria (< 20 ml/h in the adult) or an increase in BUN and CR is to review the history (episodes of hypoperfusion, operation(s), renal toxic drugs, pre-existing renal disease and severe inflammation) and physical examination (blood pressure, pulse, temperature, mentation, skin color and temperature, percussion/palpation of bladder and examination of prostate) information. Most of this information provides evidence of previous or ongoing total body hypoperfusion as well as the presence or absence of renal toxins or bladder obstruction.

## Urine specific gravity

Low urine output secondary to renal hypoperfusion is a normal physiological response to preserve sodium and water. Secretion of AVP allows tubular reabsorption of water to the maximum osmolar concentration in peritubular fluid (approximately 1200 mosmol/l) and results in a specific gravity (SG) greater than that of plasma (> 1.010, but usually < 1.030). Unfortunately, SG can be increased by other mechanisms, especially the excretion of osmotically active substances like glucose and angiogram dye, which not only increase SG but also often promote diuresis. Diuresis with increased SG (especially when > 1.030) is a clue that a large osmotically active molecule is in the urine. A physiological diuresis secondary to well-maintained hydration would more likely decrease SG. After such stress as surgery, trauma, or severe infection, the most likely cause of a large urine output with elevated SG is excretion of glucose secondary to increased blood glucose from the metabolic response to stress. A urine sugar level will rapidly determine if such is the case.

## Urine electrolytes

With normal kidney function oliguria is most often secondary to hypoperfusion, which stimulates renal preservation of sodium and water and, therefore, urine sodium concentrations of < 20 mEq/l. When urine sodium is > 40 mEq/l, the inference is that the renal tubules are injured and cannot reabsorb sodium. However, urine sodium may be elevated to allow for electroneutrality when non-physiological anions are present (e.g. penicillin). Since chloride usually follows sodium, hypoperfusion usually results in low urine chloride concentrations (< 20 mEq/l). Again, large quantities of non-sodium cations (ammonium, calcium) may increase urine chloride concentration.

The fractional excretion of sodium ( $FE_{Na}$ ) (the percentage of filtered sodium which is excreted) is considered a more accurate indication of renal hypoperfusion vs. damaged tubules.

$$FE_{Na} = \frac{U_{Na}/P_{Na}}{U_{Cr}/P_{Cr}} \times 100$$

Where $U_{Na}$ and $P_{Na}$ are urine and plasma sodium concentrations and $U_{Cr}$ and $P_{Cr}$ are urine and plasma creatinine concentrations, respectively. Values < 1.0% indicate hypoperfusion; values > 3% indicate tubular damage. However, several reports have demonstrated $FE_{Na}$ values < 1% in patients with a clinical course more consistent with tubular damage. This is seen most often in patients with intense stimuli for sodium reabsorption (e.g. congestive heart failure, cirrhosis, burns) or particular etiologies of renal damage (e.g. acute glomerular and interstitial nephritis).

## BUN and serum creatinine

BUN and creatinine levels are easily obtained estimates of glomerular filtration. Urea is a product of protein metabolism and is influenced by the amount of protein metabolized either as a result of the amount of protein administered or the metabolic capability of the liver. A diet deficient in protein coupled with a damaged liver may result in a low BUN, despite reduced glomerular filtration. High protein intake with good liver function might produce the opposite effect. Creatinine is the end product of creatine metabolism in muscle and is usually produced at a constant rate from day to day. Except with little (e.g. older, wasted patient) or excessive muscle breakdown (ischemic muscle necrosis), creatinine ranges from 0.6 to 1.0 mg/100 ml in females, and 0.8 to 1.3 mg/100 ml in males with normal glomerular filtration.

For every 50% reduction in glomerular filtration, serum creatinine doubles (Figure 1). Therefore, beginning with normal function small increments in creatinine represent significant decreases in glomerular filtration. Subsequent similar increments represent less percentage loss of function. BUN is also reabsorbed indirectly proportional to the rate of urine flow. Therefore, in oliguric states with preserved tubular function (hypoperfusion), BUN will rise more than creatinine and increase the normal BUN : CR ratio of 10–15:1 to 20–50:1. Therefore, the BUN : CR ratio can assist the recognition of hypoperfusion states.

## Urinalysis

Urinalysis is particularly useful for determining SG, the presence of glucose, and for evidence of acute renal cell injury (casts, tubular cells, eosinophils).

## DRUGS

### Diuretics

The drugs used most commonly to directly influence urine output are diuretics, which either work as a filtered osmotic load (e.g. glucose, mannitol) or interrupt sodium reabsorption (e.g. furosemide, hydrochlorothiazide, zaroxolyn). In either case, more sodium and water are excreted than otherwise, with a urine sodium concentration of 30–70 mEq/l, result-

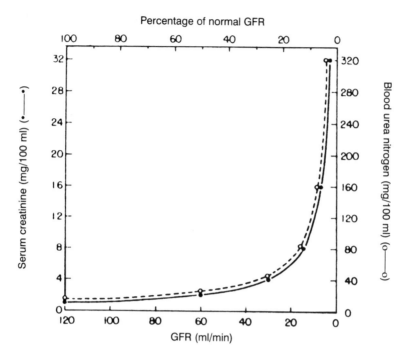

**Figure 1** Graphic representation of the increase in creatinine as glomerular filtration (GFR) decreases. Once GFR is approximately 30% of normal, small reductions in GFR may result in marked creatinine elevation. Reproduced with permission from Kassirer JP. Current concepts: clinical evaluation of kidney function – glomerular function. *N Engl J Med* 1971;285:385–89

ing in the loss of more water than sodium. Drugs that inhibit sodium reabsorption promote potassium excretion.

Acetazolamide is a carbonic anhydrase inhibitor which diminishes proximal tubular reabsorption of bicarbonate. This is particularly effective in patients with metabolic alkalosis (*vide infra*). Spironolactone inhibits aldosterone and will diminish sodium reabsorption and potassium loss. Neither of these agents promote much water loss.

## FLUID AND ELECTROLYTES

### Body fluid compartments
With the introduction of radioactive isotopes around the time of World War 2, the measurement of body fluid spaces and electrolytes became

### TABLE 2 TOTAL BODY WATER AS PERCENTAGE BODY WEIGHT

| Sex | Age (years) | Body water (%) |
|-----|-------------|----------------|
| Male | 16–30 | 58.9 |
| Male | 31–60 | 54.7 |
| Male | 61–90 | 51.6 |
| Female | 16–30 | 50.9 |
| Female | 31–90 | 45.2 |

### TABLE 3 DISTRIBUTION OF TOTAL BODY WATER AS PERCENTAGE OF BODY WEIGHT

| Sex | ICF | Total ECF | Plasma |
|-----|-----|-----------|--------|
| Male | 30.9 | 23.6 | 4.2 |
| Female | 25.9 | 22.7 | 4.2 |

ICF, intracellular fluid; ECF, extracellular fluid

scientifically more exact. Tables 2 and 3 show the water spaces in the body as percentages of body weight. A similar table of the total electrolyte composition of the body is not clinically useful, except for the recognition that the sodium ion is predominantly extracellular and potassium ion predominantly intracellular. This allows for the sodium ion to be used as a measure of the extracellular fluid space and the potassium ion to be used as a measure of the intracellular fluid space which has been termed the body cell mass. The body cell mass corresponds to functioning cells and has been shown recently to correlate well with definitions of malnutrition and response to nutritional therapy.

## Basic fluid and electrolyte therapy

*Reasons for fluid administration*
The primary reason fluids are administered is to maintain intravascular volume and thereby maintain a good circulation. As mentioned in Chapter 2, The circulation; Hypoperfusion states, a good-to-excellent circulation is a key to successful outcomes in critical illness. Therefore, as is described below, recognition and management of fluid alterations depends largely on the recognition and management principles related to the circulation. In addition, fluid and electrolyte therapy is directed at correcting specific acid–base and electrolyte disorders. Often these disorders are linked to

circulation deficits which must be corrected if the fluid/electrolyte therapy is to be successful.

*A basic approach*
The approach outlined below is designed to provide a simple method of determining the fluid and electrolyte requirements of most surgical patients. It is based on the concept that the unstressed patient lying in bed requires a baseline amount of water, sodium and potassium to provide an adequate volume and electrolytes for normal urine output, sweating and insensible loss. To this are added losses that may be measured losses, which are usually external, and unmeasured losses, which are internal.

Once these three components are estimated, the total fluid and electrolyte needs of the patient for a 24-hour period can be determined. Baseline requirements are determined, measured losses are added to these and replaced with an appropriate solution, any unmeasured losses are estimated and replaced accordingly. Baseline sodium, water and potassium requirements are 75 mEq, 25–30 ml/kg and 40 mEq, respectively, for a patient lying unstressed in bed. In general, water requirements decrease as age increases. There is an obligatory loss of potassium in the urine. Sodium loss is both by urine and by sweating. Baseline water is required for insensible loss and to provide an adequate volume for urinary excretion of metabolites.

The most common losses measured are those of gastrointestinal secretions, with gastric losses the most frequent of these. Table 4 lists the average electrolytes of intestinal secretions. Upwards of 10 l/day of total secretions are produced by the intestinal tract with no more than 100–200 ml excreted in the stool. Common volumes to encounter from gastric secretions are 1000–1500 ml/day. Biliary secretions are character-

**TABLE 4   ELECTROLYTES OF GASTROINTESTINAL SECRETIONS (MEAN VALUES)**

| Source | $Na^+$ (mEq/l) | $K^+$ (mEq/l) | $Cl^-$ (mEq/l) | $HCO_3^-$ (mEq/l) |
|---|---|---|---|---|
| Saliva | 60 | 20 | 16 | 50 |
| Gastric | 59 | 9.3 | 89 | 0–1 |
| Upper small bowel | 105 | 5.6 | 99 | 10 |
| Lower small bowel | 112 | 5.0 | 106 | 15–20 |
| Bile | 145 | 5.2 | 100 | 50 |
| Pancreas | 142 | 4.6 | 77 | 70 |

## TABLE 5   ELECTROLYTES OF INTRAVENOUS FLUIDS (MEQ/L)

| Solution | $Na^+$ | $K^+$ | $Ca^{2+}$ | $Cl^-$ | $HCO_3^-$ |
|----------|--------|-------|-----------|--------|-----------|
| Ringer's | 130 | 4 | 2.7 | 109 | 28 |
| Normal saline | 154 | | | 154 | |
| Half-normal saline | 77 | | | 77 | |
| Quarter-normal saline | 38.5 | | | 38.5 | |

istically 500 ml/day. However, all intestinal secretions will increase dramatically if there is distal obstruction.

Table 5 shows the electrolytes of intravenous fluids. A liter of 5% dextrose (D5) + half-normal (0.45%) saline has the equivalent of the baseline sodium requirements (5% dextrose has an osmolality close to plasma and may be administered without electrolytes to provide water. It is added to avoid hypo-osmolality when the sodium concentration is low and hypotonic). Two liters of D5 + quarter-normal (0.225%) saline have not only the baseline sodium requirements, but also the baseline water requirements of a patient. If 20 mEq of potassium is added to each liter of D5 + quarter-normal saline, then 2000 ml of fluid contains 77 mEq of sodium and 40 mEq of potassium. This closely approximates the baseline water, sodium and potassium needs of a 70-kg patient.

The next task is to add to this the measured losses, depending on the site of the loss. Since the most common loss is that of gastric secretions with the predominant electrolyte being chloride, it can be seen by reviewing Tables 4 and 5 that a liter of D5 + half-normal saline with 40 mEq of KCl/l will provide well for the sodium, chloride and potassium loss. Therefore, if our hypothetical patient lost 1 l of gastric secretions, his intravenous fluids for the day might read 2000 ml of D5 + quarter-normal saline with 20 mEq KCl/l plus 1000 ml D5 + 0.45% saline with 40 mEq KCl/l.

A much harder estimate is that of internal, unmeasured losses. The most common internal losses seen in general surgery are related to the trauma of surgery and the dysfunction of the gastrointestinal tract that follows abdominal trauma. Whenever tissues are injured, either by disease or by surgery, bleeding and fluid exudation may occur. Following severe tissue injury and/or infection systemic inflammation ensues, resulting in a total body increase in capillary permeability. When bleeding is minimal the exuded fluid contains the same levels of electrolytes as plasma, both at the local tissue injury site and in the rest of the body. The small bowel, when irritated enough to produce an ileus, will become distended with fluid which also has electrolytes close to the concentration of those in plasma.

The bowel wall becomes edematous with fluid with the same electrolytes as plasma. Interruption of cell membrane function allows interstitial fluid to migrate into the intracellular space. Once again, since interstitial fluid has the same electrolytes as plasma, the 'loss' consists of electrolytes which have the same concentration as the plasma.

It can be seen from this discussion that internal, unmeasured losses usually represent fluids with electrolytes of plasma. Replacing these fluids with solutions with lower concentrations of sodium will lead to hyponatremia. For this reason, any patient undergoing major trauma (or suffering from severe inflammation), either from disease or from surgery, should have fluids replaced primarily with solutions that have the same electrolytes as plasma, especially during the initial fluid sequestration phase of their trauma, which lasts at least 24 h. Providing such patients with D5 and 0.225 normal saline may lead rapidly to hyponatremia.

*Monitoring fluid therapy*
The first and foremost method for monitoring fluid therapy is to monitor the circulation as described in Chapter 2, The circulation; Hemodynamic monitoring. In essence, therefore, a patient with recent major trauma and/or severe inflammation should receive intravenous fluids with electrolytes similar to those of plasma until the initial fluid sequestration phase has been completed and concerns about maintaining intravascular volume and a good circulation are less pressing.

Subsequent to the fluid sequestration phase, the concept of baseline fluid requirements plus replacing measured losses will usually suffice to maintain adequate fluid and electrolyte balance. This will not work well in cases in which internal losses continue or in which excessive volumes of external losses are produced and cannot be measured easily. Under these circumstances obtaining input and output measurements, obtaining serum electrolyte levels and determining the concentrations of electrolytes in fluids lost from the body are all helpful. For instance, when measured losses are large (i.e. 3000 ml of gastric losses) aliquots of the solutions drained should be sent for electrolyte determinations to help to prepare fluid and electrolyte therapy.

**Common electrolyte abnormalities**
The purpose of this section is to outline the etiologies and the therapy for common electrolyte abnormalities seen in surgery. This also requires a discussion of acid–base disturbances. The most common pure electrolyte abnormality is hyponatremia. The etiologies of hyponatremia are the

gaining of water in excess of sodium (e.g. due to inappropriate secretion of AVP), the loss of sodium in excess of water (e.g. due to adrenal insufficiency), or a combination of the two (e.g. due to trauma and surgery with resultant internal and external losses, congestive heart failure, cirrhosis with ascites, diuretics). The most common cause of hyponatremia in surgery is a combination of having increased AVP production from trauma and losses of sodium both into the 'third space' (the sequestration of fluid as mentioned above), and external losses such as nasogastric suction. Increased AVP secretion may be secondary to hypoperfusion as well as other 'stress' stimuli.

Hyponatremia will not occur in the postoperative surgical patient unless the intravenous fluid therapy is inappropriate. The fundamental pathophysiology for the development of hyponatremia is within the patient. However, with appropriate intravenous fluid therapy hyponatremia will be avoided. The most common cause of hyponatremia in surgery, therefore, is hypotonic intravenous solutions.

Etiologies of hyponatremia which are laboratory values only and not true physiological values include hyperglycemia (for each 100 mg% above a glucose of 100, expect a decrease of 1.6 mEq/l sodium) and hyperproteinemia.

The etiologies of hypernatremia are desiccation (most often in burns), osmotic diuresis, high output renal failure, drainage of hypotonic fluids and diabetes insipidus. Hypernatremia is unusual in surgical patients except for burn and head trauma victims.

Before continuing with common electrolyte disturbances, a discussion of acid–base physiology is in order.

**Acid–base physiology**

The hydrogen ion concentration in body fluids is proportional to the distribution of buffer bases and the concentration ([ ]) of base to acid. This is described in the Henderson equation when the $HCO_3^-$ is the bicarbonate level. Since the carbonic acid level is proportionate to the dissolved carbon dioxide in the blood, the Henderson equation may be expressed as:

$$[H^+] = \frac{K_a\,[H_2CO_3]}{[HCO_3^-]}$$

$$[H^+] = \frac{24 \times PCO_2}{[HCO_3^-]}$$

pH is the negative log of the concentration of hydrogen ions and is expressed as the Henderson–Hasselbach equation:

$$pH = \frac{pK_a + Log[HCO_3^-]}{[H_2CO_3]}$$

An interesting empiric correlation between hydrogen ion concentration and pH has been found. For the pH range 7.10–7.50:

pH 7.40 = $[H^+]$ of 40 nmol/l

Each change of $[H^+]$ of 1 nmol/l = inverse change in pH of 0.01 pH unit:

pH 7.38 = 42 nmol/l $[H^+]$
pH 7.39 = 41 nmol/l $[H^+]$
pH 7.40 = 40 nmol/l $[H^+]$
pH 7.41 = 39 nmol/l $[H^+]$

This means that for the pH range of 7.10–7.50 the change in pH associated with a change in hydrogen ion concentration is almost linear. This allows for determination of the status of a patient's acid–base condition by looking at the pH and $P_{CO_2}$.

An acute respiratory acidosis should cause a change in hydrogen ion concentration of 0.8 times the change in $P_{CO_2}$.

Acute respiratory acidosis:

$\Delta [H^+] = 0.8 \, \Delta \, P_{CO_2}$

Chronic respiratory acidosis:

$\Delta [H^+] = 0.3 \, \Delta \, P_{CO_2}$

Acute respiratory alkalosis:

$\Delta [H^+] = 0.8 \, \Delta \, P_{CO_2}$

Chronic respiratory alkalosis:

$\Delta [H^+] = 0.17 \, \Delta \, P_{CO_2}$

Metabolic acidosis:

$1.1 \, \Delta [HCO_3^-] = \Delta \, P_{CO_2}$

Metabolic alkalosis:
variable response, no formula available.

Thus, a corresponding pH drop should follow. That is, if the change in $P_{CO_2}$ is 10 mmHg, then the change in hydrogen ion concentration would be 8 nmol/l. This should cause a normal pH of 7.40 to drop to 7.32. If presented with such a patient with a pH of 7.25, one would assume under those circumstances that both a respiratory and a metabolic acidosis were present. In addition, there is the expected drop in $P_{CO_2}$ for each 1.1 mEq change in bicarbonate level during a metabolic acidosis.

From an understanding of these numbers, it is possible to determine whether a patient has a pure type of acid–base abnormality or a combined type. This becomes especially important for patients on a respirator where the $P_{CO_2}$ value may be more dependent on ventilator settings than other acid–base phenomena.

*Metabolic acidosis*
Table 6 lists the common etiologies of metabolic acidosis. The initial evaluation of metabolic acidosis requires calculation of the anion gap: anion gap = $Na^+ - Cl^- - CO_2$, followed by breaking up the etiologies of metabolic acidosis into those groups which produce an increase in the anion gap and those which produce a normal anion gap. The most common cause of metabolic acidosis seen in surgery is lactic acidosis. As stated in Chapters 2 and 3 (Hemodynamic monitoring and Pathologic

### TABLE 6  COMMON ETIOLOGIES OF METABOLIC ACIDOSIS

*Elevated anion gap*
Lactic acidosis
Ketoacidosis
Uremia
Toxins
   salicylate
   paraldehyde
   ethylene glycol
   methyl alcohol

*Normal anion gap*
Diarrhea
Pancreatic fistula
Small intestine fistula
Ureterosigmoidostomy
Renal tubular acidosis
Carbonic anhydrase inhibitor
Exogenous HCl

Anion gap = $Na^+ - Cl^- - CO_2$, normal range 8–12

systemic inflammation sections, respectively), an elevated lactic acid can be secondary to either or both a deficit in the circulation or severe inflammation.

The treatment of metabolic acidosis is as follows:

(1) Treat the underlying cause;

(2) Treat if pH ≤ 7.0;

(3) Treat gradually if possible (no life-threatening arrhythmias or cardiac dysfunction, no severe hyperkalemia);

(4) Maintain bicarbonate levels 15 mEq/l or greater.

The first line of therapy should always be directed at the underlying cause (treat the circulation, treat the inflammation). However, severe cardiac arrhythmias and cardiac dysfunction, along with hyperkalemia leading to cardiac dysfunction, will develop if acidosis persists. Therefore, correction of acidosis *per se* is useful, especially when the pH is less than 7.0.

When acidosis appears to be secondary primarily to bicarbonate loss (pancreatic fistula, renal tubular acidosis) and when a patient is not suffering from severe cardiac dysfunction, a gradual correction of the pH is desired. This leads to fewer problems with changes in the cerebral spinal fluid acid–base ratio as the pH is corrected. For such cases, the bicarbonate space is usually considered to be 50% of body weight. Therefore, the weight in kg multiplied by 50% multiplied by the desired increment in bicarbonate concentration is used to estimate the initial bicarbonate dose. Again, the overall plan would be to correct the acidosis gradually, usually over many hours.

*Metabolic alkalosis*
The most common acid–base and electrolyte abnormality in surgery is hypochloremic metabolic alkalosis. The following factors promote this disturbance: (1) the common use of nasogastric suction in the post-operative period which removes chloride; (2) the trauma of surgery and hypoperfusion which stimulate aldosterone and cortisol release, which potentiate the loss of potassium and chloride; (3) the in-hospital use of loop diuretics which interfere with proximal tubule sodium reabsorption; and (4) patients who are already potassium and chloride depleted prior to the critical illness (chronic diuretic use). The most common type of hypochloremic metabolic alkalosis is the chloride responsive type; however, chloride responsive alkalosis will not occur until the $Na^+ - Cl^-$ difference is ≥ 39–40 mEq/l. Table 7 shows the etiologies of metabolic alkalosis.

### TABLE 7   ETIOLOGIES OF METABOLIC ALKALOSIS

*Chloride responsive*
Gastric suction
Diuretics
Villous adenoma of colon
Posthypercapnic alkalosis

*Chloride resistant*
Hyperaldosteronism
Adrenal hyperplasia
Barter's syndrome
Licorice ingestion
Severe $K^+$ depletion

Chloride responsive urine chloride concentration < 10–20 mEq/l; chloride resistant urine chloride concentration > 10–20 mEq/l

In difficult cases, the urine chloride concentration may help determine whether the metabolic alkalosis fits into the chloride responsive or resistant type. Alkalosis associated with hypochloremia is not based simply on the absolute chloride concentration, but rather on the chloride concentration relative to the concentration of sodium. For instance, a person with a serum sodium of 145 mEq/l will likely be alkalotic with a chloride of 105 mEq/l even though the chloride is normal. Similarly, a patient with a chloride of 90 mEq/l but a serum sodium of 120 mEq/l will not be alkalotic even though the chloride is low. This is because the difference between the sodium and chloride is important, not the absolute level of the chloride itself.

A relative deficit in chloride can result in the phenomenon of paradoxical aciduria. The mechanism of paradoxical aciduria is as follows:

(1)  Sodium usually absorbed with chloride in proximal tubule;

(2)  With chloride deficit, excess sodium is presented to the distal tubule;

(3)  Usual state of stress leads to increased aldosterone and cortisol levels;

(4)  Increased sodium–hydrogen and sodium–potassium exchange in the distal tubule;

(5)  Excretion of acid urine rich with potassium.

Since sodium must be reabsorbed with chloride in the proximal tubule, a significant chloride deficit will interfere with proximal sodium reabsorption and the excess sodium is presented to the distal tubule. When avidity for sodium is high (i.e. elevated aldosterone) the increase in sodium in the distal tubule promotes sodium–hydrogen and sodium–potassium exchange, leading to paradoxical aciduria with potassium loss and accentuation of the metabolic alkalosis.

The treatment of hypochloremic hypokalemic metabolic alkalosis includes: decreasing the physiological stimulus for aldosterone and/or cortisol secretion; the administration of chloride and potassium usually as NaCl and KCl; and sometimes carbonic anhydrase inhibition. Most often, replacing chloride as NaCl and KCl is adequate for the therapy. Inhibition of bicarbonate reabsorption with acetazolamide is very effective when potassium chloride or other chloride salts cannot be administered.

*Hyperkalemia*

Hyperkalemia (>5.0 mg/l) can cause an acute, life-threatening situation, the etiologies are metabolic acidosis, renal failure, hemolysis, muscle injury and intravenous or oral intake of potassium. The diagnosis of life-threatening hyperkalemia often depends on a high index of suspicion and recognition of changes in the cardiogram including peaked T waves, prolonged QRS and cardiac standstill. Table 8 outlines the treatment of hyperkalemia. The fastest onset of action is seen with the infusion of calcium (gluconate or chloride), which directly antagonizes the effect of potassium on the myocardium.

The underlying etiology must be treated directly. This may require dialysis or debridement of dead muscle or other necrotic tissue. Chronic therapy is directed at the removal of potassium via the gastrointestinal tract with Kayexalate® (Sanofi Pharmaceuticals, NY, USA). The hyper-kalemia associated with renal failure is best treated with dialysis.

### TABLE 8   TREATMENT OF HYPERKALEMIA

| Drug/treatment | Dose | Onset |
|---|---|---|
| Calcium gluconate or calcium chloride | 1–4 g IV | 1–5 min |
| Sodium bicarbonate | 44–88 mg | 15 min |
| $D^{50}W$ + insulin | 50 ml + 10 u | 15–30 min |
| Kayexalate | 15 g PO or 50 g per enema | ≥ 2 h |
| Peritoneal dialysis | | ≥ 2 h |
| Hemodialysis | | 15 min |

IV, intravenous; $D^{50}W$, 50% dextrose in water; PO, by mouth

*Osmolarity*

In surgery, conditions may arise that increase or decrease the serum osmolarity so that the consequences of this must be dealt with from either a fluid or electrolyte aspect or from a renal aspect. Serum osmolarity may be calculated by the formula:

$$mosmol/l = 2 \, [Na^+] \, mEq/l + \frac{[Glu \, mg/100]}{20} + \frac{[BUN \, mg/100]}{3}$$

Where Glu is glucose and BUN is blood urea nitrogen. The normal range is 285–295 mosmol/l. Common etiologies of hyperosmolarity are hyperglycemia, elevated BUN, alcohol ingestion leading to inhibition of AVP, desiccation (loss of $H_2O$ in excess of sodium), mannitol, intravenous and angiogenic contrast agents and calcium. The consequences of an osmotic load are:

(1) Elevation in serum osmolarity;

(2) Shift of intracellular fluid into interstitial space (hyponatremia – early);

(3) Central nervous system dysfunction;

(4) Diuresis with urine sodium 50 mEq/l (loss of more water than salt);

(5) Volume contraction and hypernatremia – late

In the intensive care unit, the most common etiologies of hyperosmolarity will be the use of intravenous contrast agents and hyperglycemia. When renal function is intact the hyperosmolarity may be aggravated by an osmotic diuresis, which causes the loss of more water than sodium. When the hyperosmolarity is secondary to hyperglycemia, insulin and the use of hypotonic intravenous solutions may be used. In non-ketotic hyperosmolar coma the insulin requirements may be much less than when a patient has acidosis.

## RENAL FAILURE AND SELECTED METABOLIC DISTURBANCES

### The effects of circulation on renal function

A decrease in blood flow and oxygen supply to the kidneys results in varying degrees of alterations in and damage to renal function, which depends largely on the magnitude of the reduction in flow or oxygen. Decreased blood flow and/or pure hypoxia can result in a transient reduction in glomerular filtration when the insult is neither severe nor prolonged. Decreased blood flow (prerenal state) can occur from one or more of the etiologies listed in Table 9.

**TABLE 9   ETIOLOGIES OF PRERENAL STATE**

*Decreased cardiac output*
Hypovolemia
Cardiogenic

*Decreased regional blood flow*
Increased abdominal pressure
?Increased pressure in Gerota's fascia
Decreased microvascular perfusion

Decreased cardiac output results in a constriction of renal afferent arterioles and a reduction in glomerular capillary pressure. The other mechanisms in the table have also been implicated as etiologies of reduced glomerular filtration. When a perfusion deficit has not been sufficient to damage renal cells the response to hypoperfusion is to release renin from the juxtaglomerular apparatus. This results in increased aldosterone secretion and increased distal renal tubule absorption of sodium. Since decreased cardiac output also stimulates AVP release, tubular reabsorption of water is also enhanced. Therefore, urine with a high specific gravity, high osmolality and low sodium will be excreted.

When renal hypoperfusion has been sufficiently severe, renal cell damage ensues. This results in tubular damage (acute tubular necrosis), which is the most common cause of 'renal' failure in surgical patients. The tubular damage may result in both obstruction of the tubules and back leak of filtrate into the renal interstitium.

Preglomerular constriction and reduced glomerular filtration rate can continue after the tubules recover, however, and implicate a microvascular insult which can aggravate the initial ischemic insult. The mechanism of continuing microvasculature constriction may be ischemia-induced thromboxane production, since prostacyclin has been shown to diminish the renal damage induced by ischemia.

**The effects of inflammation on renal function**
Renal malfunction is a common feature of the multiple organ dysfunction syndrome which accompanies the systemic inflammatory response syndrome. Therefore, the association between severe inflammation and renal malfunction is well documented. Hemodynamic alterations associated with severe inflammation, particularly hypotension, are associated with renal malfunction in these cases. However, humans with a well-maintained hyperdynamic circulation may also develop renal

malfunction, which suggests that inflammation may cause renal insults without marked reductions in renal arterial flow.

Local effects that may develop during inflammation are:

(1)  Decreased regional/microvascular blood flow;

(2)  Plugging of capillaries with leukocytes;

(3)  Alterations in cellular metabolism;

(4)  Glomerulonephritis;

(5)  Direct tubular damage.

Acute renal failure may be caused or aggravated by such inflammatory events as polymorphonuclear leukocyte activation, superoxide generation, complement activation, elevated platelet-activating factor, cytokine release and activation of endothelin.

The renal effects of severe inflammation may result in increased renal excretion of protein with, or frequently without, other evidence of renal malfunction. This association of severe inflammation with proteinuria was described by Meleney in 1924. The proteinuria may be secondary to both glomerular and tubular alterations and can parallel the course of the severe inflammation. This association may provide a simple clinical tool for assessing the presence or absence of severe inflammation.

**Renal failure**
Traditionally the etiologies of renal failure in surgical patients are listed under three categories (Table 10). The most common etiologies are

### TABLE 10   ETIOLOGIES OF RENAL FAILURE

*Prerenal (hypoperfusion)*
Hypovolemic
Cardiogenic
Regional

*Renal*
Acute tubular necrosis
Acute interstitial nephritis
Acute glomerulonephritis

*Postrenal*
Urethral obstruction
Bilateral ureteral obstruction

prerenal and the 'renal' category acute tubular necrosis (ATN). ATN has a number of proposed etiologies which are categorized broadly into three etiologies, afferent arteriolar constriction, leaking tubular cells and obstructed tubules. Usually no single etiology can be ascertained, with ATN considered secondary to multifactorial insults including severe hypoperfusion, severe inflammation, nephrotoxic antibiotics, intravenous or intra-arterial contrast, muscle necrosis, increased abdominal pressure and hemolysis.

Acute interstitial nephritis is seen most often secondary to drug allergy, particularly antibiotics. An elevated peripheral eosinophil count and urine eosinophils help support this diagnosis. Management includes a search for the offending agent and discontinuing its use.

The distinction between prerenal and renal etiologies of worsening renal function is important for both therapeutic and prognostic considerations. The common tests used to separate prerenal from renal are listed in Table 11. All are based on the normal response to hypoperfusion which results in renal release of renin followed by angiotensin and aldosterone excretion, as well as increased AVP secretion. Consequently, small volumes of urine are excreted which are concentrated and relatively sodium free.

The renal failure index (RFI) is calculated using the following formula:

$$RFI = \frac{Urine\ sodium \times Plasma\ creatinine}{Urine\ creatinine}$$

Confounding variables with renal tests include diuretic administration and osmotic diuresis (glucose, mannitol, urea). Limitations and instances

**TABLE 11   COMMON TESTS USED TO SEPARATE PRERENAL FROM RENAL ETIOLOGIES**

| Test | Prerenal | Renal |
|---|---|---|
| Specific gravity | > 1.020 | 1.008–1.012 |
| Urine sodium | < 20 mEq/l | > 40 mEq/l |
| Urine osmolality | > 500 mosmol | < 350 mosmol |
| Urine/plasma osmolality | > 1.2 | < 1.2 |
| Urine/plasma creatinine | > 15 | < 15 |
| Urine/plasma urea | > 10 | < 10 |
| Renal failure index* | < 1 | > 1 |
| Fractional sodium excretion* | ≤ 1 | ≥ 3 |
| Urine sediment | normal | casts, eosinophils, epithelial cells |

*See text for formula

of ATN with several of these indices in the prerenal range have been documented. More commonly, a prerenal state is not appreciated because of conditions that result in larger amounts of urinary sodium and/or more dilute urine than a normal physiological response. For example, high BUN levels, usually greater than 80 mg/100 ml, can promote an osmotic diuresis, which will result in a large clear-looking urine output that will have more sodium (usually 30–50 mEq/l) because obligatory water excretion decreases the concentration of sodium in the proximal tubule, where sodium reabsorption is concentration gradient limited (see Basic physiology section).

### Hemodynamic management of renal failure

Prerenal renal failure is managed by reversing hypoperfusion, usually in a total body rather than a regional (renal vascular reconstruction) fashion. This requires determining the etiology of hypoperfusion and providing appropriate therapy (see Chapter 2, The circulation; Hypoperfusion states). Physical examination can assist in the evaluation of the circulation rather than in any specific findings related to renal failure.

The same hemodynamic management principles are appropriate for 'renal' kidney failure. The injured kidney is not benefited by hypoperfusion and may respond with more urine output when well perfused. The kidneys, in general, are worth the expense and possible complications associated with pulmonary artery catheter placement. Logical manipulation of hemodynamic variables to attain increased total body oxygen delivery is the best method of treating the injured kidney besides removing potential toxins. No arbitrary formula or use of such parameters as fluid balance and body weight can predict the intravascular volume status and the best method of improving cardiac output in critically ill surgical patients. Most importantly, resuscitation of the circulation should not be abandoned because 'renal' kidney failure is present.

The infusion of dopamine may improve renal perfusion more effectively than other measures used to improve the circulation. More controversial is the use of systemic vasoconstrictors such as neosynephrine and norepinephrine for the management of oliguria associated with the hyperdynamic low systemic resistance circulation of severe systemic inflammation. As described in Chapter 3 (Pathological systemic inflammation section), therapy that increases systemic resistance but does not decrease cardiac output may improve the circulation to organs with increased resistance either from macrovascular (atherosclerosis) or microvascular narrowing. Reports of increased urine output and creatinine clearance suggest that this approach is rational when cardiac index is excellent.

**Management of 'renal' kidney failure**

Besides hemodynamic optimization, other management concerns in 'renal' kidney failure, besides dialysis, are shown in Table 12. Nephrotoxic antibiotics, particularly aminoglycosides, are commonly part of the multi-factorial etiology of renal failure in critically ill patients. Measuring blood levels to ensure non-toxic concentrations is required if therapy necessitates continuing the drug. Serum myoglobin may be elevated in patients with crush or ischemic injury to muscle and may prove toxic to the kidneys. Mechanism of injury and/or brown discoloration of the urine should prompt urine and serum myoglobin measurement. Inducing a diuresis (mannitol, loop diuretics) along with alkalinization of the urine (sodium bicarbonate) is designed to reduce tubular myoglobin concentration and precipitation. Massive muscle injury is also associated with more rapid elevation in serum creatinine (> 1 mg/100 ml/day), hyperkalemia and markedly elevated serum creatine phosphokinase (CPK). Free hemoglobin, usually secondary to hemolysis, is less renal toxic than myoglobin and is characterized by red urine, but the management principles are the same. Drugs excreted primarily via the kidneys must be adjusted to avoid toxic levels. Metabolic acidosis and hyperkalemia may

**TABLE 12   MANAGEMENT OF 'RENAL' KIDNEY FAILURE**

*Optimize renal perfusion*

*Remove renal toxins*
Nephrotoxic antibiotics
Myoglobin
Hemoglobin

*Adjust drugs for renal failure*
Antibiotics
Digoxin
Antiarrhythmics
Muscle relaxants

*Serum electrolytes*
Serum potassium
Metabolic acidosis
Hyperphosphatemia
Hypocalcemia

*Nutrition*

be severe and diminish cardiac function. Hyperphosphatemia is partly responsible for the metabolic acidosis and hypocalcemia. Even with dialysis hyperphosphatemia is difficult to control and often requires administration of aluminium hydroxide to bind phosphate in the intestinal tract. Symptomatic hypocalcemia is uncommon in critically ill patients, even when ionized calcium is low. Rarely does hypocalcemia require direct therapy. Proper nutritional management of renal failure patients is controversial. Some argue for sophisticated regimens of essential amino acids or amino acid precursors; others for standard nutritional support. With dialysis nutritional management is somewhat simplified.

The use of diuretics for 'renal' renal failure is controversial. Of greatest concern is the possibility that a response to a diuretic will result in decreased intravascular volume, hypoperfusion, and an additional insult to already damaged kidneys. Therefore, if a diuretic is used, it should be used with careful hemodynamic monitoring.

**Renal replacement techniques: dialysis and continuous hemofiltration**
The relative indications for mechanical renal replacement therapy in acute renal failure are:

(1) Congestive heart failure;

(2) Metabolic acidosis;

(3) Hyperkalemia;

(4) 'Uremia';

(5) Toxin removal

(6) Aggressive nutritional support.

Dialysis methods used include hemodialysis, peritoneal dialysis and continuous veno–venous hemofiltration. As stated previously, total body sodium and water excess does not guarantee increased intravascular volume. However, when excessive, increased vascular volume may be removed with dialysis and improve cardiac function. In such patients dialysis may also assist nutritional therapy, allowing several liters of intravenous or intestinal food to be administered. Metabolic acidosis and hyperkalemia are effectively treated by dialysis, although phosphate is poorly dialyzed and often continues to require intestinal binding. 'Uremia' is an ill-defined syndrome which may include altered mental status, pleural and pericardial effusions, and is associated with blood urea levels close to 100 mg/100 ml. Certain toxins (antibiotics, salicylates) may be removed only by dialysis.

Hemodialysis (usually over 3–4 h) is the most common method used in chronic renal failure and is used frequently in acute renal failure. Hemodialysis in critically ill surgical patients is often accompanied by hemodynamic instability resulting in administration of fluids and/or drugs to maintain cardiac output. In addition, worsening hypoxemia may be noted. The etiology of these alterations is unclear, but may relate to vasodilatation in the setting of normal or low intravascular volume. Hemodialysis may also aggravate inflammation. Replacing acetate (a vasodilator) with bicarbonate in the dialysate appears to diminish adverse hemodynamic events.

Peritoneal dialysis via insertion of a catheter into the abdominal cavity is a slower, continuous method of dialysis which does not require vascular access and results in less hemodynamic variation. Unfortunately, abdominal surgery often precludes use of this method. Complications include inadvertent viscus injury and peritoneal infection.

The development of biocompatible 'high flux' synthetic membranes with greater permeability than conventional hemodialysis membranes made the development of continuous arteriovenous hemofiltration (CAVH) and continuous renal replacement therapy (CRRT) possible in the late 1970s. Several membrane types are presently available. None ignite the inflammatory response as do older dialysis membranes. The addition of a pump into the circuit makes continuous veno–venous hemodiafiltration (CVVH) practical in many patients and can permit the application of hemofiltration in patients with a narrow arteriovenous pressure gradient. CVVH renal replacement therapy is becoming the method of choice for the management of renal failure in the critical care environment.

The techniques are straightforward. Vascular access is gained using a large two-lumen venous dialysis catheter for veno–venous diafiltration or large bore femoral arterial catheterization along with a large venous return line for arteriovenous treatment. The hemofilter of choice is connected with an in-line pump (including a bubble detector) if necessary. Anticoagulation with heparin or citrate is usually necessary.

Solute clearance may be either convective (filtration) or diffusive (dialysis). If ultrafiltration alone is desired, excess fluid and electrolyte losses must be replaced. Fluid flux may be impressive: removal of more than a liter per hour is not unusual. Sodium, bicarbonate, calcium and magnesium replacement require special attention and all electrolytes require careful monitoring.

When dialysis is the predominant form of solute clearance (CAVHD or CVVAHD), the composition of the dialysate can make electrolyte balance easier to control. The semipermeable dialysis membrane permits diffusion of solute in both directions. A steady state is eventually approached. Transmembrane pressure differences drive fluid movement but solute clearance depends on the size of the pores in the filter membrane. Molecules smaller than 10 000 Da pass readily, while molecules larger than 60 000 Da do not pass. Any drugs within these limits are filtered, including vasoactive amines, antibiotics and Dilantin® (Parke-Davies, NJ, USA). Close pharmacokinetic monitoring is advocated where possible to ensure proper therapeutic dosing of these drugs.

CRRT permits full nutritional support including full protein repletion even in severely catabolic stressed or septic patients. Amino acids are filtered in a flow-dependent manner, typically 10% of the administered solution. Nitrogen balance studies, including the nitrogen removed in the effluent fluid (FUN) as well as any excreted urinary urea nitrogen (UUN), can guide the nutrition support plan.

Complications of CRRT can be divided into the following three categories: access complications, equipment problems and process complications. Access complications include hematomas, aneurysms and arteriovenous fistulae. Infection at access sites occurs as it does with any invasive lines. Large-bore catheters are associated with vessel thrombosis. CAVH (D) has the particular requirement for a driving pressure (arterial–venous pressure gradient) of at least 60 mmHg. An on-line pump can assist extracorporeal circulation.

Equipment problems include line kinking and line disconnection with dramatic bleeding. Air embolism can be minimized by an in-line bubble detector. Filter membranes gradually clog and their efficiency deteriorates over time. They may also clot and anticoagulation with heparin, citrate or other anticoagulant is routine in the absence of contraindications.

Problems with the process of CRRT include errors in fluid and electrolyte balance. Continuous renal replacement often involves liters of fluid flux. Careful attention to detail can avoid major problems. Hypothermia can be expected with extracorporeal blood circulation. Warming of the circuit and the patient is often necessary. Depletion of other circulating molecules, such as phosphate, has been reported. Coagulopathies and monocyte activation may also occur.

Other applications of CRRT have not been proved in practice but results to date have been promising. CRRT can be used to treat congestive heart failure, and fluid removal is most clearly beneficial when congestive heart failure physiology is governing hemodynamics. CRRT may result in the additional benefit of decreasing severe inflammation. For instance, gas exchange in patients with the acute respiratory distress syndrome has been improved on CRRT. In fact, many of the mediators of inflammation are molecules readily removed by continuous hemodiafiltration. CRRT may allow removal of large volumes of sequestered fluid in severely inflamed patients. However, since CRRT may provide an anti-inflammatory therapy, the clinician should be aware that clinical improvement associated with removal of fluid may be secondary to decreased inflammation, which allows fluid to be removed without hemodynamic compromise, rather than the presumed 'beneficial' effect of removing fluid *per se*. In addition, such toxins as myoglobin are filterable and many drugs are cleared which may be useful when toxic levels are present.

## Adrenal insufficiency

As discussed in detail in Chapter 3, Pathological systemic inflammation section, systemic inflammation is common in critical illness and is usually secondary to such etiologies as infection, direct tissue damage and ischemia/reperfusion. Inflammation resulting from any of these causes may have effects that are both positive (e.g. activation of host defenses and wound healing) and negative (e.g. suppression of host defenses, organ malfunction). Severe, persistent systemic inflammation (systemic inflammatory response syndrome) is associated with the malfunction of many organs and an increased risk of death.

Many recent studies have investigated factors that promote (hypoperfusion, tumor necrosis factor production, interleukin-1 production) and decrease (improved perfusion, antagonists which inhibit cytokine release or function) severe systemic inflammation. As part of the stress response, blood levels of the endogenous glucocorticoid cortisol are characteristically increased in critical illness and are usually greater than 30 $\mu$g/100 ml. Cortisol exerts both metabolic and anti-inflammatory effects. Since absolute adrenal insufficiency decreases survival following acute insults, the effects of a physiological increase in cortisol concentration are presumably beneficial.

Severe adrenal insufficiency during critical illness has been reported, usually associated with adrenal hemorrhage, infarction or unrecognized adrenal suppression from prior steroid administration. However, over the past two decades several reports have suggested that lower than expected blood cortisol concentrations may be present during critical illness without anatomical disruption or previous suppressive therapy. Administration of cortisol to these patients using physiological rather than pharmacological doses appears to improve clinical status. Such reports suggest that critical illness and severe inflammation can sometimes be associated with low or 'normal' rather than the expected increased blood cortisol concentrations. The reasons for this response are unclear, but suggest that severe inflammation may inhibit an endogenous negative-feedback mechanism and thereby result in an ongoing, unregulated and potentially destructive process.

Pharmacological doses of steroids (i.e. 30 mg/kg methylprednisolone) severely limit inflammation and may interfere with the desired effects. Physiological doses of hydrocortisone (150–300 mg/day) in patients exhibiting a less than expected adrenal response to stress may limit the detrimental systemic effects of inflammation by replacing a deficit in an endogenous-feedback system. While this logic is intriguing and would allow an inexpensive therapy for destructive inflammation, further study is needed to define the incidence, possible mechanisms and potential benefits of this therapy.

Clues that adrenal insufficiency may be present are:

(1) Eosinophilia;

(2) Hyperkalemia without renal failure or acidosis;

(3) Hyponatremia;

(4) Ongoing evidence of systemic inflammation (fever, tachycardia, fluid sequestration).

Eosinophilia (total eosinophil count > 450) is uncommon in critical surgical illness and unless an allergic cause or interstitial nephritis is apparent, should prompt investigation of adrenal status. Hyperkalemia is rare without accompanying renal failure or acidosis and may indicate adrenal insufficiency. Hyponatremia is fairly common and by itself would be least suggestive.

Clinical evidence of ongoing systemic inflammation after assessment and treatment of usual inflammatory diseases (i.e. pneumonia, intra-abdominal abscess) may be the most common prompt to investigate adrenal function. Patients who continue to exhibit such symptoms as fever, tachycardia, fluid sequestration and respiratory failure after usual therapy is administered may have inadequate adrenal function contributing to the ongoing inflammatory state.

The assessment of adrenal function includes a baseline serum cortisol followed by an ACTH stimulation test (injection of $\alpha$-cortitropin 0.25 mg with repeat cortisol 30 and 60 min later). Low-baseline cortisol with increased cortisol following ACTH would indicate pituitary malfunction.

Low-baseline cortisol and no response to exogenous ACTH would indicate adrenal malfunction.

Table 13 lists degrees of adrenal malfunction which may be encountered. Therapy should be 'physiological' doses of hydrocortisone (300 mg/day maximum) with tapering to normal daily adrenal output (25 mg in the morning, 12.5 mg in the evening) as the stress state of the patient

**TABLE 13   DIAGNOSIS OF ADRENAL INSUFFICIENCY DURING CRITICAL ILLNESS**

| Adrenal deficit | Baseline cortisol ($\mu g/100$ ml) | Response to ACTH ($\mu g/100$ ml) |
|---|---|---|
| Severe | < 10 | none |
| Moderate | 10–19 | < 30 |
| Mild | 20–30 | < 30 |
| None | > 30 | >> 30 |

ACTH, adrenocorticotropic hormone

**TABLE 14   ETIOLOGIES OF HYPOMAGNESEMIA**

*Gastrointestinal loss*
Malabsorption
Nasogastric suctioning
Diarrhea
Fistula
Pancreatitis

*Iatrogenic*
Total parenteral nutrition
Osmotic diuresis
Gentamicin
Other diuretics

*Other*
Hypercalcemia
Alcohol ingestion
Protein-calorie malnutrition
Renal loss
Hyperthyroidism
Hypothyroidism
Phosphate deficiency

decreases. Often a dramatic improvement in patient status is noted. If the patient survives the critical illness, repeat studies near the time of discharge may demonstrate a return to normal or higher serum cortisol concentrations both at baseline and in response to ACTH indicating that the adrenal malfunction was transient, and that prolonged adrenal support will not be necessary.

### Hypomagnesemia

Hypomagnesemia may develop insidiously in critically ill patients secondary to the etiologies listed in Table 14. The clinical consequences are: (1) cardiovascular including tachyarrhythmias and digitalis-toxic arrhythmias, and (2) non-cardiovascular including hypocalcemia, mental status change and hypokalemia. Magnesium may be provided as magnesium sulfate or magnesium chloride. Sulfate binds calcium and should be avoided with hypocalcemia.

### Hypocalcemia

Hypocalcemia (defined as decreased ionized calcium) is common in critical illness and is associated with the conditions listed below:

(1)  Hypovolemic hypoperfusion;

(2)  Severe inflammation;

(3)  Multiple blood transfusions;

(4)  Renal failure;

(5)  Albumin resuscitation.

Importantly, the magnitude of decrease in ionized calcium is indicative of the severity of illness. Patients with the lowest ionized calcium levels at the time of intensive care unit admission are more likely to die, even though they die many days later. Hypocalcemia in this setting is associated with increased parathyroid hormone (parathormone) levels.

Proposed etiologies of this hypocalcemia are listed in Table 15. Symptomatic hypocalcemia (i.e. perioral numbness, carpopedal spasm) is rare in critical illness and implies a different physiology for hypocalcemia in critical illness, as compared to that seen after removal of the parathyroid glands. Increasing evidence demonstrates migration of extracellular calcium into the intracellular space, particularly following inflammatory insults such as pancreatitis or sepsis. In humans an increase in red cell calcium has been documented during sepsis, which implies that the red cell can serve as a readily accessible tissue assay for this phenomenon.

## TABLE 15    PROPOSED ETIOLOGIES OF HYPOCALCEMIA

| |
|---|
| *Extracellular sequestration* |
| Citrate infusion |
| Parathyroidectomy |
| Renal failure |
| Albumin resuscitation |
| *Inadequate PTH secretion* |
| *Intracellular migration* |
| Hypoperfusion |
| Severe inflammation |
| Drugs |

PTH, parathyroid hormone

The association of increased mortality risk with the lower ionized calcium levels is in keeping with the concept that a defect in cellular metabolism is responsible for this abnormality which is reflective of the severity of cellular injury.

Increased intracellular migration may improve cellular function. For example, the effect of digitalis on cardiac performance is mediated, at least in part, by increased calcium migration. However, intracellular calcium in high concentrations may be toxic to cellular function, especially mitochondria. If intracellular migration is an important etiology of hypocalcemia during critical illness, the advisability of exogenous calcium administration or drugs which promote intracellular calcium accumulation (i.e. epinephrine) is uncertain, especially when symptomatic hypocalcemia is not present.

Most reports of improved hemodynamics following calcium administration describe clinical or experimental conditions favoring extracellular sequestration or decreased mobilization from bone (i.e. infusion of sodium citrate, removal of parathyroid glands). Under these circumstances calcium administration may provide physiological therapy to overcome the extracellular sequestration. If the primary etiology of hypocalcemia is intracellular migration, then calcium administration may be more pharmacological (normally calcium administration increases blood pressure) than physiological. Such pharmacological therapy may be toxic. Therefore, administration of exogenous calcium to critically ill patients should proceed only when clear evidence of extracellular sequestration or inadequate parathormone levels are present.

As a corollary to the concept that critical illness results in intracellular migration of calcium, there are reports of hypercalcemia occurring in critically ill patients. This has been shown to develop in patients who previously had many episodes of hypocalcemia and at a time when the severity of critical illness is decreased. When this hypercalcemia develops parathormone levels are low. This suggests that previous intracellular migration of calcium results in a pool which then migrates out of the cells when the illness is resolving and cellular metabolism improves.

# THE GASTROINTESTINAL/ NUTRITIONAL SYSTEM

Gastrointestinal dysfunction
    Effects of hypoperfusion
    Effects of severe inflammation on the gastrointestinal tract
    Esophageal hemorrhage
    Stomach and duodenum
    Liver and biliary tree
    Pancreas
    Diarrhea
    Intra-abdominal abscess
    The GI tract as a reservoir for infection and/or inflammation
        in the critically ill surgical patient
Nutritional physiology
    Stress vs. starvation
    Common nutritional deficiencies
    Immunological function and nutrition
    Measures of nutritional status
Nutritional therapy
    Requirements during stress
    Methods/types of nutritional support

## BASIC GASTROINTESTINAL PHYSIOLOGY

Gastrointestinal (GI) physiology will be presented as it relates to surgical critical care only.

### Stomach

Gastric physiology most germane to surgical critical care encompasses primarily gastric acid production and mucosal cell integrity. Hydrochloric acid is secreted by the parietal cells which are located in the fundus and body of the stomach. The regulation of acid secretion depends largely on the synergistic interaction of vagal innervation and the hormone gastrin. Factors that stimulate and inhibit vagal and gastrin stimulated acid secretion are listed in Table 1. The secretion of pepsinogen is activated primarily from vagal stimulation and to a lesser degree by gastrin. Pepsinogen is converted to pepsin, most rapidly at a pH $\leq$ 2.0 and pepsin is most active as a proteolytic enzyme at pH 1–3.

The stomach's primary mechanism for protection against mucosal acid injury is the mucosal permeability barrier. Variables that serve as protective mechanisms are:

(1)   Mucosal blood flow;

(2)   Secretion of acid and production of an 'alkaline tide' in the mucosa and submucosa;

### TABLE 1   GASTRIC ACID SECRETION

| Phase | Stimulation | Inhibition |
|---|---|---|
| Cephalic phase | sight, smell, thought of food | sleep |
| Gastric phase | antral distension, peptides, peptones, alkalinity | empty stomach, no food, acid, pH $\leq$ 2.0 |
| Intestinal phase | food in duodenum | acid in duodenum, enterogastric reflex |
| | others: histamine, acetylcholine, calcium | others: $H_2$ blockers, atropine, prostaglandin E and A |

$H_2$, histamine receptor

(3)   Carbonic anhydrase;

(4)   Prostaglandins;

(5)   Mucus secretion.

Most important is adequate mucosal blood flow which allows metabolic protection mechanisms to function.

The digestive functions of the stomach serve to mix food with water and acid, digest some protein, and gradually empty food into the duodenum. Proper motility of the stomach depends on intact vagal innervation which allows relaxation of the body and fundus with the ingestion of food, mixing and propulsion by the antrum, and passage of food into the duodenum. Gastric emptying is slowed by solids, increased or decreased osmolality compared to extracellular fluid, intraduodenal acid, fatty acids and hypo- or hyperthermic substances. It is increased by liquids.

**Small intestine**
The primary function of the small intestine is to further digest and absorb food and liquids. During digestion large molecules in the diet are broken down into molecules which can be absorbed by the enterocytes. In addition, fat is converted from being water insoluble to water soluble. With absorption the intraluminal contents are transported from the enterocytes to the portal vein or the lymphatics. The steps in the process of fat, carbohydrate and protein digestion and absorption are listed in Tables 2, 3 and 4, respectively.

Another important function of the small and large bowel is the absorption of water and electrolytes. An estimated 8 l of secretions and ingested fluid reach the proximal small bowel every 24 h. The small bowel absorbs about 7 l, the colon 800–900 ml, leaving only 100–200 ml in the stool. Water is primarily absorbed passively after the absorption of sodium and chloride, mechanisms for which are:

(1)   Coupling to absorption of organic solutes: glucose, amino acids, water soluble vitamins and bile salts (ileum);

(2)   'Neutral process' inhibited by increased cyclic-AMP in the cell. Sodium extruded from the cell on the serosal side by an ATP-dependent pump;

(3)   Electrogenic mechanism in distal small bowel secondary to low intracellular sodium concentration maintained by the Na–K-ATPase pump;

## TABLE 2   FAT DIGESTION AND ABSORPTION

*Emulsion formation*
Antral mixing
Bile salts

*Hydrolysis by lipase*
Lingual lipase (mostly medium- and short-chain triglycerides, 8–12 or
  ≤ 7 carbons, respectively)
Pancreatic lipase
Pancreatic phospholipase A$_2$
Pancreatic cholesterol esterase

*Micelle formation (not needed for short- and medium-chain triglycerides)*
Bile salts
Fatty acids
Monoglycerides

*Micelle migration to brush border*

*Release of free fat molecules for passive absorption*

*Formation of chylomicrons*
Resynthesis of triglycerides
Outer coat of β-lipoprotein

*Passage of chylomicrons into lymphatics (short- and medium-chain
  triglycerides pass into portal system)*

---

(4)   Colonic active absorption of Na$^+$ and Cl$^-$ against high concentration
  gradients.

While the small and large intestine absorb water and electrolytes, each area of the small and large bowel also secretes liquids. Electrolyte compositions are described in Chapter 5, The renal system; Fluid and electrolytes.

**Pancreas**
The pancreatic physiology that results in the most common surgical problems is the physiology of exocrine secretion. Stimulation of the duodenal mucosa with food results in the release of cholecystokinin-pancreozymin (CCK-PZ), which in turn stimulates the release of trypsinogen and chymotrypsinogen, the inactive precursors of the

**TABLE 3   CARBOHYDRATE DIGESTION AND ABSORPTION**

*Hydrolysis*
Salivary amylase – minimal
Pancreatic $\alpha$-amylase
Brush border enzymes
   isomaltase
   glucoamylase
   sucrase
   lactase

*Transport of monosaccharides*
Active (coupled with sodium)
   glucose
   galactose
Facilitated diffusion
   fructose

*Transport of disaccharides*

*Transport to portal blood*

**TABLE 4   PROTEIN DIGESTION AND ABSORPTION**

Initial breakdown to a few amino acids and peptides in stomach by acid
   pH and pepsins

Further breakdown to amino acids and peptides in small bowel by
   pancreatic proteolytic enzymes

More digestion by brush border and cytoplasmic amino-oligopeptidases

Active amino acid transport (sodium dependent) across intestinal mucosa

Transport of dipeptides, tripeptides and tetrapeptides across intestinal
   mucosa

Transport to portal blood

proteolytic enzymes, trypsin and chymotrypsin, as well as other proteolytic enzymes (e.g. carboxypeptidase, amino peptidase), lipase for digestion of fat and amylase for digestion of carbohydrate. Proteolytic precursors are activated by enterokinase in the duodenal mucosa, as well as bacterial growth. Acid in the duodenum stimulates the release of secretin which results in the secretion of water, bicarbonate and other electrolytes. The pancreas secretes 500–1200 ml/day with a pH of 8.

## Biliary tree
The biliary tree delivers and stores bile which aids in the digestion of fat. The gallbladder also concentrates bile (about tenfold) and expels it in response to food-stimulated release of CCK-PZ. Bile flow normally ranges from 600 to 1000 ml/day. Bile salts are reabsorbed in the intestine (primarily in the ileum) and then travel in the portal circulation to the liver where they are resecreted. About 10% of bile salts secreted are lost each day in the stool. Liver disease may result in diminished removal of bile acids from portal blood and the pruritus seen with liver disease or obstructive jaundice may be from elevated blood bile salt levels.

## Liver

### *Bilirubin metabolism*
Bilirubin is a breakdown product of heme and is derived primarily (75%) from old red cells destroyed in the reticuloendothelial system. Bilirubin circulates bound to albumin, is taken up by the hepatocyte, is conjugated with glucuronide and secreted into the bile canaliculi. Conjugated bilirubin is not bound to albumin and can be filtered by the renal glomeruli and excreted, resulting in a positive urine test for bilirubin. Urobilinogen results from intestinal bacterial metabolism of bilirubin, is partly absorbed by the intestinal mucosa and excreted in the urine (a positive test for urobilinogen, not bilirubin or bile). With complete biliary tract obstruction no bile gets into the intestine, no urobilinogen is formed and none can be excreted in the urine.

### *Protein metabolism*
The liver is the most active site of protein metabolism in the body. Protein synthesis activities that commonly relate to surgical critical care are the synthesis of acute phase reactants (i.e. haptoglobin) and coagulation proteins. Breakdown of protein to urea and the metabolism of 'toxic' protein-related materials (e.g. ammonia) are important functions which may be altered in critical illness.

*Carbohydrate metabolism*
The liver is the primary site of glycogen storage and gluconeogenesis. Epinephrine, glucagon and cortisol promote glycogen lysis and gluconeogenesis. The amino acid alanine is a primary substrate for gluconeogenesis.

*Lactic acid metabolism*
Lactic acid produced in non-hepatic tissues is metabolized by the liver. Severe hepatic malfunction may result in an elevated lactic acid level even when peripheral production of lactic acid is normal.

## GASTROINTESTINAL MONITORING

### Physical examination
Physical examination of the abdomen is presented broadly here with more details to follow in each of the appropriate disease state sections. Examination begins with observation and noting such factors as patient motion, the degree of abdominal distension, changes in skin color or texture, and masses. Auscultation assesses bowel activity (e.g. normoactive, hypoactive, hyperactive bowel sounds) and the presence or absence of arterial bruits. This is followed by percussion to elicit tympany, dullness and/or pain to percussion. Next, light palpation is used to assess the presence of voluntary vs. involuntary guarding. Deeper palpation may follow in areas with little tenderness to discover referred tenderness, enlarged organs and/or masses.

### Measurement of gastric pH
Gastric pH is usually measured using litmus paper. The accuracy of pH measurement with this method has been questioned, but in one study this technique proved very accurate, as compared with an intragastric pH probe.

### Measurement and evaluation of intestinal output
Because intraluminal and extraluminal tubes and/or stomas are often present in surgical patients, much gastrointestinal monitoring is accomplished by the measurement of output from various sites. Whatever the site, important information includes the quantity and, when excessive, the electrolyte composition. The evaluation of intestinal output frequently includes determination of the presence or absence of gross or occult blood from monitored sites.

## Measurement of intestinal mucosal pH

GI mucosal cells are subject to a variety of insults which may diminish cellular function (see Gastrointestinal dysfunction section). The pH of the gastric mucosal cells, rather than the pH of gastric secretions, appears to be a sensitive and specific indicator of such a decrease in function. A device called a tonometer can be placed in the lumen of the stomach and/or the colon to measure the mucosal pH. As stated in Chapters 2 and 3, the use of this device as an indicator of illness has been advocated to evaluate not just the gastrointestinal tract, but also the overall state of illness in individual patients.

## Liver tests

The most common liver tests are bilirubin, alkaline phosphatase, gamma glutamyl transpeptidase (GGT), aspartate amino transferase (AST), alanine amino transferase (ALT), prothrombin time, prealbumin, ammonia and urea. Bilirubin elevations are common with all liver insults. Alkaline phosphatase and GGT relate primarily to diseases related to the bile ducts, both intrahepatic and extrahepatic. AST and ALT relate more to hepatocyte damage than bile duct insults. Prothrombin time and prealbumin relate to the protein synthesis capabilities. Ammonia relates to protein detoxification and urea to protein breakdown. Lactic acid elevation from liver malfunction is usually a preterminal event.

## Pancreas tests

Amylase and lipase blood levels are used to assist the evaluation of inflammatory diseases of the pancreas. Blood glucose levels are commonly elevated in critical illness, as is endogenous insulin. Therefore, an elevated glucose rarely indicates pancreatic endocrine insufficiency secondary to damaged or missing pancreatic tissue.

## GASTROINTESTINAL MEDICATIONS

The most common GI medications used in surgical critical care are used to reduce the secretion of or diminish the effect of gastric acid.

## Antacids

Antacids diminish the concentration of intraluminal gastric acid and increase pH. Ordinary fasting gastric contents have a concentration of 0.1 N hydrochloric acid. An increase in pH to 3.5 results in a 99.9% reduction in acid and decreased pepsin activity. Therefore, it is unnecessary to neutralize gastric pH to the 'physiological' level of 7 to achieve significant reductions in gastric acid.

The neutralizing capacity of several antacids and the sodium concentrations of each are listed in Table 5. The magnesium-containing antacids (e.g. Maalox®, Novartis Consumer, NJ, USA; Mylanta®, Johnson and Johnson/ Merck, PA, USA) produce intraluminal magnesium chloride of which about 15–30% is absorbed and excreted via the kidneys. Patients in renal failure may develop magnesium toxicity with these agents. Magnesium also is a cathartic and may produce or aggravate diarrhea. Aluminium hydroxide (Amphogel®, Wyeth-Ayerst, PA, USA) is preferred for patients in renal failure because there is no magnesium and aluminium binds intraluminal phosphate, which reduces hyperphosphatemia. Amphogel is constipating and has been associated with intestinal obstruction.

### $H_2$ receptor blockers
The parietal cell proton pump may be stimulated by three distinct mechanisms: acetylcholine, histamine and gastrin. Although each mechanism is different, synergistic interdependence allows therapy directed at one mechanism to significantly alter overall secretion. Therefore, histamine blockade at the $H_2$ receptor inhibits acid secretion from all three stimuli. $H_2$ receptor blockers bind competitively to gastric $H_2$ receptors. The clinical evidence supporting the effectiveness of $H_2$ blocker therapy is best documented for duodenal ulcer, with ulcer healing rates of 85–95% by 8 weeks.

$H_2$ receptors are also present on many other tissues. The side-effects of $H_2$ blockers may be secondary to interactions at these other sites (Table 6).

### Sucralfate
Sucralfate is a complex of sulfated sucrose and aluminium hydroxide which is minimally absorbed and minimally effective against acid. Sucralfate adheres to ulcers and promotes a proteinaceous exudate at the ulcer site which may be a barrier to hydrogen ions. Sucralfate also adsorbs bile, decreases pepsin activity, stimulates mucosal regeneration, promotes thicker mucous production and may stimulate endogenous production of prostaglandin $E_2$, a cytoprotective substance. Side-effects include constipation, aluminium toxicity and hypophosphatemia.

Claims have been made that sucralfate does not alter intraluminal gastric pH and, therefore, will limit the growth of organisms in the stomach, as compared with acid-limiting therapies. However, some studies have demonstrated an increase in gastric pH which suggests that sucralfate effects may not be limited to cytoprotection.

**TABLE 5   ANTACID NEUTRALIZING CAPACITY AND SODIUM CONCENTRATION OF VARIOUS ANTACIDS**

| Antacid | Neutralizing capacity (mEq/l) | Sodium (mg/ml) |
|---|---|---|
| Mylanta II | 4.1 | 0.386 |
| Maalox | 2.6 | 0.434 |
| Mylanta | 2.4 | 0.328 |
| Amphogel | 1.9 | 0.621 |
| Gelusil | 1.3 | 1.07 |

**TABLE 6   ADVERSE EFFECTS OF $H_2$ RECEPTOR BLOCKERS**

| Receptor site | Adverse effect |
|---|---|
| Brain | agitation, confusion, mental depression |
| Bone marrow | agranulocytosis, thrombocytopenia |
| Liver enzymes | increased transaminases, decreased hepatic blood flow, decreased metabolism of drugs – lidocaine, propranolol |
| Hormone receptors | increased prolactin, galactorrhea, gynecomastia |

**Proton-pump inhibitors**

Omeprazole is an inactive substance which in the presence of acid is converted to an active agent that can bind and inhibit the gastric mucosal enzyme pump, which is responsible for the secretion of hydrogen ions into the gastric lumen. It is very effective in decreasing acid secretion and has proved most useful for esophagitis secondary to acid reflux. Significant toxicity is rare.

**Prostaglandin $E_1$ analogs**

Prostaglandin $E_1$ is part of the gastric mucosal barrier system and reduces gastric acid secretion. Misoprostol, a prostaglandin $E_1$ analog, has been used with success to control gastric acid in critically ill surgical patients. The main side-effect is diarrhea.

## GASTROINTESTINAL DYSFUNCTION

### Effects of hypoperfusion

Hypoperfusion secondary to any etiology characteristically results in decreased perfusion of the GI tract, liver and pancreas. Similar to the effects of decreased cardiac output on renal blood flow, perfusion to the organs of digestion decreases more than perfusion to the brain, heart and lungs. Arginine vasopressin and angiotensin II have been suggested as important determinants of this proportional decrease in splanchnic blood flow.

Gastrointestinal hypoperfusion during disease states does not require a reduction in cardiac output. Severe inflammation may result in a regional decrease in splanchnic blood flow despite increased total body perfusion. In addition, the microcirculation may suffer a decrease in flow despite maintenance of flow in named vessels. Once in place, hypoperfusion may result in the alterations listed in Table 7.

### Effects of severe inflammation on the gastrointestinal tract

Severe inflammation may result primarily in a global or regional decrease in perfusion to the splanchnic organs. Following hypoperfusion, super-oxide generation from activated inflammatory cells may result in new or further damage to all of the organs mentioned in Chapter 2, The circulation; Hypoperfusion states.

Despite evidence of decreased blood flow during inflammation, severe inflammation appears to affect the liver differently from severe hypoperfusion alone. Microscopic examination of liver tissue of patients suffering from severe inflammation often demonstrates intrahepatic cholestasis rather than the centrilobular necrosis which is characteristic of severe hypoperfusion by itself. Several experimental studies have documented altered hepatic metabolism following ischemia/reperfusion and severe inflammatory insults which develop despite well-maintained or increased regional blood flow. Therefore, severe inflammation may result in hepatic insults which are not primarily blood-flow induced.

As discussed in more detail in the Gastrointestinal dysfunction section, severe inflammation may interfere with the mucosal barrier function of the GI tract, which prevents the migration of microorganisms and the breakdown products of microorganisms from gaining access to extra-luminal sites (e.g. peritoneal cavity, lymph nodes draining the GI tract, portal blood). Many insults that result in inflammation (e.g. ischemia/reperfusion, burns, endotoxin, infusion of live bacteria) increase the migration of intestinal organisms across the lumen (collectively termed

**TABLE 7  GASTROINTESTINAL ALTERATIONS SECONDARY TO HYPOPERFUSION**

| Location | Alterations |
| --- | --- |
| Stomach/duodenum | gastritis/duodenitis, ulcer, bleeding, perforation, ? translocation |
| Gallbladder | acalculous cholecystitis/necrosis |
| Liver | centrilobular necrosis |
| Pancreas | pancreatitis |
| Small bowel | translocation, ischemic necrosis/partial or full thickness |
| Large intestine | ischemic necrosis/partial or full thickness |

translocation as listed in Table 7). Hemorrhagic hypoperfusion may also cause translocation and the mechanism(s) responsible for translocation continue to be investigated. Regardless of the specific mechanism(s), the GI tract may provide a reservoir of microorganisms and related substances which repeatedly seed tissues outside the lumen with the potential of initiating or aggravating hypoperfusion and/or severe inflammation.

Severe inflammatory diseases, such as calculous acute cholecystitis, cholangitis and acute diverticulitis can affect the GI tract more directly. These conditions are usually more evident and require less understanding of the influence of hypoperfusion and remote inflammatory insults upon GI tract function.

**Esophageal hemorrhage**
Esophageal varix hemorrhage occurs most often in patients with severe liver disease and results in further deterioration of the metabolic, hemodynamic, hematological and renal alterations already present. Most authorities advise against emergency surgery in these patients and support the use of temporizing measures to at least acutely arrest hemorrhage, and to allow for metabolic, hemodynamic, hematological, renal and possibly nutritional improvement. The non-operative management options for esophageal variceal bleeding include the following:

(1)  Intravenous vasopressin;

(2)  Intravenous octreotide;

(3)  Sclerosis;

(4)  Varix banding;

(5)  Sengstaken-Blakemore or Minnesota tube for tamponade of gastric and esophageal varices;

(6)  Transjugular portal–systemic shunt

Most often intravenous octreotide or vasopressin will arrest hemorrhage, and balloon tamponade is less frequently necessary. The non-operative intervention of a transinternal jugular portal–systemic shunt (TIPS) has the advantage of decompressing the portal venous system without the potential deleterious effects of major abdominal surgery. Therefore, this type of decompression may be considered appropriate even in the emergency setting. The TIPS procedure, which usually alters the anatomy of the intrahepatic portal vein, does not disturb the extrahepatic portal system which then improves the technical feasibility of subsequent liver transplantation. The complications of these measures are listed in Table 8.

Mallory-Weiss tear hemorrhage is usually controlled with conservative measures which may include vasopressin.

**Stomach and duodenum**
As stated above, following any etiology of hypoperfusion and severe inflammation the entire intra-abdominal GI tract supplied by the celiac axis and the superior and inferior mesenteric arteries suffers insults which may be disproportionally large, as compared to the heart, lungs and brain. Since the GI mucosa is the most actively metabolic layer, the mucosa suffers the most from metabolic insults. This damaged mucosa becomes more susceptible to other insults such as acid, steroids, non-steroidal anti-inflammatory drugs and possibly components of bile and/or pancreatic secretions. In the stomach and duodenum this mucosal damage can be clinically manifest as gastritis, duodenitis, gastric ulcers and duodenal ulcers. These alterations can result in upper intestinal bleeding and are seen at the time of diagnostic upper endoscopy. However, stress damage is not necessarily limited to the mucosa. Full-thickness damage and perforation are also possible.

The most convincing evidence that acid promotes the 'stress' injury in the stomach and duodenum is that controlling gastric pH significantly

**TABLE 8  COMPLICATIONS OF MEDICAL MANAGEMENT OF VARICEAL HEMORRHAGE**

| | Complications |
|---|---|
| Vasopressin | severe vasoconstriction, coronary ischemia, water retention |
| Balloon tamponade | aspiration, migration of tube and airway obstruction, rupture of esophagus |
| Transinternal jugular portal–systemic shunt | extraluminal hemorrhage, encephalopathy, thrombosis of stents |
| Sclerotherapy/banding | esophageal rupture, mediastinitis |

reduces upper GI bleeding in critically ill surgical patients. Aggressive gastric pH control requires frequent (sometimes hourly when a patient is bleeding) gastric pH measurement and therapy designed to keep gastric pH $\geq$ 4. Whatever regimen is used to control acid (antacids, $H_2$ blockers, proton-pump inhibition) an arbitrary regimen of therapy without gastric pH measurement is inadequate.

The concept of mucosal protection rather than aggressive acid control is the usual logic applied to the use of sucralfate for protection of the stomach and duodenum. As stated in the 'Gastrointestinal medication' section of this Chapter, the mechanism of action of sucralfate is not perfectly understood, but this agent is an acceptable alternative.

Potential complications of acid control are:

(1)  Antacids causing changes in stomach volume resulting in distension or aspiration, excess absorption/binding of sodium, magnesium and albumin, and/or diarrhea/constipation;

(2)  $H_2$ blockers causing mental status alterations, thrombocytopenia, leukopenia and/or jaundice;

(3)  Increased growth of microorganisms.

**Liver and biliary tree**

*Jaundice*
Jaundice is quite common after major surgical illness and may be secondary to many factors including multiple blood transfusions, liver

hypoperfusion, hematoma resorption, drugs, hepatitis, severe inflamma-tion and extrahepatic biliary obstruction. The measurement of common liver tests usually provides an indication of whether the jaundice is associated with evidence of significant hepatocellular injury (marked AST and ALT elevations). Hepatocellular damage is more consistent with severe hypoperfusion ('shock' liver) and hepatitis. Acute infectious hepatitis is not common in surgical critical care, but drugs, including alcohol, may cause direct hepatocellular insults.

Jaundice without significant AST/ALT elevation is quite common and may or may not be associated with increased alkaline phosphatase and GGT levels. An elevation primarily in unconjugated bilirubin without an elevation in alkaline phosphatase or GGT would suggest hemolysis as a cause of jaundice. This can be further supported by measuring decreased haptoglobin levels and increased urine free hemoglobin. Jaundice with an elevated conjugated bilirubin and an increase in alkaline phosphatase and GGT suggests cholestasis of extrahepatic origin. This is especially true when alkaline phosphatase and GGT have increased to a similar degree as total bilirubin (i.e. a bilirubin of 7 mg/dl is associated with a seven-fold increase in alkaline phosphatase). When conjugated bilirubin increases rapidly without a significant increase in alkaline phosphatase or GGT, this is often a manifestation of intrahepatic cholestasis secondary to severe inflammation remote from the liver and biliary tree (i.e. pneu-monia, necrotizing soft-tissue infection).

Regardless of the pattern of bilirubin and/or alkaline phosphatase elevation, evaluation of the biliary tree using a non-invasive approach like ultrasound is reasonable to assess the possibility of extrahepatic obstruc-tion in any critically ill jaundiced patient. However, except for the occurrence of acalculous acute cholecystitis, there is little reason to expect an extrahepatic biliary tree disease in most critically ill surgical patients who develop jaundice without a prior injury or surgical disease related to the liver or biliary tract.

*Manifestations of liver failure*
Liver failure may be the predominant manifestation of hypoperfusion/severe inflammation-induced organ failure. However, liver failure sufficient to result in life-threatening alterations is much more likely when severe hypoperfusion/inflammation impinge on a liver already diseased. The magnitude of pre-existing liver disease is frequently categorized using Child's criteria (Table 9). Any patient with Child's class C liver disease or who develops this class in the hospital is likely to die from

**TABLE 9   CHILD'S CRITERIA FOR THE CLASSIFICATION OF LIVER DISEASE**

| Child's class | Bilirubin (mg/dl) | Albumin (g/dl) | Ascites | Nutrition | Encephalopathy |
|---|---|---|---|---|---|
| A | <2.0 | >3.5 | none | excellent | none |
| B | 2–3 | 3–3.5 | little | good | little |
| C | >3.0 | <3.0 | marked | poor | marked |

hepatic failure. Other manifestations of severe liver disease are coagulopathy (prothrombin time unresponsive to vitamin K, prolonged partial thromboplastin time), hypoglycemia, elevated lactic acid, hepatorenal syndrome and hypoxia. Inability of the liver to synthesize coagulation factors and glucose and to metabolize lactic acid are usually preterminal determinations.

*Hepatorenal syndrome*
The hepatorenal syndrome is also usually considered preterminal unless the liver recovers or a liver transplant is performed. Some authors describe 'reversal' of the hepatorenal syndrome without specific therapy for the liver and, therefore, there is some discrepancy in definitions. To simplify, patients with severe liver disease often become oliguric. The oliguria is characterized by urinary indices most indicative of a prerenal state, such as low urinary sodium concentration, low fractional excretion of sodium ($FE_{Na}$), and high urine osmolality. Reportedly, kidneys in this condition can be transplanted and function normally. However, this prerenal condition can progress into frank renal failure which requires dialysis.

The etiology of the hepatorenal syndrome is unknown. Speculation continues about possible toxic effects of bilirubin, high aldosterone levels, elevated endothelin-1 levels, increased intra-abdominal pressure and renal hypoperfusion from hypovolemia. Interventions that simultaneously increase intravascular volume and reduce the intra-abdominal pressure from ascites (e.g. peritoneal–venous shunts, TIPS) have been reported to 'reverse' the hepatorenal syndrome. As stated above, such claims depend on the definition of the condition. However, measures that ameliorate a prerenal, hepatorenal syndrome-like clinical condition may improve patient status significantly, regardless of the definitions. One test advocated for distinguishing a prerenal state from 'true' hepatorenal syndrome is the urine/plasma creatinine ratio. Values >30 suggest hepatorenal syndrome (indicative of profound water retention), as compared with values <30.

Patients with liver disease-associated alterations in renal function may suffer significant further deterioration secondary to a variety of other insults, such as acute intravascular volume depletion, severe inflammation, non-steroidal anti-inflammatory agents, intravenous contrast and aminoglycosides. Therefore, the fundamental principles (described in Chapter 5, The renal system; Renal failure and selected metabolic disturbances) of protecting the renal circulation and decreasing exposure to renal toxins apply equally as well to the liver failure patient with oliguria. As mentioned above, peritoneal–venous shunting and/or portacaval shunting may be the only effective method for protecting the renal circulation in some patients.

*Ascites*

Intractable ascites is also a manifestation of liver failure and is usually treated medically with salt and water restriction, bed rest, aldosterone inhibition (spironolactone) and diuretics. Peritoneal–venous shunting is useful for the management of intractable ascites, as are portosystemic shunts, particularly of the side-to-side variety, like the TIPS. The peritoneal–venous-shunt tubing will remain patent longest when the ascitic fluid is not protein rich, and therefore will less likely produce a fibrin clot in the tubing. Besides clotting the tubing, most of the complications of peritoneal–venous shunting (congestive heart failure, acute respiratory distress syndrome and coagulopathy) are secondary to proteins and protein break-down products in the ascites. Thus far coagulopathy has been the main reason for interrupting the shunt postoperatively. Coagulopathy can usually be avoided if the ascitic fluid is discarded in the operating room and the peritoneal cavity is irrigated with saline to reduce the concentration of tissue plasminogen activator in the ascites which can result in fibrinolysis.

*Hepatic encephalopathy*

Encephalopathy is another manifestation of severe liver malfunction and can develop during severe, acute liver failure in patients with previously normal livers, or in patients with chronic liver disease as that disease worsens. In general, encephalopathy in the setting of acute liver failure portends a worse prognosis.

Generally, hepatic encephalopathy is considered to be secondary to neuroactive substances that originate in the GI tract but are no longer detoxified by the liver. Portosystemic shunts, particularly those that decompress the portal vein proper, aggravate these detoxification difficulties by shunting blood with neuroactive substances away from the liver as well as diverting hepatic blood flow, which may be especially essential to protect the damaged liver from further insult. Under such circumstances acute severe liver malfunction may develop in patients with chronic liver disease, and often results in hepatic encephalopathy accompanied by the hepatorenal syndrome.

As a marker for this deficit in detoxification, arterial blood ammonia levels are usually, but not always, elevated when hepatic encephalopathy is present. Therefore, encephalopathy should still be considered in any patient with severe acute or known severe chronic liver disease who exhibits an altered mental status despite normal ammonia levels.

Many acute insults may precipitate or aggravate hepatic encephalopathy, including hypovolemic hypoperfusion, severe inflammation, GI hemorrhage, hypokalemia, renal failure, sedatives/analgesics, portosystemic shunt and zinc deficiency. Management includes measures taken to ameliorate these conditions, as well as the traditional restriction of protein (especially by mouth), laxatives, enemas and lactulose administration. Cerebral edema is more common in the hepatic encephalopathy associated with acute liver failure, as compared with chronic liver failure. Measures to monitor intracranial pressure and treat elevations may be particularly important, especially to preserve brain tissue in anticipation of a liver transplant.

*Acute acalculous cholecystitis*
Another manifestation of the 'stress' injury to the GI tract is acute acalculous cholecystitis (AAC). Decreased mucosal blood flow, increased inflammatory mediator production and decreased gallbladder contractile function have all been associated with AAC.

Most often seen in males who have been injured, AAC may become clinically evident several days after an insult, with a spectrum ranging from vague clinical manifestations, such as fever and jaundice, to frank right upper-quadrant peritonitis. Usually the diagnosis requires a high index of suspicion in critically ill patients who are often sedated and/or paralyzed. This disease is primarily a condition that results from direct damage to the gallbladder wall rather than indirectly from pressure increasing in the gallbladder lumen. Therefore, an accurate diagnosis often requires direct inspection of the gallbladder wall rather than the use of less-invasive techniques. As a consequence, ultrasound and cholecystographic scans are not as useful as in calculous acute chole-cystitis. Both are subject to a high false-positive rate in critical illness. A normal scintigraphy scan, however, makes the diagnosis extremely unlikely.

Since the diagnosis is best discerned based on the appearance of the gallbladder wall, a high index of suspicion may require direct inspection of the gallbladder. This can be accomplished with laparoscopy when a patient can tolerate general anesthesia, or can be accomplished by a minilaparotomy under local anesthesia. With either technique, if the gallbladder looks normal, no intervention is needed. If the gallbladder wall looks viable but the gallbladder is markedly distended, a chole-cystostomy tube can be placed. If the gallbladder is abnormal, the gallbladder should be removed.

Some authors (e.g. Werbel *et al.*, 1989) advocate radiographically directed percutaneous drainage of the distended gallbladder in the critical care setting, and claim that this is a treatment for acalculous cholecystitis. Since the specific diagnosis of acalculous cholecystitis requires inspection of the gallbladder wall, it is difficult to interpret the sensitivity and specificity claims of such reports. If the gallbladder wall is severely diseased, simple decompression is inadequate therapy and cholecystectomy is required. Therefore, any patient subjected to percutaneous gallbladder drainage who does not improve as expected should have the gallbladder directly visualized to assess this diagnosis and the effects of the tube decompression.

## Pancreas

### Pancreatitis

Pancreatitis may produce marked physiological disturbances which require ICU management. The common etiologies of pancreatitis are alcohol, gallstones and trauma, while the potential etiologies frequently encountered in the ICU setting are cardiopulmonary bypass and major abdominal aortic surgery. Hypoperfusion of the pancreas can result in pancreatitis and may be the etiology related to cardiopulmonary bypass and major aortic surgery.

The severity of pancreatitis is the major determinant of associated physiological disturbances and has been categorized by Ranson's clinical criteria (Table 10). Severe pancreatitis may require ICU monitoring and therapy for any or all of the following problems: hypoperfusion, respiratory failure, renal dysfunction, peritoneal lavage, early diagnosis of infected pancreatic necrosis and postoperative support. Management of hypo-perfusion, respiratory failure and renal dysfunction follow the same principles described in previous Chapters.

**TABLE 10   RANSON'S CRITERIA OF PANCREATITIS SEVERITY**

*At the time of admission*
Age >55 years
Glucose >200 mg/dl
WBC>16 000 cmm
LDH >700 IU/l
AST >250 U/l

*At 48 h*
Calcium <8 mg/dl
BUN increase >5 mg/dl
HCT fall >10
Base deficit >4 mEq/l
Arterial $Po_2$<60 mmHg (room air)
Fluid sequestration >6 l

WBC, white blood cell count; LDH, lactic dehydrogenase; AST, aspartate amino transferase; BUN, blood urea nitrogen; HCT, hematocrit

Hypovolemic hypoperfusion and resultant renal malfunction early in the course of severe pancreatitis are associated with increased mortality risk, especially in older patients. Hypoperfusion not only damages important organs like the kidneys, but also may aggravate the pancreatitis itself. No other single disease more clearly illustrates the intimate association of inflammation and hypoperfusion described in the opening Chapters of this manual. The common clinical sequelae of severe pancreatitis (e.g. fluid sequestration, increased pulmonary shunt, hypocalcemia, increased lactic acid) emphasize this point further. Therefore, optimal management demands precise and aggressive management of the circulation and efforts to limit the effects of the severe inflammatory disease as well.

One such method advocated to limit the amount of inflammatory alterations is peritoneal lavage. Severe pancreatitis usually results in the accumulation of free brown fluid in the abdominal cavity, which contains inflammatory cells. Continuous lavage of the abdominal cavity with peritoneal dialysis solution to remove this fluid for 7 days may diminish the early hemodynamic and pulmonary alterations and decrease the risk of eventual infectious complications. While several studies suggest that the early manifestations of severe pancreatitis may abate with lavage, the claim that infectious complications and mortality are decreased is more controversial. However, short of emergency surgery to debride the pancreas, little else but peritoneal lavage is available to ameliorate the inflammation early in this disease.

*Pancreatitis infectious complications*
Patients who survive the early phase of severe pancreatitis are at risk for developing infectious complications in the region of the inflamed pancreas, namely infected pancreatic necrosis and/or an infected pancreatic pseudo-cyst. Of these the easiest to diagnose and treat is the infected pseudocyst. The fibrotic capsule forming as the wall of a pseudocyst can provide a well-circumscribed collection which can be recognized readily by ultrasound or computed tomography (CT) scan. Drainage externally by percutaneous techniques is usually successful. Infected pancreatic necrosis is present when necrotic pancreatic tissue or, more commonly, inflamed peripancreatic tissue becomes infected. Ultrasound and CT cannot distinguish infection of such tissue as different from a sterile inflammatory mass. Under these circumstances, needle aspiration of the phlegmon with organisms seen on Gram stain or grown in culture is usually sufficient to make the diagnosis. With this diagnosis surgical debridement, rather than drainage, is indicated and may require multiple trips to the operating room for resolution.

**Diarrhea**
Many potential small bowel and colon problems (e.g. obstruction, fistula, anastomotic leak) may be encountered in the surgical ICU. Most of these relate to the underlying surgical disease or surgical intervention. Both accurate diagnosis and expeditious management of these conditions are important to surgical critical care, but are better discussed in the context of the specific diseases and surgical interventions. However, a GI problem particularly vexing in the surgical ICU is diarrhea, particularly when it inhibits the use of the GI tract for nutrition.

The potential etiologies of diarrhea on the ICU are listed in Table 11. Differentiating a secretory vs. an osmotic diarrhea is usually simple. If diarrhea continues after stopping intestinal feeding, the diarrhea is secretory. *Clostridium dificile* colitis is becoming a more common cause of secretory diarrhea and stool titers should be obtained to confirm the diagnosis. The first line of treatment is with metronidazole; if that fails, oral vancomycin is usually effective.

**TABLE 11   POTENTIAL ETIOLOGIES OF ICU DIARRHEA**

*Secretory*
Intraluminal inflammation
  pseudomembranous colitis
  antibiotic-associated diarrhea
  inflammatory bowel disease
Extraluminal disease
  partial small bowel obstruction
  intra-abdominal abscess
Short gut – inability to absorb endogenous secretions

*Osmotic*
Bowel edema – low serum albumin
Ischemia
Severe inflammation
Diminished small bowel surface
Diminished large bowel surface
Decreased fat absorption

Extraluminal disease, especially partial small bowel obstruction, may produce a secretory diarrhea. Attention to abdominal physical findings and abdominal X-rays should establish this diagnosis, and the disease is usually treated by nasogastric decompression. Diarrhea may be the clue that an intra-abdominal abscess is developing. Diarrhea in this setting may result either via direct irritation of adjacent small or large bowel, or by producing a partial obstruction. Drainage of the abscess is the primary treatment.

Osmotic diarrhea is evident primarily when intestinal feeding is used. Since the bowel is supplied by the systemic circulation, bowel edema can develop because of hypoalbuminemia. Therefore, if systemic capillary leaking is not considered likely, the provision of albumin may help reduce osmotic diarrhea. Any process that interferes with mucosal function, such as ischemia, will enhance an osmotic diarrhea. Diminished small and large bowel surface may be adequate to absorb endogenous secretions but not tolerate the addition of feedings. Decreased fat absorption from diversion of the bile and pancreatic secretions or ileal resection and the consequent reduction in bile salt secretion may result in malabsorption, which can be treated by eliminating long-chain triglycerides from the diet and using medium-chain triglycerides and carbohydrate as the main caloric sources.

Management of an osmotic diarrhea usually requires adjustment of the types, concentrations and rates of foodstuff administered. For instance, an elemental diet may be better tolerated by a patient with deficient pancreatobiliary secretions. In addition, medications that inhibit intestinal motility may decrease an osmotic diarrhea by allowing more time for absorption of liquids and solids.

## Intra-abdominal abscess

Surgical patients commonly have disease and/or procedures that result in contamination of the abdominal cavity with intestinal tract or, on occasion, extra-intestinal organisms. The risk factors for developing an intra-abdominal abscess are the degree of contamination, hypovolemic hypoperfusion, severe inflammation, age >55 years, cancer, steroids, inadequate debridement, intra-abdominal hematoma, diabetes and malnutrition. This list reads like a description of all risk factors related to infection, except that the surgical fundamentals of adequate debridement and hemostasis must be used even in the healthiest patients if the risk of infection is to be diminished following intra-abdominal operations.

Once the patient is recognized to be at risk, vigilance for early detection of new or recurrent intra-abdominal infection is necessary to allow prompt intervention. Clinical clues that suggest such infection are (1) persistent fever and/or hypothermia, (2) persistent fluid sequestration, (3) elevated white blood cell count with immature forms, (4) new organ malfunction and (5) glucose intolerance, and are non-specific as to origin (i.e. pneumonia could result in the same findings). History and physical examination are the first tools to use when evaluating the possibility of new infection from any location, and may suggest an abdominal focus (e.g. new onset of abdominal pain, abdominal distension, absent or decreased bowel sounds, localized tenderness). Few routine tests are discriminative for an intra-abdominal abscess; plain X-ray evidence consistent with an abscess includes pleural effusion, gas bubbles that do not move with changing position, mass displacing abdominal contents and partial bowel obstruction; a multiorganism bacteremia is also suggestive. Except for surgical exploration, the study that yields the best false-positive/false-negative rate is the abdominal CT scan. CT also provides sufficient anatomic definition to discern if percutaneous, rather than operative drainage, is possible.

Drainage is the primary therapy for intra-abdominal abscess. The method of drainage should be individualized to a patient's disease. If a well-localized abscess is diagnosed by CT and can be approached percutaneously, this is preferred as it allows treatment without general anesthesia and manipulation of intra-abdominal viscera. Surgical intervention is indicated when the diagnosis is highly suspected but cannot be localized, when multiple collections make percutaneous drainage impractical, or when significant visceral injury is likely via a percutaneous route.

Antibiotic therapy alone is inadequate therapy for an intra-abdominal abscess. Antibiotics treat the surrounding cellulitis and may decrease the systemic sequelae of an abscess. Once the abscess is drained, the surrounding cellulitis usually abates rapidly (within 72 h). There is no arbitrary duration of antibiotic therapy for an intra-abdominal abscess. Antibiotic therapy should be continued until there is evidence that the surrounding cellulitis and systemic sequelae have abated, which usually occurs when the patient is afebrile and the leukocyte count is normal or approaching normal. Prolonged antibiotic therapy after resolution of cellulitis will not provide any therapeutic advantage and may augment the growth of resistant organisms both at the abscess site and elsewhere.

The type of antibiotics used depends first on the knowledge of the likely source of contamination and the usual flora of that site; subsequently, the sensitivities of organisms cultured at the drainage procedure should dictate antibiotic therapy.

### The GI tract as a reservoir for infection and/or inflammation in the critically ill surgical patient

The GI tract is frequently the location of an initial disease process which results in an episode of severe hypoperfusion and/or severe inflammation. Intestinal hemorrhage, severe pancreatitis, perforated diverticulitis and penetrating intestinal injury are examples of such intestinal insults. However, such primary intestinal processes are not the only mechanism responsible for intestinal participation and potential augmentation of illnesses which cause hypoperfusion and inflammation from other foci (i.e. ruptured abdominal aortic aneurysm resulting in ischemia to the sigmoid colon). The potential for the intestine to serve as a reservoir for infection and/or inflammation can be catalogued as listed in Table 12.

Patients who have undergone surgery on the intestinal tract which included closure of intestinal wounds or anastomosis(es) are at risk for developing a wound breakdown and fistula which may or may not result

## TABLE 12   THE GI TRACT AS A RESERVOIR FOR INFECTION/INFLAMMATION DURING CRITICAL ILLNESS

*Intestinal leaks/perforations*
Anastomoses
Stress ulcers
Perforated diverticulitis

*Intestinal ischemia*
Aortic surgery
Low cardiac index
Embolism
Pancreatitis
Acalculous cholecystitis

*Translocation*
Decreased mucosal barrier function
Decreased local immunocompetence
Overgrowth of abnormal flora

*Aspiration of stomach contents*
Gastric ileus
Alkaline pH
Tubing in esophagus

in an intra-abdominal abscess. If the patient received a course of antibiotics during and following the initial surgical intervention, at least some of the organisms responsible for the new infection are likely to be resistant to the previous antimicrobial therapy. Depending on such surgical features as the use of drains, intraluminal tubing and open-wound management, new infections may include flora that arise from both the patient (i.e. common intestinal bacteria and fungi) as well as the ICU environment (i.e. *Staphylococcus epidermis*, resistant enterococcus, *Pseudomonas, Serratia, Enterobacter*). The recovery of *S. epidermidis*, enterococcus, *Candida* species, and a nosocomial Gram-negative rod as a single organism or in various combinations from the abdomen in these patients has been termed tertiary peritonitis; it is distinguished from primary peritonitis as seen in cirrhotics with ascites and secondary peritonitis as seen with *de novo* perforated diverticulitis, for instance. As is discussed later, culture of these organisms from the abdominal cavity does not necessarily require gross anatomical disruption of the intestinal wall. Therefore, a clinical syndrome more consistent with an intra-abdominal abscess without a fistula may be the presentation of the tertiary peritonitis.

Patients who receive high-dose steroid therapy in a critical care setting, usually for respiratory disease, may develop perforated diverticulitis. In the past, steroids were more commonly associated with peptic perforations of the stomach and duodenum. Effective prophylaxis for stress ulcer has decreased the prevalence of such events. In recent years a severe acute intestinal insult in such a patient is more likely related to the colon and will behave more like a 'secondary peritonitis' from a microbiological perspective.

Ischemia sufficient to produce partial or full-thickness necrosis of the intestinal wall will result in a continuing inflammatory insult, regardless of whether microorganisms and/or breakdown products traverse the bowel wall into nearby tissues or the bloodstream. Such ischemia may be secondary to anatomical alterations in the macrovasculature (e.g. ligation of the inferior mesenteric artery, embolism to the superior mesenteric artery) or decreased global perfusion (e.g. low cardiac index, vaso-constrictor administration). The ileocecal region is particularly prone to ischemic insults secondary to a low cardiac index. Evidence of ongoing inflammation (e.g. fever, abnormal white blood cell count, decreasing platelets) with abdominal pain, sometimes localized tenderness, bowel movements containing blood (gross or microscopic) and metabolic acidosis are common associations with ischemic intestine. When suspected, several methods may be used to discern the presence, location and severity of ischemia including endoscopy, arteriography, laparoscopy, peritoneal lavage and exploratory laparotomy. The details related to the surgical and medical treatment of intestinal ischemia/infarction are beyond the scope of this manual.

As discussed in the 'Liver and biliary tree' and the 'Pancreatitis' sections, the gallbladder and pancreas may become inflammatory organs secondary to an episode of severe regional or global hypoperfusion. In addition, severe inflammation may injure the gallbladder. Therefore, either of these organs may become the focus of new or continuing inflammation.

As mentioned previously in this Chapter, the migration of micro-organisms or related byproducts from the intestinal lumen to extraluminal tissues is called translocation. Normally the gut provides an essential barrier function, which prevents organisms and toxic substances from gaining access to the internal milieu. Evidence that this barrier function can be deficient, especially in the small intestine, without gross anatomical disruption of the intestine is extensive in experimental literature and suggestive in human studies. Translocation may develop as a consequence of the following three mechanisms: deficient mucosal barrier, decreased host defenses at the intestinal site, and overgrowth of aerobic organisms.

Mucosal barrier function may decrease secondary to both decreased total body perfusion and/or systemic inflammatory insults. As with each discussion about cellular injury presented in this manual, separating the effects of decreased oxygen delivery from the potential of direct toxic effects to cells is difficult, if not impossible, as it relates to both hypo-perfusion and inflammation. The function of the mucosal barrier appears to also be strongly influenced by the nutrition of the mucosal cell. The amino acid glutamine is consumed primarily by the small intestine. Glutamine supplementation, either via feeding the intestinal tract or with total parenteral nutrition, improves barrier function.

IgA, an immunoglobulin secreted into the lumen of the GI tract, is decreased in models of experimental critical illness. Such models also exhibit a global suppression of cellular defense mechanisms and the GI tract is not immune from this suppression. Therefore, local humoral and cellular functions which would inhibit translocation are impaired.

Antibiotic therapy often results in the growth of endogenous or exogenous organisms in the lumen of the GI tract which are resistant to the previously used antibiotics. The endogenous organism *Candida* is particularly prone to emerge. But devices that pass from the environment into the lumen of the GI tract (e.g. nasogastric tubes, jejunal feeding tubes) promote the colonization of the upper GI tract with nosocomial organisms such as resistant *S. epidermidis*, enterococcus and *Pseudomonas*. High concentrations of these organisms may migrate across a normal intestine. Therefore, any significant impairment of mucosal barrier or host defenses at the GI level will augment translocation once the intraluminal concentrations of these organisms increase.

Translocation may result in ongoing evidence of inflammation without positive blood cultures (organisms trapped in nearby tissues, such as lymph nodes, liver and spleen) or with positive blood cultures. The upper GI tract may also act as a reservoir for organisms that result in pneumonia, urinary tract infection, wound infection and empyema, as well as the 'tertiary' peritonitis mentioned above. The epidemiological association of ICU pneumonia with organisms cultured in the stomach is supported by many studies. More controversial is whether altering such aspects as the pH of the stomach or attempts to sterilize the upper intestine using antimicrobial agents is effective in reducing the incidence of pneumonia and the other infectious complications listed above. Further study is needed to resolve these controversies.

General management principles that serve to limit the upper intestinal tract as a source of ongoing and recurrent inflammation are:

(1)   Treat hypoperfusion;

(2)   Treat pathological inflammation;

(3)   Use limited antibiotics for specific therapeutic indications;

(4)   Provide adequate nutrition – usually via GI tract.

While efforts to maintain an excellent circulation and to treat severe inflammation are underway, antibiotic therapy should be as limited and specific as possible. This is especially important regarding therapy directed at anaerobic organisms. Because such therapy appears to particularly augment translocation, the clinician should use antibiotics effective against anaerobic organisms only when documented as present, or when the primary site of disease is expected to contain high concentrations. For instance, perforated diverticulitis is much more likely to contaminate the peritoneal cavity with large numbers of anaerobes, as compared to acute cholecystitis. In addition, clear endpoints for discontinuing antibiotics should be applied by the following methods: careful application of prophylaxis vs. therapeutic principles, and stopping antibiotics when clinical signs of infection have abated, rather than giving an arbitrary dosage for surgical diseases.

Adequate nutrition assists mucosal barrier function. Most studies have demonstrated a superiority of enteral nutrition over parenteral nutrition for this assistance. The mechanics of providing parenteral nutrition may add additional infectious and non-infectious risk (see Nutritional therapy section). Gaining access to the proximal small bowel for feeding during intra-abdominal surgery for critically ill patients is an often overlooked opportunity, which may not only provide a convenient and safe long-term method of providing nutrition, but may also decrease the risk of further infectious complications.

## NUTRITIONAL PHYSIOLOGY

The nutritional physiology of importance in surgical critical care pertains mostly to the differences in nutritional needs of patients under stress as compared with simple starvation, common deficiencies in surgical patients, the dependence of immunological function on nutrition, recognition of the depleted patient, assessing nutritional depletion and the response to therapy.

## Stress vs. starvation

Estimates of the baseline nutritional requirements, especially protein, of non-stressed humans are difficult to determine but generally considered to be in the range shown in Table 13. Following ingestion of a meal, insulin levels rise to a level that inhibits mobilization of fatty acids and promotes migration of glucose and protein into skeletal muscle. Movement of glucose into the liver is not insulin dependent, but insulin inhibits hepatic glycogenolysis and gluconeogenesis. Interestingly, hepatic extraction of glucose is greater with oral as compared to intravenous administration of glucose, even with similar insulin levels and with intraportal vein infusion of glucose. Glycogen is synthesized from glucose in the liver and skeletal muscle, with skeletal muscle representing the largest glycogen storage area. However, skeletal muscle lacks the enzyme glucose-6-phosphatase, which converts the largest breakdown product of glycogen, glucose-6-phosphate, to glucose. Therefore, glucose cannot be released from the myocyte to other cells.

During the usual postabsorptive state, which lasts several hours, insulin levels fall and glucagon levels increase and promote glycogenolysis and gluconeogenesis. Glucagon enhances lipolysis, allowing delivery of fatty acids to tissues that can use this energy source. While insulin levels are lower than they are after ingestion, enough remains to inhibit amino acid release from muscle and fatty acid release from adipocytes.

During early starvation without other stress (e.g. injury or infection), glycogen stores in the liver (about 150 g, or 600 kcal) are depleted rapidly to provide glucose to the brain (about 144 g/day) and other glycolytic tissues (e.g. erythrocytes, leukocytes, bone marrow, renal medulla, peripheral nerves). Once glycogen is depleted, glucose is synthesized in the liver from lactate, pyruvate, glycerol and gluconeogenic amino acids. Other body tissues (e.g. heart, renal cortex, skeletal muscle) can use fatty acids or ketone bodies (e.g. acetoacetate or $\beta$-hydroxybutyrate). The liver can also derive its energy from the oxidation of fatty acids to acetyl-CoA. However, early in starvation insulin levels are high enough to inhibit lipolysis.

If prolonged, this insulin inhibition of fatty acid release would eventually result in protein catabolism, primarily of muscle, to provide

**TABLE 13    BASELINE NUTRITIONAL REQUIREMENTS**

*Protein (1 g/kg/day)*
Essential amino acid rich or 'high quality' (0.8 g/kg/day)
Non-essential amino acids (0.2 mg/kg/day)

*Energy needs*
Males (30–50 kcal/kg/day)
Females (25–45 kcal/kg/day)
Carbohydrate 75% of energy needs
Fat 25% of energy needs

*Essential fatty acids*
2–4% calories as linoleic acid
7.7 g/day linoleic acid

*Micronutrients*
Zinc 2.5 mg/day
Copper 0.5 mg/day
Chromium 0.01–0.02 mg/day
Manganese 1.0 mg/day
Phosphate 20–25 mEq/1000 kcal
Selenium
Iodine 150 μg/day
Iron 10 mg/day
Magnesium
Vitamins

gluconeogenic amino acids, especially alanine. However, with prolonged starvation, insulin levels diminish while glucagon levels remain the same or increase, fatty acids are released and metabolized, and the brain begins to use ketone bodies, thereby sparing protein from gluconeogenesis. In addition, liver gluconeogenesis proportionally uses more lactate, pyruvate and glycerol. In this manner the energy from fat oxidation supports liver metabolism, provides ketones to the brain, and supports the creation of glucose in the liver for tissues that cannot use fat. After 30 days, the kidney uses glutamine from skeletal muscle via the glutamine cycle to produce about half of the synthesized glucose. Plasma levels of amino acids during prolonged starvation demonstrate lowering of all types, including branched-chain (BCAA), aromatic (AAA) and sulfur-containing (SCAA) amino acids (Table 14).

The metabolic response to stress results in a markedly different interaction of carbohydrate, fat and protein. Catecholamines (e.g. epinephrine from the adrenal medulla, norepinephrine from the sympathetic nervous system) stimulate gluconeogenesis and glycogenolysis in the liver, lactate release from skeletal muscle and fatty acid mobilization. Norepinephrine inhibits insulin release from the pancreas; epinephrine enhances it but not usually enough to result in normal glucose levels. Epinephrine also increases glucagon secretion, and glucagon often remains elevated throughout the injury period into recovery. Therefore, hyperglycemia is common with stress.

### TABLE 14   AMINO ACID TYPES

*Branched chain*
Valine*
Leucine*
Isoleucine*

*Aromatic*
Phenylalanine*
Tyrosine

*Sulfur containing*
Taurine
Cystine
Methionine*

*Other*
Alanine
Aspartic acid
Glutamic acid
Proline
Glycine
Serine
Threonine*
Lysine*
Histidine
Tryptophan*

*Essential amino acid

Adrenocorticotropic hormone (ACTH) increases with stress and results in not only the release of cortisol, but also the release of fatty acids and insulin, and decreased deamination of amino acids. Cortisol stimulates hepatic gluconeogenesis, mobilization of amino acids from muscle and synthesis of protein in the liver.

Growth hormone also increases and offsets some of the other hormonal effects by promoting the intracellular transport of amino acids and protein synthesis. However, growth hormone reduces the response of insulin to hyperglycemia and promotes oxidation of fat.

The overall effect of stress (e.g. trauma and/or especially severe infection) promotes muscle protein breakdown for gluconeogenesis and produces acute phase reactant proteins in the liver. Elevated or normal insulin levels are insufficient to maintain normoglycemia and promote peripheral protein synthesis, but are sufficient to inhibit a ketotic state. Tissues that might adapt to ketosis and reduce protein breakdown cannot because of high blood glucose and few ketones.

Plasma amino acid concentrations are different in stress as compared to starvation. There is an increase in the AAA phenylalanine and tyrosine as well as the SCAA taurine, cystine and methionine. BCAA remain normal and the ratio of BCAA to total amino acids may decrease. Essential amino acids, glutamine and alanine are released from skeletal muscle and presumably serve as substrates for metabolism in the liver.

**Common nutritional deficiencies**

The common nutritional deficiencies seen in critically ill surgical patients before and after surgical intervention are listed in Table 15. Preoperative protein-calorie malnutrition is common, especially in patients with chronic disease such as chronic steroid use, inflammatory bowel disease, renal failure, alcohol abuse, any of which may be associated with micronutrient deficiencies from inadequate intake or malabsorption. Postoperative protein-calorie malnutrition may develop even in previously healthy patients secondary to the metabolic changes mentioned above. Micronutrient inadequacies emphasized in the early experience of patients receiving only intravenous nutrition have been essential fatty acid, zinc and phosphate deficiencies (described in more detail in the Nutritional therapy section of this Chapter).

**Immunological function and nutrition**

Common sense supports the concept that normal immunological function depends on adequate nutrition. Scientific evaluation of nutrition and

## TABLE 15   COMMON NUTRITIONAL DEFICIENCIES

*Preoperative*
Calorie
Protein
Micronutrient
   iron
   folate
   vitamin K
   thiamine

*Postoperative*
Calorie
Protein
Fat
Micronutrient
   magnesium
   zinc
   phosphate
   water-soluble vitamins
   fat-soluble vitamins

immunological function has demonstrated that cellular immunity, dependent upon T lymphocytes, appears to be most affected by protein-calorie malnutrition. Functions of T lymphocytes that may be depressed are blast formation and participation in humoral antibody production, and less 'helper cell' activity. In addition, polymorphonuclear leukocytes (PMN) demonstrate decreased *in vitro* bactericidal and fungicidal activity. The functions of macrophages, the B lymphocytes for humoral immunity and the complement system do not appear to be as markedly altered by protein-calorie malnutrition. Interleukin-1 release from macrophages may be decreased following protein malnutrition.

Since cellular immunity is critical to delayed hypersensitivity, skin testing for 'recall' antigens (mumps, *Candida*, trichophytin, tuberculin purified protein derivative (PPD) and streptokinase/streptodornase) has been used to assess nutritional status in surgical patients and the response to nutritional repletion. Unfortunately, delayed hypersensitivity may be depressed by many factors besides nutrition (e.g. trauma, cancer, sepsis), and serves best to indicate which patients are at greater risk for postoperative morbidity and mortality, rather than indicating which patients suffer primarily from malnutrition.

## Measures of nutritional status

Several measures of nutritional status are listed in Table 16. The clinician uses the history, physical examination and laboratory tests to assess the nutritional status of patients, or at least to assess the likelihood that a patient is nutritionally depleted and the effect this may have on planned interventions, such as surgery. Measured body weight below 80% of ideal weight suggests significant malnutrition, but body weight may be maintained by expansion of the extracellular fluid despite severe malnutrition, especially with depleted protein as seen in kwashiorkor. An acute loss (within 3 months) of 10% or more of body weight increases the risk of significant protein-calorie depletion. Physical examination may demonstrate loss of body fat, gross evidence of skeletal muscle wasting (temporal and interosseous muscles), as well as ascites and/or peripheral edema, which may indicate inadequate protein concentrations. While history and physical examination may be considered less objective than other measures, excellent correlation between clinical nutritional assessment and objective testing has been documented, which then also correlates with postoperative morbidity risk. Therefore, the use of a more sophisticated system such as the prognostic nutritional index may be of little additional value to careful clinical evaluation.

Objective measures may be more valuable in evaluating the response to nutritional therapy. The standard method of evaluating overall nutritional therapy is nitrogen balance, which, when positive, argues that a patient is receiving adequate calories and protein, but does not indicate if visceral protein synthesis and immunological status have been improved. Visceral proteins that have relatively short half lives (e.g. transferrin, 9 days; pre-albumin, 24 h; retinol-binding protein, 10 h) allow evaluation of visceral protein synthesis. Re-evaluation of cutaneous delayed hypersensitivity response determines if immunological status has changed. Measurement of albumin synthesis and body cell mass are research techniques that help delineate which nutritional regimens are best for various clinical conditions, but cannot be used routinely to evaluate nutritional therapy.

Potassium is most concentrated in the intracellular compartment. Measurement of total body potassium has been used as a measure of lean body mass. Alterations in intracellular potassium may occur quickly following starvation and/or refeeding and appear to correlate with muscle cell function. Nitrogen loss and gain under these circumstances appears

## TABLE 16   MEASURES OF NUTRITIONAL STATUS

*History and physical examination*
Weight loss
Chronic disease
Dietary habits
Anorexia
Vomiting
Diarrhea
Jaundice
Cheilosis
Glossitis
Loss of subcutaneous fat
Evidence of muscle wasting
Ascites and peripheral edema

*Measures of caloric and protein reserve*
Anthropometric assessment of body fat
Anthropometric assessment of body protein
Creatinine excretion and creatinine/height index
3-methyl histidine excretion

*Circulating protein status (visceral protein)*
Total protein
Albumin
Transferrin
Prealbumin
Retinol-binding protein

*Serial nutritional assessment*
Transferrin
Prealbumin
Retinol-binding protein
Albumin synthesis
Measurement of body cell mass

*Prognostic nutritional index* – the risk of postoperative morbidity and/or mortality

*Nitrogen balance*

*Total exchangeable potassium*

*Skeletal muscle function*

---

Prognostic nutritional index % = 158 – (16.6 × albumin) – (0.78 × triceps skinfold) – (0.20 × serum transferrin) – (0.58 × delayed hypersensitivity to any of three recall antigens (mumps, streptokinase/streptodornase, *Candida*)

to respond more slowly. Therefore, measures of muscular function may provide useful information about the effect of nutritional depletion and repletion. Clinically, such events as successful weaning from a ventilator may represent evidence that nutritional therapy is effective.

## NUTRITIONAL THERAPY

### Requirements during stress
While calorie, protein and essential nutrient requirements have been reasonably determined for healthy non-stressed adults, the requirements for varying degrees of stress remain controversial. The depletion of muscle so characteristic of severe illness has prompted numerous attempts to measure metabolism and adjust nutritional formulations of carbohydrate, fats, amino acids and trace elements, striving to achieve positive nitrogen balance and improve visceral and muscle protein mass. Most such attempts have been unsuccessful. Nutritional therapy, per se, during stress primarily decreases the loss of functional tissues. Resolution of the catabolic state requires therapy directed at the primary underlying metabolic derangement rather than more precise nutritional formulations. Curiously, the type(s) and route of administration of food stuffs may assist in the therapy of the underlying disease process without necessarily correcting specific nutritional deficits.

Table 17 lists nutritional requirements which can serve as a starting point for nutritional management. Recommendations for specific amounts of vitamins and minerals are readily available. Usually, the clinician will adjust the calories (quantity and type) and protein therapy more than the vitamin and mineral supplementation.

The use of direct or indirect measurement of resting energy expenditure along with oxygen consumption and carbon dioxide production to adjust nutritional (especially calorie administration) therapy is controversial. Energy expenditure without exercise (resting energy expenditure) is characteristically increased in most patients following hypoperfusion and/ or inflammatory insults. However, the magnitude of this increase which is secondary to disease is difficult to ascertain, since measurement of resting energy expenditure can be influenced by such variables as fever, sedation and catecholamine. In addition, the most severe states of inflammation may be associated with a decrease in resting energy expenditure, suggesting deficits in cellular metabolism sufficient to interrupt oxygen use.

Measuring oxygen consumption and carbon dioxide production can be useful for assessing the potential value of adjusting the caloric source

**TABLE 17    INITIAL ESTIMATES OF NUTRITIONAL
REQUIREMENTS (adapted from DeBiasse and Wilmore)**

*Calories (provide 80% of estimate)*
25–30 kcal/kg/day for most
40–45 kcal/kg/day severe burns and trauma

*Protein*
1.5 g/kg/day for most
2.0 g/kg/day severe burn and trauma
  type of proteins
  essential amino acids
  glutamine
  alanine

*Ratio of non-protein calories to nitrogen*
150 kcal : g nitrogen

*Carbohydrate/fat*
Carbohydrate no greater rate than 4–5 mg/kg/min
Carbohydrate/fat ratio 70 : 30
Must include essential fatty acids

*Vitamins/minerals*
Vitamin A
Vitamin D
Vitamin E
Vitamin K
Vitamin $B_1$ (thiamine)
Vitamin $B_2$ (riboflavin)
Vitamin $B_6$ (pyridoxine)
Vitamin $B_{12}$ (cyanocobalamin)
Niacin
Pantothenic acid
Biotin
Folid acid
Vitamin C
Selenium
Zinc

(carbohydrate vs. fat). Patients with a high ventilatory dead space to tidal volume ratio (VD/VT >50%) may have particular difficulty weaning from a ventilator when carbohydrate is used as the primary caloric source. Carbohydrate metabolism results in more carbon dioxide production as compared to fat, and this may provide an additional respiratory stress which can be diminished if more fat calories are used. Patients with a relatively low VD/VT ratio should not experience this difficulty.

Overfeeding of calories has several potential adverse effects including hyperglycemia, deposition of fat in the liver, excess carbon dioxide production and hypertriglyceridemia. Of these, hyperglycemia is common, even when excess feeding is not provided. However, provision of excess carbohydrate calories and the required insulin does not improve nutritional well being and promotes deposition of fat in the liver. Such deposition may be sufficient to alter hepatic function.

## Methods/types of nutritional support
The two fundamental methods of nutritional support are enteral and parenteral. These methods are not mutually exclusive and benefits may be accrued by using both in some patients. The considered benefits of enteral and parenteral nutritional support are listed in Table 18. In general, the use of enteral feeding is preferred, and access for feeding during intra-abdominal procedures should be a high priority for any patient considered critically ill during the operation or expected to be critically ill after the surgery. Placement of a tube in the jejunum, either directly or via the stomach, is the most practical since the small intestine is more likely to function than the stomach during critical illness.

Disease states that make use of the small intestine problematic are:

(1)   High small bowel fistula;

(2)   Small bowel obstruction;

(3)   Severe small bowel ileus;

(4)   Ischemic small bowel;

(5)   Hypoproteinemia;

(6)   Massive small bowel resection (short gut).

A proximal small bowel fistula (but still distal to the ligament of Trietz) makes enteral feeding less useful unless access to the small intestine can be obtained distal to the fistula. A distal small bowel fistula is not a

### TABLE 18    COMPARATIVE BENEFITS OF ENTERAL VS. PARENTERAL NUTRITIONAL SUPPORT

*Enteral*

Avoid complications of central vein access

Improved mucosal barrier function

Improved GI host defense function

    cellular

    humoral

Provision of substrate to improve host defenses and diminish inflammatory state

    glutamine

    omega-3 fatty acids

    nucleotides

*Parenteral*

Does not require GI function

Does not require GI tract access

---

contraindication for enteral feeding, since much of the feeding may be absorbed and the host defense benefits may still be realized. An obstructed or severely paralyzed small intestine will not benefit from enteral feeding. Severe small intestine ileus is rare compared to ileus of the stomach and colon.

Patients with either marked global or regional hypoperfusion may suffer sufficient ischemia to the small intestine to make enteral feeding both impractical and potentially dangerous. Absorption of food increases small intestine oxygen utilization and enteral feeding may become a 'stress' test of the ischemic small intestine, promoting further ischemic insult.

During and following resolution of severe inflammation, decreased serum albumin concentrations are common. Edema in tissues supplied by the systemic circulation (which includes the GI tract) is common. Edema of the small intestine has been implicated as an etiology of osmotic diarrhea in critically ill patients. Such edema may be aggravated by hypoalbuminemia. Therapy with albumin may decrease systemic, and thereby small intestine, edema, but only following resolution of severe systemic inflammation and the accompanying increase in total body capillary permeability. Providing albumin during severe systemic inflammation does not significantly decrease systemic edema formation.

Several enteral formulations have been developed which appear to improve the host defense functions of the GI tract and potentially alter the systemic inflammatory response during critical illness. This has been best documented in experimental and clinical studies of burn patients. The addition of glutamine, omega-3-fatty acids, increased branched-chain amino acids, arginine, nucleic acids and other nutrients also appears to improve outcome in trauma patients. As compared to parenteral nutrition, the additional expense of these enteral formulations may be of little consequence, especially if morbidity and mortality are reduced.

# 7

# THE CENTRAL NERVOUS SYSTEM

## INTRODUCTION

Central nervous system (CNS) dysfunction in critical surgical illness is usually secondary to metabolic disturbances and/or trauma, and less frequently secondary to cerebrovascular accident or CNS infection. Depressed mental status (stupor to coma) with or without focal neurological findings is common and an organized approach to physical examination and laboratory studies serves well to attain a rapid diagnosis and begin treatment. The following sections discuss anatomy and pathophysiology related primarily to coma and the corresponding physical examination findings.

## ANATOMY

Knowledge of the anatomy of the cerebral cortex, with sensory and motor loci is important for assessing focal sensory and motor deficits. However, many etiologies of depressed mental status produce global alterations in cortical function and may or may not be associated with localized findings. Important for assessing altered mental status is an understanding of the

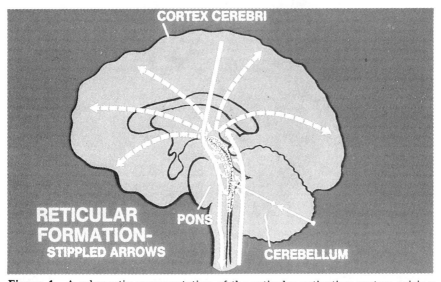

**Figure 1** A schematic representation of the reticular activating system arising from the brainstem and projecting impulses cephalad throughout the cortex. Reproduced with permission from ACS Committee on Trauma. *Advanced Trauma Life Support – Student Manual,* 1997 edn. Chicago: American College of Surgeons

anatomy of the reticular activating system (RAS), a diffuse group of neurons which extend along the central brainstem from the medulla to the thalamus (Figure 1). The RAS is stimulated by every major somatic and special sensory pathway and serves to activate the cerebral cortex. Since the RAS arises in the brainstem, knowledge of the anatomy of the brainstem is useful for evaluating the status of the RAS.

The brain is enclosed in a hard rough chamber which while protective can be responsible for direct or 'counter-coup' injury (Figure 2). The medial temporal lobe is positioned close to the midbrain, the path of the third cranial nerve, and cerebral blood vessels (Figure 3). Medial displacement of the temporal lobe is particularly likely to interrupt the function of first, the third cranial nerve, then the midbrain and, subsequently, larger areas of the brainstem (Figure 4).

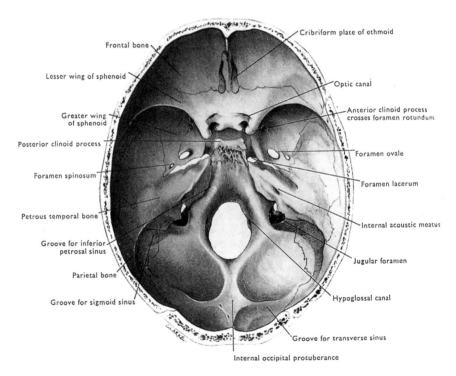

**Figure 2** The interior of the base of the skull illustrating the bony prominences which can result in direct or counter-coup injury to the brain. Reproduced with permission from Romanes GJ. *Cunningham's Manual of Practical Anatomy.* 14th edn. Oxford, UK: Oxford University Press, 1978:146

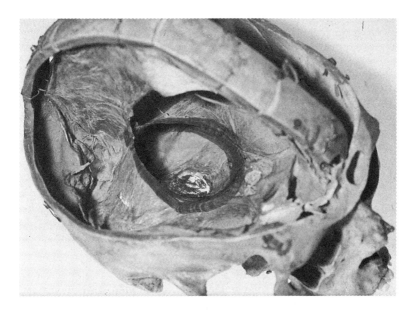

**Figure 3** An open skull depicting the tentorium and the position of the midbrain in juxtaposition to the medial, anterior tentorium and adjacent to the location of the temporal lobe. Reproduced with permission from ACS Committee on Trauma. *Advanced Trauma Life Support – Student Manual*, 1997 edn. Chicago: American College of Surgeons

The brainstem is divided into midbrain, pons and medulla (Figures 5 and 6). Brainstem or cranial nerves that are evaluated in stupor and coma include the following:

(1) The third for innervation of the medial rectus and parasympathetic innervation to the pupil;

(2) The fifth for sensation to the cornea;

(3) The seventh for motor to the eyelids;

(4) The sixth for innervation of the lateral rectus;

(5) The eighth for innervation of the vestibular apparatus;

(6) The medial longitudinal fasciculus connecting the eighth to the sixth and the third;

(7) The course of the sympathetic nervous system through the entire brainstem.

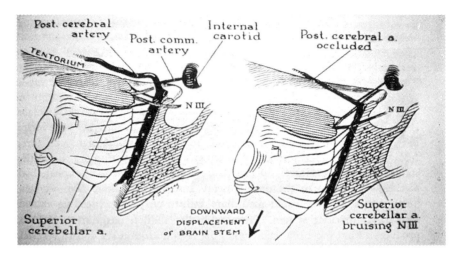

**Figure 4** A schematic representation further depicting the close apposition of the tentorium and, therefore, the temporal lobe to the midbrain, the oculomotor nerve and the brainstem circulation

## PHYSIOLOGY

Consciousness requires cortical function and is not lost unless cortical function is diffusely diminished. Diffusely diminished cortical function may result either from direct, global disruption of cortical function or from disruption of the RAS in the brainstem. Since the cortex is more sensitive to metabolic disturbances than the brainstem (i.e. hypoglycemia, hypoxia), 'cortical coma' is much more likely to be 'metabolic', whereas 'brainstem coma' most often is secondary to structural damage to the brainstem.

Much of the physical examination evaluation of the stuporose or comatose patient is dependent upon eliciting brainstem and/or posturing reflexes. The pupillary reflex depends upon intact sympathetic (dilatation from noxious stimuli) and parasympathetic (constriction from light) innervation (Figure 7). The sympathetic nervous system arises in the hypothalamus, above the brainstem, runs through the brainstem, exits from the thoracic spinal cord and follows the arterial supply to the eye. Constriction of the pupil is secondary to parasympathetic innervation which arises in the midbrain and accompanies the oculomotor nerve to the eye. Corneal reflexes represent sensation by the fifth and motor response by the seventh nerve, both in the pons. Oculovestibular and oculocaloric reflexes (Figure 8) result from stimulation of the vestibular apparatus innervated by the

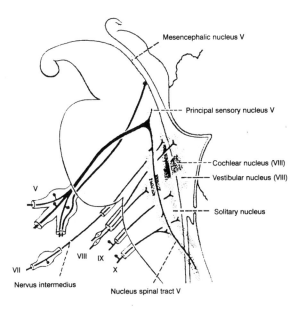

**Figure 5** A schematic representation of the sensory nerves of the brainstem with the midbrain devoid of major sensory nerves, the pons with the fifth nerve, important for the corneal reflex, and the eight nerve at the pontomedullary junction, important for the oculovestibular and oculocaloric reflexes. Reproduced with permission from *Gray's Anatomy*, 28th edn. Baltimore: Lea & Febinger, 1968

eighth nerve at the pontomedullary junction with response by the sixth and third nerves connected to the eighth nerve via the medial longitudinal fasciculus. Decorticate rigidity (arms point towards the cortex; Figure 9) to noxious stimuli represents loss of cortical-spinal innervation either from cortical or internal capsule malfunction. Decerebrate rigidity (arms point away from the cortex; Figure 10) usually represents at least partial, bilateral separation of midbrain function from higher centers.

### Physiology of cerebral blood flow, oxygen metabolism and intracranial pressure

The brain requires a continuous supply of oxygen and glucose to support the aerobic glycolysis necessary to maintain the integrity of brain neurons. The brain is proportionally more sensitive to decreased delivery of oxygen compared to decreased delivery of glucose. The cerebral metabolic rate of oxygen ($CMRO_2$) is a useful measure of brain metabolism and is calculated as follows:

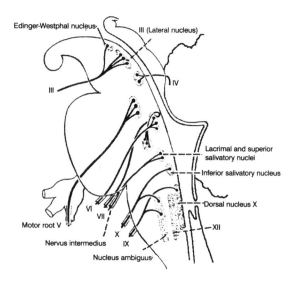

**Figure 6** A schematic representation of the motor nerves of the brainstem, with the midbrain contributing the Edinger-Westphal nucleus for parasympathetic innervation of the pupil, and the third nerve which is important for oculovestibular and oculocaloric reflexes. The pons contributes the sixth nerve, also important for oculovestibular and oculocaloric reflexes, as well as the seventh nerve which is important for the corneal reflex. Reproduced with permission from *Gray's Anatomy*, 28th edn. Baltimore: Lea & Febinger, 1968

$$\text{CMRO}_2 = \text{CBF} \times \text{C(a} - \text{v)O}_2$$

where CBF is cerebral blood flow, C is oxygen content and a and v are arterial and venous, respectively.

In awake adults CBF approximates to 50 ml/100 g tissue at $Pa_{CO_2}$ of 40 mmHg. $\text{CMRO}_2$ is about 3.2 ml/100 g under these conditions. $\text{CMRO}_2$ may increase with such activity as seizures and decrease with drug induced coma. Usually, CBF adjusts to meet alterations in $\text{CMRO}_2$. However, severe brain injury may lead to disruption of the autoregulation of CBF such that too much or too little CBF may be provided for the metabolic demands of the brain.

CBF is primarily determined by cerebral perfusion pressure (CPP) which is the difference between mean arterial pressure (MAP) and intra-cranial pressure (ICP), as well as the arteriolar vascular resistance in the brain tissue. Therefore, CBF will increase if CPP increases and/or arteri-olar resistance decreases and CBF will decrease if CPP decreases and/or

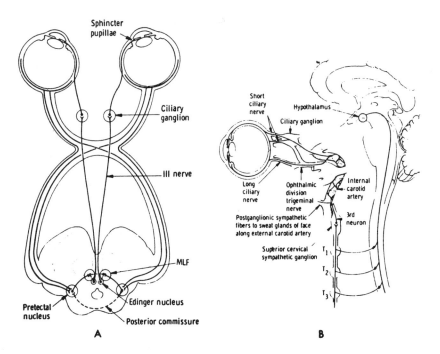

**Figure 7** A schematic representation of the anatomy of the parasympathetic, pupillary constriction, innervation of the pupil (A), and the anatomy of the sympathetic, pupillary dilatation, innervation of the pupil (B). Note that the parasympathetic system originates in the midbrain. The sympathetic system originates in the hypothalamus, above the brainstem, and courses through the brainstem before exiting via the thoracic spinal cord to follow the arterial supply to the eye. (MLF, medial longitudinal fasciculus). Reproduced with permission from Plum F, Posner JB. *The Diagnosis of Stupor and Coma*, 3rd edn. Philadelphia: FA Davis Company, 1982

arteriolar resistance increases. When CBF falls sufficiently that more oxygen cannot be extracted (< 23 ml/100 g), then $CMRO_2$ will decrease. First synaptic function ceases then cell death ensues unless the normal metabolic demand of brain cells is reduced. The equation for $CMRO_2$ shown above can be rearranged to the following:

$$C(a-v)O_2 = \frac{CMRO_2}{CBF}$$

This demonstrates that alterations in arteriovenous content are secondary to alterations in $CMRO_2$ or CBF or both. Recently, alterations in venous

CONDITION: OCULAR REFLEXES IN UNCONSCIOUS PATIENTS

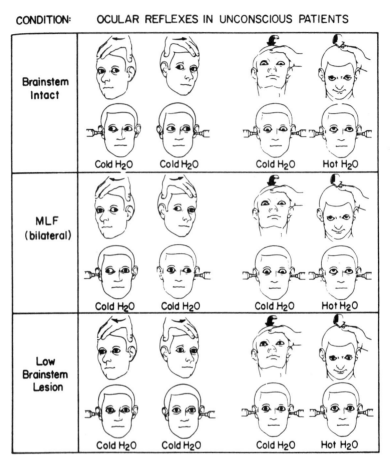

**Figure 8** A representation of normal oculovestibular and oculocaloric reflexes for a comatose patient with an intact brainstem. The stimulus to the vestibular system innervated by the eighth nerve sends impulses to the sixth nerve in the pons and the third nerve in the midbrain, which then results in conjugate medial and lateral deviation of both eyes. Note that when coma is present cold stimulation of the tympanic membrane results in deviation of the eyes towards the cold stimulus. Reproduced with permission from Plum F, Posner JB. *The Diagnosis of Stupor and Coma*, 3rd edn. Philadelphia: FA Davis Company, 1982

saturation rather than content have been argued to more accurately reflect brain oxygen status, especially when venous oxygen saturation is low indicating marked oxygen extraction. Measurement of jugular oxygen

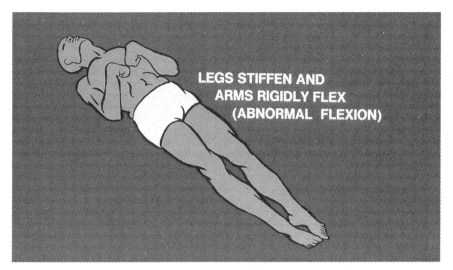

**Figure 9** A representation of decorticate posturing, with flexion of the upper extremities as the lower extremities extend

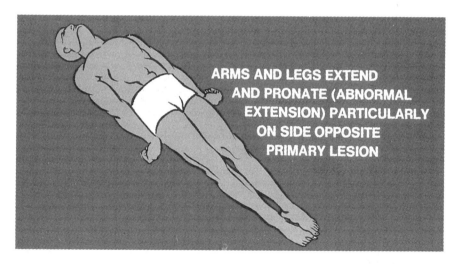

**Figure 10** A representation of decerebrate posturing, with extension of both upper and lower extremities. Figures 9 and 10 reproduced with permission from ACS Committee on Trauma; *Advanced Trauma Life Support – Student Manual*, 1997 edn. Chicago: American College of Surgeons

content or saturation as well as measurement of CBF are necessary for these calculations. To date, measurement of these variables has not become a common clinical undertaking.

ICP (normally < 15 mmHg) is determined by cerebrospinal fluid (CSF) volume, cerebral blood volume (CBV) and brain cell volume. ICP may be increased by any of the following:

(1) Increased CSF volume due to:
    (a) Obstructed flow – occlusion of third ventricle;
    (b) Obstructed reabsorption – occluded arachnoid granulationes.

(2) Increased brain cell volume due to:
    (a) Trauma – contusion;
    (b) Hyponatremia;
    (c) Hypoxia – hypoperfusion;
    (d) Infection – Reye's syndrome;
    (e) Mass lesions
        (i) trauma – hemorrhage, epidural, subdural, intraparenchymal;
        (ii) tumors.

(3) Increased cerebral blood volume due to:
    (a) Increased CBF;
    (b) Intracerebral vasodilatation.

The measurement of ICP and the use of CPP as well as oxygen related monitors to manage severe head trauma are discussed in the head trauma section.

## PHYSICAL EXAMINATION

As with all conditions, physical examination of the patient with neurological malfunction begins with vital signs. Vital signs may also alert the clinician to the presence of underlying neurological injury. Most critically ill patients are tachycardic. Bradycardia is unusual, especially in trauma patients, and may indicate increased ICP. Similarly, hypertension is less common than hypotension, and may also result from increased ICP. Since many critically ill surgical patients are assisted by a ventilator, respiratory status is a less useful indicator of neurological function, except for the broad categories of present or absent.

Neurological physical examination begins with an assessment of overall neurological activity. The Glasgow Coma Scale (Table 1) is often used for this purpose, but does not describe well the evaluation of the barely responsive or unresponsive patient. The physical examination includes

## TABLE 1   GLASGOW COMA SCALE (GCS)

| Physical examination | Points |
| --- | --- |
| *Eye-opening response* | |
| Spontaneous | 4 |
| To speech | 3 |
| To pain | 2 |
| None | 1 |
| *Verbal response* | |
| Oriented | 5 |
| Confused, still answers | 4 |
| Inappropriate words | 3 |
| Incomprehensible sou..ids | 2 |
| None | 1 |
| *Motor response* | |
| Obeys | 6 |
| Localizes | 5 |
| Withdraws | 4 |
| Abnormal flexion | 3 |
| Abnormal extension | 2 |
| None | 1 |

GCS, best eye-opening and best verbal and best motor response (maximum 15)

assessment of vital signs, Glasgow Coma Scale, pupil reflexes, corneal reflexes, oculocaloric or oculovestibular reflexes, posturing response, gross motor (upper and lower extremity), gross sensory (upper and lower extremity) and deep tendon and Babinski reflexes. Precise documentation of these aspects of the neurological examination is mandatory. Potentially confusing terminology such as 'doll's eyes' should be avoided. More useful is the statement 'oculovestibular reflex: medial and lateral rectus function bilaterally', which describes precisely the test and the results.

## ETIOLOGIES OF COMA

Coma is categorized broadly into cortical and brainstem etiologies (Table 2). As mentioned previously, the brainstem is much more resistant to metabolic derangements and requires severe metabolic insults (i.e. cardiopulmonary arrest) to malfunction. Most brainstem dysfunction is

## TABLE 2    ETIOLOGIES OF COMA

*Cortical*
Metabolic
   hypoglycemia
   hypoxia
   hypercapnia
   hyperglycemia
   hyponatremia
   hypercalcemia
   narcotics
   barbiturates
   diazepam
   severe inflammation
   liver failure
   renal failure
Infectious
   meningitis
   encephalitis
Traumatic
   diffuse contusion
   subarachnoid bleed

*Brainstem*
Metabolic
   severe hypoxia – brainstem infarct
   severe drug overdose
Traumatic
   supratentorial mass
   infratentorial mass
   direct injury

secondary to trauma or basilar artery occlusion. Broadly speaking, if physical examination is consistent with an intact brainstem (e.g. normal pupils, normal corneal reflexes, normal extraocular movements), the patient most likely has a cortical and, therefore, a metabolic coma (diffuse cortical trauma may cause similar findings). On the other hand, if any brainstem reflex is abnormal (e.g. one pupil larger and less reactive than the other, diminished corneal reflexes, absence of an extraocular movement), the patient is more likely to have a mass lesion pushing on the brainstem, or direct brainstem injury.

## CNS MALFUNCTION

### Effects of hypoperfusion on CNS function

Depending on the magnitude and duration, decreased oxygen delivery to brain tissue can cause alterations in CNS function, ranging from agitation to brain death. The sudden cessation of cerebral circulation results in coma in 6–7 s, with the cerebral cortex suffering from lack of oxygen before the brainstem. Therefore, the initial state of coma is a cortical coma. The exact duration of absent circulation that will cause irreversible cortical and subsequent brainstem death is controversial. In addition, reperfusion of ischemic brain may be attenuated by a no-reflow phenomenon (post-ischemic hypoperfusion) secondary to cerebral vascular vasospasm. Mechanisms such as extracellular potassium accumulation, intracellular calcium migration, activation of phospholipase $A_2$, products of arachidonic acid metabolism and superoxide radical generation have all been implicated in this postischemic hypoperfusion state. Several of these mechanisms are important in inflammatory conditions and, therefore, severe brain ischemia appears to result in activation of inflammation as does ischemia to other tissues.

Compared with total cessation of blood flow, electroencephalograph abnormalities have been documented to develop when CBF decreases to a range of 30–50% of normal. Patients suffering from hemorrhagic hypoperfusion are often agitated and combative. Such alterations in CNS function may be an important clinical clue that there is a deficit in the circulation. When the brain is traumatized hemorrhagic hypoperfusion may result in a sustained decrease in CBF even after systemic blood flow is restored. This suggests that a no-reflow mechanism is possible which does not require complete cessation of blood flow if the brain tissue is directly injured.

The relationship between the Glascow Coma Scale and the $CMRO_2$ in severe head trauma patients can be broadly characterized as shown in Table 3 (Glascow Coma Scale < 8 = coma). Since $CMRO_2$ is primarily determined by CBF, the association of a marked decrease in brain oxygen metabolism with severe neurological malfunction following trauma suggests that decreased CBF may aggravate brain cell dysfunction after trauma and result in 'secondary' brain injury.

### Effects of inflammation on CNS function

The intimate relationship between alterations in the circulation and inflammation is well illustrated by disease states which result in either systemic inflammation or inflammation in and around the brain (i.e.

### TABLE 3    RELATIONSHIP OF GLASCOW COMA SCALE TO CEREBRAL METABOLIC RATE OF OXYGEN ($C_{MRO_2}$)

| $C_{MRO_2}$ *(ml/100g tissue)*<br>*(normal 3.2)* | *Glascow Coma Scale*<br>*(normal 15)* |
| --- | :---: |
| 0.6 | 3.0 |
| 1.3 | 4–5 |
| 1.7 | 6–7 |

trauma). Severe systemic inflammation has been associated with reduced CBF. In addition, the mechanisms considered as etiologies of post-traumatic and post-ischemic hypoperfusion actively participate in the physiology of inflammation. Therefore, the relationship between inflammation and alterations in CBF is the best documented potential mechanism for depressed CNS function at the time of systemic and/or local inflammation. Alterations in cerebral function secondary to other potential metabolic disturbances during systemic inflammation (e.g. changes in serum amino acids) are less well documented and supported, although these concepts are not necessarily without merit.

**Head trauma**

Head trauma, especially with coma, requires careful attention to the ABCs of resuscitation, as well as an orderly diagnostic approach. This may be difficult when confronted with other major injuries and the hemorrhage and unsightly appearance associated with head injury. The basic initial clinical approach to the patient with head injury, which may begin at the scene of injury and continue into the intensive care unit (ICU) should include (1) ABCs of resuscitation, (2) determination of level of consciousness (Glasgow Coma Scale), (3) examination of the brainstem, (4) examination of the skull and face, (5) C-spine X-rays, and (6) computed tomography (CT) scan. As described in detail below, the injured brain is particularly susceptible to further insults which decrease CBF or increase the local inflammatory reaction. In addition, the brain does not tolerate hypoxia secondary to inadequate pulmonary function. Therefore, rapid and aggressive attention to the ABCs of trauma and continuing attention to oxygenation and resuscitation of the circulation are as, if not more, important with brain injury as with any other injured tissues. Previous ideas that brain injury could be limited by providing minimal resuscitation of the circulation are not supported by epidemiological studies, which demonstrate an increased risk of death and neurological disability in brain-injured patients who suffer hypotension anytime during the early post-injury period.

In the comatose patient an intact brainstem indicates a cortical coma, with little immediate threat to life from the head injury. At the opposite extreme, bilateral mid-position fixed pupils, absent corneal reflexes and no extraocular movement indicate a severely damaged brainstem with little chance of survival, let alone regaining consciousness.

The head trauma patient who deserves the most rapid evaluation and/or treatment is the patient who demonstrates some brainstem dysfunction, such as one pupil larger and less reactive, diminished or absent corneal reflex on one side, or loss of an extraocular movement. In addition, unilateral motor and/or sensory deficits should prompt aggressive diagnostic and management intervention. Until proved otherwise by diagnostic studies, these patients should be considered to have a supratentorial mass lesion producing compression of brainstem nerves or nuclei. In most hospitals much of this initial evaluation and subsequent therapy will be undertaken before the patient arrives on the ICU. On the ICU more attention will be directed at continuing to assess the level of consciousness and brainstem function as indicators for further diagnostic and/or therapeutic measures. However, the same principles apply and the ICU team should also be alert to the possibility of associated facial and cervical spinal injury.

The most common types of supratentorial head injury are cerebral contusion, diffuse axonal injury, epidural hematoma, subdural hematoma and intraparenchymal bleeding. The most common types of subtentorial head injury are cerebellar contusion and/or hemorrhage, and brainstem contusion and/or hemorrhage. Any of the supratentorial lesions may result in compression of the brainstem, either laterally (temporal lobe herniation) or symmetrically downward ('coning'). Coma may be secondary to diffuse cortical injury or interruption of the RAS in the brainstem. With subtentorial lesions coma is usually secondary to direct brainstem injury, but cerebellar enlargement may compress the pons producing indirect malfunction. Patients with no direct brainstem injury and little or no cortical injury (e.g. mild cerebral contusion, evacuated epidural hematoma) have the best prognosis.

Today, most patients with documented or suspected brain injury will have a cranial CT scan before or shortly after ICU arrival. However, even with a 'normal' CT scan, significant brain injury may be present and may require a follow-up CT scan for documentation. In addition, documented

CT abnormalities may change despite little clinical difference. Therefore, repeat CT scan is often useful in the routine evaluation of head trauma patients.

**Physical examination of the patient with head trauma**
The basic physical examination of the comatose patient was described in the CNS section. This section will further describe 'classical' findings with particular injuries.

*Temporal lobe herniation*
The temporal lobe sits on the tentorium in proximity to the midbrain and the oculomotor nerve. Supratentorial mass lesions (e.g. epidural, subdural, intraparenchymal) push the temporal lobe medially, first compressing the third nerve outside the brainstem, and resulting in an ipsilateral dilated, laterally deviated pupil (the 'blown' pupil; Figure 11). This may be associated with contralateral paralysis. Similar findings may be present with early compression of the mid-brain proper. Unfortunately, maximum pupillary dilatation and lateral deviation are not always present. A pupil may be slightly larger or sluggish, and loss of medial deviation may require testing of extraocular movements. A slightly larger pupil with good medial deviation of the eye argues against significant third nerve or midbrain malfunction.

Temporal lobe herniation does not require the presence of the loss of third nerve function. Again, any unilateral abnormality in brainstem function (e.g. loss of an extraocular movement, different pupils, loss or diminished corneal reflexes) should be considered evidence of a supratentorial mass laterally impinging upon the brainstem until proved otherwise.

*Symmetrical downward brainstem displacement 'coning'*
Symmetrical downward brainstem displacement may result from diffuse bilateral cerebral enlargement, or may follow an initial lateral displacement which subsequently interrupts cerebral circulation. Progressive loss of brainstem function from rostral to caudal is the characteristic progression, and there is little chance of function returning following therapy.

Mid-brain function is lost first. Interruption of both parasympathetic and sympathetic pupil innervation results in mid-position, fixed pupils which are often characterized as fixed and dilated. (One should remember that this is not maximal dilatation and that especially when sympathomimetic drugs are used, such as epinephrine and dopamine, maximal dilatation may be present with or without brainstem injury.) Spontaneous lateral eye deviation is rare and sixth nerve function may be elicited only

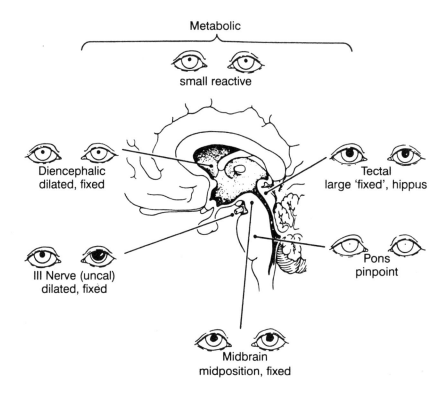

Metabolic

small reactive

Diencephalic
dilated, fixed

Tectal
large 'fixed', hippus

III Nerve (uncal)
dilated, fixed

Pons
pinpoint

Midbrain
midposition, fixed

**Figure 11** A representation of pupillary alterations, with coma affecting different regions of the brainstem. With early temporal lobe herniation the oculomotor nerve is compressed before the midbrain, which may result in the loss of parasympathetic function as well as the loss of medial deviation. This figure demonstrates the loss of parasympathetic function with sympathetic function maintained (maximal dilatation), but fails to demonstrate simultaneous lateral deviation, which may also be present. Reproduced with permission from Plum F, Posner JB. *The Diagnosis of Stupor and Coma*, 3rd edn. Philadelphia: FA Davis Company, 1982

with oculovestibular or oculocaloric reflexes. Corneal reflexes will be present. Pontine function is lost next as evidenced by no corneal and no extraocular movement. Subsequently medullary centers are destroyed with loss of gag reflex and respiration.

### Basilar skull fracture
Physical examination is usually sufficient to diagnose basilar skull fracture based on battle sign ecchymosis behind the ear, hemotympanum, bilateral

periorbital ecchymosis and/or CSF mixed with blood. CSF mixed with blood from either the nose or an ear is determined by placing the liquid on a piece of filter paper. CSF will migrate more rapidly than blood, producing a 'ring' around the blood. Patients with basilar skull fractures have a communication of CSF with the environment and are at greater risk of developing a CSF infection. Also, with evidence of frontal sinus fracture, passage of nasogastric or nasotracheal tubes should be avoided or performed with great care to prevent intracranial passage of these devices.

*ICP monitoring – maintenance of CPP*
ICP monitoring is a commonly used tool to assist in the diagnosis and management of head trauma. The different methods and their respective benefits and limits will not be discussed. Instead, indications and general measures used to reduce ICP will be presented. The indications for ICP monitoring in head trauma are Glascow Coma Score < 8, early warning of potentially reversible new mass lesion, and reduction in secondary brain injury. In general, ICP monitoring is of little use once severe brainstem injury has occurred, and is used instead to indicate the possibility of new, reversible supratentorial bleeding or to institute therapy in an attempt to avoid secondary brain injury from decreased CBF. By itself, ICP monitoring may provide prognostic information. When aggressive attempts are used to manage ICP, poor outcome correlates directly with the highest ICP as well as the percentage of time the ICP is > 20 mmHg. Successful lowering of the ICP using surgical intervention and/or medical therapy is associated with a better outcome than either no therapy or therapy that is not successful.

Methods used to reduce ICP are generally used for ICP >20 mmHg and include:

(1) Elevating head of bed;

(2)· Hyperventilation, $P_{CO_2}$ about 25 mmHg;

(3) Increasing serum osmolality with
    (a) Mannitol,
    (b) ?Hypertonic saline;

(4) Dehydration by
    (a) Water restriction,
    (b) Diuretics;

(5) Barbiturate coma;

(6) Paralysis;

(7) CSF drainage.

Of those listed, prolonged therapy with mannitol and hyperventilation may have deleterious side-effects. Both are more useful for the acute change in ICP that may stimulate further investigation and/or management and not as a long-term management tool. Dehydration, elevating the head of the bed and use of loop diuretics are not recommended. Barbiturate coma and paralysis for ICP control are advocated by some. Drainage of CSF will be discussed further as part of a regimen advocated to keep CPP ≥ 70 mmHg.

While methods used to lower ICP may have therapeutic benefit, monitoring techniques that are directly applicable to the concept of maintaining excellent oxygen delivery to the injured brain are gaining acceptance. As described above, measurement of CBF, $C_{MRO_2}$ and jugular venous saturation are used both in experimental and clinical research to evaluate cerebral oxygen metabolism.

The measurement of CPP is most commonly available, compared with more sophisticated monitoring techniques. Since CBF is determined by both CPP and cerebrovascular resistance, CPP does not provide a direct monitor of CBF or oxygen metabolism. However, the concept of maintaining CPP ≥ 70 mmHg to diminish secondary brain injury is gaining acceptance and obviates the necessity of more sophisticated monitoring.

Two methods may be used to maintain/increase CPP: maintain/increase MAP, or decrease ICP. The first principle for maintaining MAP is to ensure excellent resuscitation of the circulation by providing normal intravascular volume. The fluids used for intravascular volume resuscitation following brain injury continue to be studied, but preliminary evidence suggests that hypertonic saline may be particularly beneficial for early resuscitation, and may restore intravascular volume with less edema formation in the cranial vault, especially in brain tissue that is not directly injured. As a result ICP elevation is less. In humans, resuscitating patients with head injuries at the scene of the accident with a hypertonic saline/dextran solution has resulted in better neurological outcome. The role of hypertonic saline for resuscitation of the patient with brain injury beyond the initial resuscitation time frame is uncertain. Avoiding hypotension because of new disease (e.g. severe new inflammation, hemorrhage) or iatrogenic interventions (e.g. sedative overdose) is crucial to this therapeutic plan.

If these measures do not result in an adequate CPP, Rosner and colleagues (1995) have advocated a regimen which includes volume expansion, CSF drainage, vasoconstrictor administration, and mannitol, in that order, to achieve the CPP endpoint. Clearly titration of CPP using this combination of techniques requires active participation and direction by the neurosurgery staff. Management that may cause ICP to increase must be used with caution. These include hypoventilation, overhydration, positive end-expiratory pressure, pneumatic antishock garment application and nitroglycerin administration. ICP monitoring should be considered for any severe head trauma patient receiving such interventions.

### Diabetes insipidus

Diabetes insipidus is common after severe head injury and may also be present with relatively mild head trauma. The diagnostic hallmarks are large volumes of dilute urine with low osmolality and with rising serum osmolality. The diuresis may be of a magnitude to produce hypovolemic hypoperfusion. Parenteral administration of antidiuretic hormone is the treatment of choice and may be given as a long-acting injection or as an intravenous drip. The kidneys are exquisitely sensitive to AVP and a low-dose drip allows careful titration in patients who may have fluctuating diabetes insipidus and intravascular volume.

### ICU delirium

ICU delirium is common and use of the term ICU psychosis is a misnomer, since most patients are delirious and not truly psychotic. The etiologies of ICU delirium are many (Table 4), and a careful search for an anatomic, metabolic or drug-related etiology should be undertaken. Ascribing delirium to simply the ICU atmosphere is unwise and may lead to a delay in diagnosis.

### Spinal cord injury

Spinal cord injury should always be suspected in any trauma victim and requires careful evaluation of neurological examination and radiographic information. ICU personnel may receive a patient after emergency surgery, which had precluded such evaluation preoperatively.

Neurological findings that suggest spinal cord injury include symmetrical loss of motor function, symmetrical loss of sensation, loss of sensation below the nipple line, flaccid areflexia and warm extremities with hypotension. Warm extremities with hypotension suggest interruption of sympathetic-mediated vasoconstriction, well-maintained cardiac output and low systemic vascular resistance. This 'neurogenic' shock does not represent hypoperfusion, and does not require aggressive resuscitation

## TABLE 4    ETIOLOGIES OF ICU DELIRIUM

*Anatomic*
Cerebral vascular accident
Trauma related hemorrhage
Trauma related increased intracranial pressure

*Metabolic*
Severe inflammation
Hypoxia
Hypoperfusion
Hypo- or hypernatremia
Hypo- or hyperglycemia
Hypercapnia

*Drug*
Barbiturate
Narcotic
Sedatives
$H_2$ blockers
Antipsychotics

unless there is an associated brain injury which will require measures to maintain the CPP. Under these circumstances a vasoconstrictor may be necessary. Other management concepts for spinal cord injury (steroid administration, surgical stabilization of fractures, etc.) are primarily guided by the neurosurgical and/or orthopedic physicians involved in the management of such injuries.

# THE
# INTEGUMENT/BURNS

## FUNCTIONS OF THE SKIN

The functions of the skin that are lost in burn injury are (1) prevention of loss of body fluids, (2) mechanical barrier to infection, (3) protection against environmental temperature change, and (4) barrier to toxic agents. Loss of the stratum corneum allows the evaporative loss of water from normal (0.1–0.5 ml/cm$^2$/h) to 10–12 ml/cm$^2$/h (2 liters/24 h for a 50% burn). Electrolytes and protein are also lost from the vascular volume into the burn wound and subsequently into dressings. After a burn injury bacteria and fungi may colonize injured tissues that often have either a poor blood supply or are frankly necrotic. The thermoregulatory function of the skin is lost, which allows greater heat loss by evaporation and convection. The most common possibly toxic substances encountered on the burn patient's skin are topical antibiotics, which are discussed later in this Chapter.

## THE EFFECTS OF HYPOPERFUSION ON BURN INJURY

Prior to the 1960s, severely burned patients often suffered organ injury and death secondary to prolonged hypoperfusion. Beginning in the mid-1960s aggressive resuscitation with large quantities of crystalloid solutions avoided early death from a grossly inadequate circulation. However, as with any severe inflammatory insult, alterations in the microcirculation may develop which appear to respond only to a hyperdynamic circulation rather than simply to the restoration of normal circulatory dynamics.

Alterations in the microcirculation occur primarily at the burn site, but, depending on burn size, capillary permeability and capillary hydrostatic pressures may increase in a total body fashion. Many mediators of inflammation have been identified in the burn wound (e.g. histamine, cytokines, complement activation, prostaglandins, leukotrienes, serotonin, superoxide radicals) and may influence capillary permeability and hydrostatic pressures both in the burn wound and systemically. In addition, the tissue adjacent to permanently damaged cells (zone of stasis vs. zone of coagulation) has the potential to survive if worsening regional hypoperfusion does not develop.

Cellular malfunction may develop as a local and systemic consequence. Therefore, cells not directly injured may exhibit deficiencies in membrane pump activity, which allows interstitial fluid to migrate into the cells. Inadequate resuscitation will aggravate this local and diffuse cellular malfunction and possibly result in increased cell death both at the site of injury and systemically.

While burn wound edema may be considered potentially damaging to the viable nearby partially injured skin, a deficit in perfusion to these tissues is more detrimental. Therefore, early burn resuscitation is optimal when both global and regional circulation is restored. Edema formation, particularly during the first 24 h, is an unavoidable consequence of the tissue injury and the achievement of adequate resuscitation. The various formulae used for resuscitation may influence local and total body edema formation, but should never be used in a fashion that would diminish total body tissue perfusion.

## THE EFFECTS OF INFLAMMATION ON BURN INJURY

As previously stated, inflammatory mediators are generated after a burn injury as with any injury to tissues. Deleterious local and systemic effects, such as regional and systemic hypoperfusion, immunosuppression and pulmonary malfunction, can develop from mediator activity. Therapies that limit mediator activity (e.g. antioxidants, plasma exchange, inhibition of thromboxane and leukotriene formation, administration of a serotonin antagonist) suggest that the local and systemic hemodynamic, as well as other, manifestations of large burns are influenced by the severity of burn wound inflammation. However, attempts to limit the deleterious effects of this inflammatory response are not clinically available. Limiting tissue injury by adequate resuscitation of the circulation is the mainstay for restricting this inflammatory response.

## RESUSCITATION

Resuscitation of the burn victim begins with the basic ABCs as with any critically ill patient. Patients with evidence of thermal or toxic (smoke inhalation) injury to the face, mouth or pharynx should undergo intubation, preferably before upper airway obstruction is clinically evident. Immediate difficulties with breathing (decreased arterial $Po_2$ and increased $Pco_2$) suggest either direct injury to the lung (smoke inhalation) or decreased chest wall compliance (circumferential chest burn). The former would require supplemental oxygen and possibly ventilator management. The latter may require escharotomy (usually vertical lateral incisions) to relieve the restrictive effects of the eschar. Resuscitation of the circulation begins with an estimate of the percentage of the burn (rule of nines in adults) and the patient's body weight. Recognition of partial vs.

full thickness injury is not critical for this determination. All the burned area should be considered in this calculation.

Burn injury results in hypovolemic hypoperfusion secondary to the acute depletion of intravascular volume by the following mechanisms:

(1) Sequestration of fluid in the injured tissue;

(2) Migration of fluid into the intracellular space;

(3) Interstitial edema in non-burned tissue:
    (a) Secondary to decreased plasma oncotic pressure;
    (b) Secondary to generalized increased capillary permeability;

(4) Destruction of red blood cells;

(5) Evaporative loss estimated by ml/h = (25 + % burn) × total body surface in square meters.

Loss of fluid into the burn wound is well accepted, with an increase in local capillary permeability which lasts 24–36 h. Loss of fluid into the intracellular space from decreased cell membrane function and the mechanism of interstitial edema in non-burned tissues are controversial topics. However, the infrequent incidence of acute respiratory distress syndrome (ARDS) in burns without inhalation injury argues against a marked increase in total body capillary permeability. Red cell destruction is usually not apparent early, since the hematocrit usually increases in response to the larger loss of plasma. Evaporative loss is also extensive. The magnitude of intravascular fluid loss depends on the severity and extent of the burn and associated injuries. With a major burn (> 30% surface area) fluid is lost initially at a rate of about 4 ml/kg/h, which then requires more than this rate of fluid replacement to maintain vascular volume. The additional injuries of smoke inhalation and muscle necrosis cause further fluid sequestration.

The choice of fluids most commonly advocated for intravascular volume resuscitation are listed in Tables 1 and 2. As seen in Table 2, the total amount of sodium and water is very similar over the first 48 h for a 40% burn in a 70-kg adult. Several authors recommend crystalloid only during the first 24 h of increased capillary permeability, followed by colloid to reduce fluid administration, increase serum oncotic pressure and presumably reduce edema in the burn and non-burned tissues.

Another method of providing resuscitation with less water administration is through intravenous hypertonic saline. Several studies in burns, trauma and severe inflammation demonstrate that hemodynamic resusci-

### TABLE 1    FLUID RESUSCITATION REGIMENS

| | 24 h | | 48 h | |
| --- | --- | --- | --- | --- |
| *Regimen* | *Water* | *Protein* | *Water* | *Protein* |
| Evans | 1.0 ml/kg/% burn | 1.0 ml/kg/% | 1.5 ml/kg/% burn | 1.5 ml/kg/% |
| | LR + 2000 ml $H_2O$/24 h | burn/24 h | LR + 4000 ml $H_2O$/48 h | burn/48 h |
| Brooke | 1.5 ml/kg/% burn | 0.5 ml/kg/% | 2.25 ml/kg/% burn | 0.75 ml/kg/% |
| | LR + 2000 ml $H_2O$/24 h | burn/24 h | LR + 4000 ml $H_2O$/48 h | burn/48 h |
| Parkland | 4 ml/kg/% burn | colloid PRN | 500–2000 ml $H_2O$ | colloid PRN |
| | LR/24 h | | in second 24 h | |

LR, lactated ringer solution; PRN, take as required

### TABLE 2    COMPARISON OF FORMULAE
### (40% BURN IN A 70-KG ADULT)*

| *Regimen* | *Water administered* (ml/48 h) | *Sodium administered* (mEq/48 h) |
| --- | --- | --- |
| Evans | 12 400 | 1736 |
| Brooke | 12 400 | 1694 |
| Parkland | 13 200 | 1716 |

*From Artz *et al.*, 1979

tation depends primarily on the amount of sodium administered rather than the amount of water. Using solutions with twice the concentration of sodium results in the administration of about half the amount of water given with isotonic solutions and an associated reduction in burn, and possibly non-burn, edema. Presumably, water moves out of the intracellular compartment to increase interstitial and intravascular volume. The administration of concentrated crystalloid may allow the same reduction in edema as does colloid administration but with much less cost. The indications for hypertonic saline and the duration of administration appear to be burn-center specific, with no general accepted guidelines. However, monitoring serum sodium is a must and administration of hypertonic saline is usually stopped if the serum sodium reaches 160 mEq/l. Disturbingly, a recent study, by Huang and colleagues, suggested that the use of hypertonic saline in burn shock increased the incidence of renal failure and death.

Whatever resuscitation method chosen, no formula is adequate to predict precisely each patient's requirements. Clinical parameters, such as blood pressure, pulse, mental status, skin color, urine output and hematocrit must be followed repeatedly to assess perfusion status. Low urine output (< 0.5 ml/kg/h) and rising hematocrit usually indicate intravascular volume deficits. Central venous pressure or pulmonary artery catheter monitoring is not commonly needed, except possibly in patients with known significant heart disease or associated respiratory failure. Myocardial suppression from burn injury has been described but cardiac malfunction is a rare etiology of prolonged hypoperfusion. Since burn patients are markedly susceptible to infection and venous thrombosis, central venous catheters should be avoided when possible.

Many mediators are released from white cells and platelets following burn injury and may be responsible for both the local and systemic physiological derangements. Occasionally aggressive resuscitation efforts are unsuccessful in reversing 'burn shock'. Under these circumstances measures taken to wash the blood of toxins (e.g. exchange therapy, continuous hemofiltration) may produce dramatic hemodynamic improvement. Whether such measures are beneficial in less critical situations remains to be studied.

Resuscitation is designed to improve the circulation; therefore, circumferential burns, especially to extremities, may produce sufficient compression to decrease perfusion to the compressed and more distal tissues. Escharotomy, incision of the burn wound parallel to the blood and nerve supply, is indicated whenever vascular compromise is suspected.


## INHALATION INJURY

Inhalation injury is another immediate threat to life in both burned and unburned patients. The spectrum of inhalation injury includes upper airway, smaller airways and alveolar injuries. Heat is not transmitted effectively below the vocal cords unless carried by a substance with a high specific heat, such as steam. Therefore, the respiratory 'burn' is most often secondary to the toxic products of combustion, such as aldehydes, ketones, hydrochloric acid, other acids and alkalis, inhaled with smoke. This may result in marked upper airway, smaller airway and alveolar injury alone, or in any combination. Therefore, patients may present with problems including upper airway obstruction, bronchospasm, alveolar flooding, or all three.

Inhalation injury should be suspected in any burn patient, but particularly in those burned in a closed space with much nearby material aflame. Flash burns from an explosion, for instance, are less likely to produce prolonged toxin exposure. Smoke inhalation is more likely in patients with facial burns and singed nasal vibrissae. Since the toxins are usually mixed with smoke, evidence of smoke in the tracheobronchial tree (e.g. expectorated soot, suctioned soot particles after endotracheal intubation) establishes the diagnosis. Bronchoscopy demonstrating soot, laryngeal or bronchial edema, and/or other investigation (e.g. ventilation perfusion scans, xenon washout scans) should be reserved for patients suspected of having a significant inhalation injury without other evidence. Carbon monoxide is inhaled frequently with smoke and can serve as a marker of exposure intensity. Carbon monoxide is also the most common etiology of death at the fire scene. Administration of 100% oxygen is the primary therapy for carbon monoxide intoxication and is logical for the early management of any severely burned patient.

The therapy of inhalation injury is determined by which problem(s) predominate. Upper airway obstruction requires endotracheal intubation or tracheostomy. Smaller airway injury usually requires intubation for respiratory toilet and often bronchodilators to diminish bronchospasm. Alveolar injury results in non-cardiogenic pulmonary edema and management similar to that employed for ARDS patients (see Chapter 4, The pulmonary system; Lung dysfunction). Nitric oxide inhalation and the use of high-frequency jet ventilation may have particular benefit following some inhalation injury.

The incidence of non-cardiogenic pulmonary edema with smoke inhalation is controversial. Most authors agree, however, that several days of worsening pulmonary status usually indicates infection, commonly in the burn wound itself. At this time after injury, non-cardiogenic pulmonary edema from such an insult distant from the lungs (true ARDS) is not a continuation of the smoke inhalation injury *per se*.

Pneumonia risk subsequent to inhalation injury is significant and must be considered as an etiology or deteriorating pulmonary function as should pulmonary embolism.

## INFECTION IN BURN PATIENTS

Burn injury results in several factors that promote susceptibility to infection including a break in skin barrier, necrotic tissue, depressed non-specific immunity and depressed specific immunity. Consequently, infection is the major cause of mortality in burn patients and may arise from any or all of several foci, including the burn wound, pneumonia, phlebitis and the urinary tract.

Burn wound infection may be difficult from both diagnostic and therapeutic considerations. Patients may die of burn wound infection without having documented bacteremia or fungemia, and patients may have bacteremia or fungemia without burn wound infection. The precise diagnosis of burn wound sepsis requires documentation of burn wound invasion (i.e. $\geq 10^5$ organisms/g of tissue, pathological demonstration of nearby viable tissue invaded by organisms). Simple surface cultures are inadequate. Burn wound sampling for culture and biopsy should begin by day 3 to locate invasion which will require debridement before other sites.

The best method of limiting the consequences of burn wound infection is prophylaxis. Methods used to reduce the rate of burn wound infection are:

(1) Debridement of loose, necrotic tissue;

(2) Topical antibiotics;

(3) Controlled environment;

(4) Early excision and grafting;

(5) Intestinal feeding and/or prophylactic intestinal antibiotics.

Most authorities have abandoned the use of antistreptococcal systemic antibiotics in the first 24–48 h. Initial cleansing of burned tissue of extraneous debris and loose dead skin is usually followed by the application of topical antibiotics:

(1) Silver nitrate: poor eschar penetration, must begin early, bacteriostatic, no resistant organisms, no sensitivity, painless, rapid debridement of eschar, absorption of large amounts of water from the wound, leaching of sodium, potassium, magnesium, calcium into wound and dressings;

(2) Mafenide: good eschar penetration, bacteriostatic, painful, sensitivity possible, carbonic anhydrase inhibition;

(3) Silver sulfadiazine: intermediate eschar penetration, bacteriostatic, painless, sensitivity possible, leukopenia, thrombocytopenia.

Dressings are applied to keep the antibiotic in contact with the wound and to support splints.

Once this initial care is provided, it is important for the patient's environment to be as organism free as possible. Private rooms or enclosed beds are preferred in a traffic-controlled dedicated ward separate from other critically ill surgical patients. Personnel must adhere strictly to handwashing, mask, gown and glove protocols.

The burn wound itself provides the largest potential focus for invasive infection; therefore excision of the burn wound with grafting is the most effective method of preventing burn wound infection. When burn wound infection is established, this method becomes effective therapy. Many studies have demonstrated improved immunological function following excision, which suggests that total body mechanisms for combating infection are enhanced by such local therapy. However, there are difficulties with excision and grafting in adults. Transfusions of red cells are commonly needed with each excision and have associated coagulopathies, fluid-balance difficulties and risk of disease transmission. Anesthesia risk includes hypoventilation, especially if adequate minute ventilation for these hypermetabolic patients is not provided during transport or during the procedure. Extensive burns limit the availability of autografts, and substitution with homograft (cadaver), heterograft (pig), biological dressings (amnion), or artificial skin is often necessary. Efforts at major excision and grafting require dedicated personnel and an institution committed to the care of the severe-burn patient. Care is best provided in burn centers.

The gastrointestinal (GI) tract may be the source of microorganisms in the circulation, and, therefore, since burn patients may develop infection from such organisms, the concepts of feeding the GI tract to improve the mucosal barrier to microorganisms and/or selectively decontaminating the GI tract have been studied recently. Early intestinal feeding appears to reduce the risk of infection both from the GI tract and from other sources. Selective decontamination of the GI tract remains controversial, with the exception of the effect on subsequent fungal infection (see Chapter 10, Intensive care unit infectious disease; Opportunistic infection in the ICU).

## NUTRITIONAL SUPPORT

The hypermetabolic burn-injured patient exhibits all the hormone–substrate interactions described previously as secondary to injury and/or infection (see Chapter 6, The Gastrointestinal/nutritional system; Nutritional physiology), except that caloric expenditure and protein catabolism are greater than in any other stress state. Nutritional therapy can only decrease protein catabolism until the burn injury and any subsequent infection are treated effectively, as with other less severe alterations.

Estimates of caloric need are best determined by indirect calorimetry. However, a reasonable estimate can be obtained using the following formula:

$$\text{energy requirements} = 25 \text{ kcal/kg} + 40 \text{ kcal/% BSA}$$

where BSA is burned surface area, with a maximum of 50%. Above a 50% burn, further provision of calories does not appear to improve nitrogen retention and may aggravate liver dysfunction. Glucose administration is calculated to approximate 5 mg/kg/min with the plan to administer 60% of calories as carbohydrate and the rest as fat. Protein is administered at a rate of about 2 g/kg/day. Both enteral and parenteral food administration can be used, with the enteral route preferred for the reasons above and to avoid the infectious, mechanical and thrombogenic problems with central venous access. Beginning enteral feedings in the first 2 postburn days is ideal.

Methods used to reduce energy expenditure and potentially improve protein synthesis include maintaining a warm environment to limit evaporative heat loss calorie expenditure, excellent resuscitation to reduce the neurohumoral effects on metabolism, excellent wound care to decrease inflammatory mediator influences on the hypermetabolic state, early diagnosis and therapy of infections, and maintenance of GI tract integrity (all these measures are applicable to any critically ill surgical patient).

A novel method of reducing the hypermetabolism of burn injury and improving nutritional status is the administration of growth hormone. Preliminary studies suggest that nitrogen balance and morbidity are improved following growth hormone administration. This suggests that many of the neurohumoral and mediator-induced alterations in metabolism may be diminished using a single anabolic hormone.

## MUSCLE INJURY WITH BURNS

Muscle injury with burns may occur for several reasons including ischemia, direct heat injury, other trauma and electrical burn. Ischemia from circumferential injury has already been addressed. Direct heat injury, the fourth-degree burn, may damage muscle and result in myoglobulinemia.

Clinical clues to this degree of injury as with missed injuries elsewhere (e.g. fractures, ruptured spleen) include difficulty with resuscitation (more fluid required than expected), severe oliguria, brown urine, hyperkalemia, rapidly rising creatinine and markedly elevated serum creatine phosphokinase (CPK). Debridement of necrotic muscle is necessary to eliminate a potential focus of invasive infection as well as the potentially renal toxic effects of myoglobin and life-threatening hyperkalemia.

Electrical burns are a particular problem because the extent of muscle injury may be far greater than the skin injury indicates. In addition, as the electrical current passes through the body any organ in the path may be damaged despite clear evidence of entrance and exit wounds on extremities. However, most injury occurs where the cross-sectional area is less, thereby concentrating the current. When muscle is damaged by current, edema formation in fascial compartments results in compartment syndromes and subsequent ischemic injury. Therefore, suspicion of muscle damage is managed by an early aggressive approach to explore potentially injured areas, perform fasciotomy where necessary, and debride dead muscle. This will prevent further loss of tissue from ischemia and relieve the kidneys of the myoglobin burden. Technetium 99 muscle scans may aid identification of compromised muscle which may not be clinically apparent or suspected. Concern about myocardial injury with electrical burns is related primarily to the acute insult and the development of fatal arrhythmias. Subsequent myocardial morbidity is rare.

# 9

# THE HEMATOPOIETIC SYSTEM

Normal coagulation
Effects of hypoperfusion on coagulation
Effects of inflammation on coagulation
Disorders of coagulation
Massive transfusion (>10 units of packed cells)
      Autotransfusion
Hypothermia
Transfusion of blood products
      Adverse effects of transfused blood products

## NORMAL COAGULATION

Vascular endothelium inhibits coagulation via such mechanisms as the secretion of prostacyclin, which decreases platelet function; heparin sulfate proteoglycans, which enhance the activity of antithrombin III; and thrombomodulin, which can inactivate thrombin. Injury to the vasculature results in procoagulant rather than anticoagulant activity, with the platelet as the normal first responder. Platelets adhere and aggregate, forming a plug. Platelets promote further platelet activity and the coagulation process by releasing numerous factors including ADP, serotonin, arachidonic acid products, platelet factor 4, platelet factor 5 and growth factors. Thrombin generated from platelet procoagulant activity results in further platelet activity and more thrombin generation.

Two protein/enzymatic cascades related to coagulation proteins have been described: the intrinsic system which does not require tissue proteins but only the proteins contained in plasma, and the extrinsic system which responds to tissue proteins. The factors/proteins related to the steps in these two cascades can be seen in Table 1. The prothrombin time (PT) is a test of the entire extrinsic system, the partial thromboplastin time (PTT) is a test of the entire intrinsic system.

Clinical bleeding disorders are noted secondary to platelet deficiency either in number or function as well as deficits in coagulation factors VIII, IX, X and V. Prothrombin and factors VII, IX and X are vitamin K dependent. Proteins that limit the coagulation cascade are antithrombin III, protein C and protein S, the latter two proteins being vitamin K dependent. Removal of the fibrin clot is accomplished by activation of plasminogen to plasmin by urokinase or tissue plasminogen activator. Fibrin-derived breakdown products are soluble, and one that binds to factor XIIIa is called the D-dimer which is frequently measured as an indicator of fibrinolysis.

## EFFECTS OF HYPOPERFUSION ON COAGULATION

Few experimental and clinical data address specifically the relationship between hypoperfusion and coagulation. Most clinical studies investigate the relationship between massive blood loss and coagulation deficits and some demonstrate a relationship between episodes of hypotension and the magnitude of coagulopathy. Massive transfusion is associated with prolongation of the PT and PTT but not usually to coagulopathic levels. Most often thrombocytopenia is the primary coagulation deficit following massive hemorrhage. The association of prolonged hypotension with more

### TABLE 1   COAGULATION PROTEINS/FACTORS CASCADES

*Initial step*

Intrinsic
  factor XII
  high molecular weight kininogen
  prekallikrein
  surface for activation
Extrinsic
  tissue factor
  factor VIIa
  calcium
  cell membrane

*Middle steps*

Intrinsic
  activation of factor XI
  activation of factor IX
Extrinsic
  activation of factor IX
  activation of factor X

*Final steps (common pathway)*

Activated factor X reacts with activated factor V, calcium and cell
  membranes which activates factor II
Activated factor II with calcium and cell membranes converts prothrombin
  to thrombin and then fibrinogen to fibrin

---

severe coagulopathy suggests that hypoperfusion can initiate a process which aggravates coagulopathy beyond the dilutional effect of massive resuscitation.

A fall in platelet count is characteristic of severe inflammatory states, and therefore, since hypoperfusion can elicit an inflammatory response, thrombocytopenia after massive transfusion could be secondary to both dilutional effects and sequestration. Prolongation of the PT and PTT following massive transfusion and episodes of hypoperfusion can similarly be considered secondary to dilutional effects as well as inflammation (see below). In addition, prolonged hypoperfusion of the liver may inhibit synthesis of coagulation proteins.

## EFFECTS OF INFLAMMATION ON COAGULATION

Severe inflammation characteristically results in a decreased platelet count. Platelet sequestration in the lungs secondary to thromboxane release appears to be a potent mechanism for this common phenomenon. Severe inflammation may also result in a coagulation disorder consistent with disseminated intravascular coagulation (DIC) (see below). Thrombocytopenia as well as prolongation of the clotting cascade are common features of DIC.

## DISORDERS OF COAGULATION

The types of coagulation disorders seen regularly in surgery are:

(1) Congenital disorders:
      (a) Von Willebrand disease;
      (b) Hemophilia A;
      (c) Hemophilia B;
      (d) Factor XI deficiency.

(2) Acquired disorders (pre-existing):
      (a) Thrombocytopenia;
      (b) Liver disease;
      (c) Aspirin intake;
      (d) Vitamin K deficiency;
      (e) Renal disease.

(3) Acquired disorders (acute):
      (a) Thrombocytopenia;
      (b) DIC;
      (c) Fibrinolysis;
      (d) Hypothermia.

The pre-existing disorders will not be discussed further.

Thrombocytopenia is common in critical illness and may be secondary to various etiologies including:

(1) Severe inflammation (with or without DIC);

(2) Massive transfusion;

(3) Heparin induced;

(4) Suppression of platelet production due to:
      (a) Chloramphenicol;

    (b) Ethanol;
    (c) Thiazide diuretics;
    (d) Sulfonylureas;
    (e) Estrogens;
    (f) Nutritional deficiency ($B_{12}$, folate).

(5) Increased destruction:
    (a) Quinidine;
    (b) Heparin as above.

Severe inflammation, massive transfusion and heparin-induced are the most common etiologies. Heparin-induced thrombocytopenia may occur in 5% of patients receiving the drug. With first-time exposure to heparin this condition usually becomes manifest after several days, consistent with the generation of the IgG antibody responsible for the IgG–heparin immune complex which captures platelets. Since this is an immunological rather than a toxic reaction to the drug, the potential for this disorder is not closely related to the dose. As with any IgG-mediated process, patients who had previously received heparin and receive it again may manifest this disorder more rapidly. The resultant thrombocytopenia most often is mild and results in little or no morbidity. However, in some patients acute arterial thrombosis may develop with severe sequelae (i.e. myocardial infarction, cerebrovascular accident). Therefore, repeated measurement of platelet count is indicated for any patient receiving heparin. With all the common causes of thrombocytopenia, the management of the underlying etiology is the mainstay of therapy, with platelet transfusion reserved for actively bleeding patients.

The acute disorders of DIC and fibrinolysis may be difficult to diagnose and treat. The non-hematological clinical features of DIC are fever, hypotension, acidosis, respiratory failure, renal dysfunction and neurological alterations (focal). The common clinical associations with DIC are severe inflammation, obstetric and gynecological disease, prostate disease (fibrinolysis), malignancy, cardiac surgery, vascular surgery and head trauma. The laboratory tests for DIC are listed in Table 2. Fibrinolysis is less likely to result in thrombocytopenia, as compared to DIC.

The treatment of DIC and fibrinolysis is directed primarily at the underlying disease and supportive therapy is maintained until the disease is controlled. When patients are bleeding with DIC, platelets, fresh frozen plasma and sometimes cryoprecipitate are administered. Heparin administration during active bleeding is controversial, but strongly advocated by some. When thrombosis is the major phenomenon, then heparin is

## TABLE 2 LABORATORY DIAGNOSIS OF DISSEMINATED INTRAVASCULAR COAGULATION (DIC)

|  | Normal | DIC (mean) |
|---|---|---|
| Platelets ($\times 10^3/mm^3$) | 150–400 | 52 |
| Prothrombin time | 11–13 | 18 |
| Fibrinogen (mg/dl) | 200–300 | 135 |
| Anti-thrombin III levels | normal | decreased |
| Fibrin degradation products ($\mu$g/ml) | <10 | >10* |
| D-Dimer | 0 | increased |

*greater with significant fibrinolysis

indicated. When fibrinolysis is paramount, treatment with a fibrinolytic inhibitor ($\varepsilon$-amino-caproic acid, tranexamic acid) is indicated.

## MASSIVE TRANSFUSION (>10 UNITS OF PACKED CELLS)

The frequency and magnitude of the problems related to large volumes of stored blood given rapidly are controversial. The adverse effects of a large volume of blood delivered at a fast rate are altered hemoglobin affinity for oxygen, citrate infusion, hypothermia, acidosis, electrolyte disturbance and coagulopathy. Those of a large volume of blood only include trans-mission of disease and depressed immunocompetence. Problems appear to be transient provided that the patient is rapidly resuscitated, and thereby suffering minimal hypoperfusion. However, when hypoperfusion is prolonged each of these abnormalities is accentuated by the underlying disease and probably augmented by the alterations in the administered blood products. However, this does not mean that red cells, for instance, should be avoided when a patient needs oxygen-carrying capacity and large living particles to maintain intravascular volume and deliver oxygen. Rather, careful evaluation of the necessity of each blood product should precede administration and arbitrary formulae and indications for blood products should be avoided. This has been particularly borne out with routine regimens designed to replace calcium, platelets and coagulation proteins. Only patients with medical bleeding and measured abnormalities related to massive transfusion deficiencies should receive therapy as described in Table 3.

### TABLE 3    TREATMENT OF MASSIVE TRANSFUSION DEFICIENCIES

| Treatment | Deficiencies |
|---|---|
| Calcium (for citrate toxicity-induced hypocalcemia and resultant myocardial depression) | severe hepatic dysfunction (liver transplant), hypothermia, many blood volume TX |
| Platelets (for continuing hemorrhage without a 'surgical' etiology) | thrombocytopenia (< 50 000), prolonged bleeding time |
| Fresh frozen plasma (for continuing hemorrhage without a 'surgical' etiology) | prolonged prothrombin time and partial thromboplastin time (>1.5 × normal) |
| Cryoprecipitate (for continuing hemorrhage without a 'surgical' etiology) | low fibrinogen |

TX, transfusion

**Autotransfusion**

Autotransfusion is used most frequently in cardiac, vascular and trauma surgery and in liver resection/transplantation, with cardiac surgery most predominant. When used for elective surgery in patients suffering little hypoperfusion, autotransfusion is associated with little hematological abnormality. Coagulopathies are usually mild and resolve spontaneously in 24–48 h. When used in severe hemorrhage and hypoperfusion cases coagulopathies are more frequent and difficult to attribute to the autotransfusion, although evidence suggests that thrombocytopenia and platelet dysfunction may be aggravated by autotransfusion. The critically ill patient subjected to massive hemorrhage and blood replacement is as likely to exhibit the effects associated with massive transfusion as is the patient without autotransfusion. Usually these patients also receive multiple exogenous blood products. The autotransfusion mainly diminishes the risk of hemolytic transfusion reaction and transmissible disease.

Following intra-abdominal trauma and injury to the intestine, autotransfusion has been avoided for fear of transfusing bacteria directly into the bloodstream. With modern autotransfusion devices, this may be less likely.

## HYPOTHERMIA

Hypothermia in critical illness is most often associated with accidental or surgical trauma. Severely injured trauma patients frequently arrive at a hospital hypothermic, presumably as a result of several mechanisms, such as exposure, hypoperfusion, ethanol ingestion and immobility. Patients undergoing large surgical procedures often develop hypothermia as a consequence of evaporative loss, administration of cool or cold fluids, therapeutic cooling during cardiopulmonary bypass, or decreased metabolic rate during anesthesia. The degree and duration of hypothermia correlates with outcome. Several of the adverse sequelae associated with hypothermia are coagulopathy, vasoconstriction, fluid sequestration and organ failure. However, hypothermia may be protective of cells which have high energy demands (e.g. brain) and successful resuscitation of hypothermic patients from such causes as drowning may be possible despite no evidence of neurological function at the time of presentation.

Clotting enzymes and platelets do not function normally during hypothermia. Standard tests for the coagulation cascade are usually performed at 37 °C. Therefore, it is possible for a patient to exhibit hypothermic coagulopathy despite normal laboratory values. Continued bleeding in hypothermic patients may be impossible to manage until rewarming has taken place. Temporizing measures, such as packing of major liver injuries followed by aggressive rewarming, may be more effective than continuing surgery and the administration of cool blood products.

Rewarming may be enhanced by all the following measures:

(1) Covering with warm blankets;

(2) External warming devices;

(3) Heating infused fluids and blood products;

(4) Inhalation of warmed gases;

(5) Covering all exposed tissues;

(6) Peritoneal dialysis with warm fluid;

(7) Arteriovenous rewarming (cardiopulmonary bypass or similar device).

Most effective is the use of cardiopulmonary bypass or a similar device. Use of this method should be strongly considered for severe hypothermia associated with either the threat of exsanguination or the possibility of recoverable neurological function.

## TRANSFUSION OF BLOOD PRODUCTS

### Adverse effects of transfused blood products

Potential adverse effects of transfused blood include: temperature elevation, hemolytic reaction (immunological or non-immunological) and allergic reactions (urticarial and anaphylactic). Most often an elevation in temperature is secondary to the transfusion of leukocytes, and not a 'transfusion reaction', which implies one of the hemolytic processes listed. Without other signs of an acute hemolytic transfusion reaction, i.e. fever, chills, hypotension, flushing, dyspnea, nausea, chest pain, hemoglobinuria (dark urine), little investigation or therapy is indicated simply because temperature elevation is present. Administration of antipyretics is adequate therapy.

A blood incompatibility hemolytic transfusion reaction which may be mild enough to go unnoticed and severe enough to cause death is most feared. Hypotension, DIC and renal failure accompany severe reactions. Laboratory findings in acute hemolytic transfusion reactions include anemia, hemoglobinemia, hemoglobinuria, decreased haptoglobin, a positive direct Coomb's test, increased lactate dehydrogenase, thrombocytopenia, hypofibrinogenemia and prolonged PT and PTT. When suspected the transfusion should be interrupted immediately, and patient and blood unit identification checked. The remaining blood and a new patient blood sample should be sent to the blood bank for retyping, re-crossmatch and Coomb's test. The vascular volume should be maintained and a large urine output should be maintained by enforced diuresis with care not to deplete the vascular volume. Hypoperfusion should be treated and depleted coagulation products replaced.

Allergic reactions which do not cause hemolysis may occur with urticaria most commonly, and with anaphylactic shock rarely. Therapy for urticaria includes antihistamines.

# 10

# INTENSIVE CARE UNIT INFECTIOUS DISEASE

Introduction and epidemiology
Intravascular catheter infection
'Opportunistic' infection in the ICU
> Fungal infection
> Coagulase-negative staphylococci
> Enterococcus
> Cytomegalovirus

Antibiotics
> Basic antibiotic pharmacology
> Antibiotic adjustments in renal failure
> Commonly used antibiotics

## INTRODUCTION AND EPIDEMIOLOGY

Surgical patients who arrive in a critical care setting such as the intensive care unit (ICU) may be subject to infections related primarily to the initial disease process (e.g. perforated diverticulitis). He or she may also develop infections related mainly to the combination of variables that affect the ICU patient. This Chapter concentrates on the infectious processes which develop as a consequence of the variables listed in Table 1 and which have not been addressed elsewhere (infections such as pneumonia and *Clostridium difficile* colitis are presented elsewhere).

## INTRAVASCULAR CATHETER INFECTION

As discussed in Chapter 3; Normal immunology section, epithelial barriers are important deterrents to the migration of microorganisms. Intravascular devices traverse the skin barrier and may allow skin organisms to colonize the catheter and, subsequently, become a primary source of infection. While central venous catheters have been most frequently recognized as an infectious focus, peripheral venous and arterial catheters may also promote microorganism invasion.

The organisms most frequently associated with catheter-related infection are *Candida*, coagulase-negative staphylococci, *Staphylococcus aureus, Serratia, Pseudomonas* and enterococci. These organisms are either endogenous and colonize the skin subsequent to the promotion of growth by such factors as antibiotics and gastrointestinal surgery (e.g. *Candida*, enterococcus), or ICU flora with colonization promoted by critical illness (coagulase-negative staphylococci, *S. aureus, Serratia, Pseudomonas*). Indwelling catheters may also be colonized following bacteremia and/or fungemia from other foci. Diagnosing the catheter as the primary focus requires demonstration of sequential migration of organisms from the skin to the subcutaneous portion of the catheter, followed by the catheter tip (culture of the catheter tip, subcutaneous portion, and hub all required). A positive catheter tip identifies the catheter as a colonized intravascular device, but not necessarily the primary focus. While a firm diagnosis of catheter-related infection is important for investigational study, the documentation of a quantitatively significant number of organisms (>15 colony forming units) on the catheter tip is usually sufficient to remove the catheter as a likely focus.

The risk of catheter infection is increased by catheter duration, location (venous > arterial), the placement procedure, dressing technique, line

## TABLE 1   VARIABLES RELATED TO INTENSIVE CARE UNIT (ICU) INFECTIONS

*Decreased host defenses*
Impaired cellular immunity
Impaired humoral immunity
Impaired non-specific host defenses
    decreased polymorphonuclear leukocyte function
    decreased macrophage function
Disrupted epithelial barriers
    wounds
    devices traversing the skin
    drains
    catheters
Decreased gastrointestinal tract barrier
Devices in normally sterile regions
    bladder catheters
    endotracheal tubes
    chest tubes
    intraperitoneal drains

*Exposure to ICU organisms*
ICU Gram-positive
    coagulase-positive staphylococci
    coagulase-negative staphylococci
    *Clostridium difficile*
ICU Gram-negative
    *Pseudomonas*
    *Serratia*
    *Enterobacter*
    *Klebsiella*

*Overgrowth/emergence of endogenous organisms*
Fungal
    *Candida*
    *Torulopsis glabrata*
    *Aspergillus*
Viral
    cytomegalovirus
    herpes

manipulations, infection elsewhere and depressed immunocompetence. Dedicated total parenteral nutrition lines, placed and managed according to strict protocol, need be changed only when catheter infection is likely. Triple-lumen central venous catheters with multiple connections and potential manipulations are a greater infection risk, and such catheters should be assessed whenever the catheter has been in place for several days and a patient develops clinical evidence suggestive of new infection without an obvious other focus. Such catheters can be changed over a wire, thereby saving the access site. If the catheter tip is positive on a quantitative culture, the replacement catheter can be removed and a new puncture, preferably at another site, used for access. Any catheter placed under less than ideal circumstances (e.g. emergency room, rapid access in the operating room) with poor attention to sterile technique should be removed within 24 h of placement.

## 'OPPORTUNISTIC' INFECTION IN THE ICU

Critical surgical illness is frequently associated with clinical factors such as antibiotics, central lines, gastrointestinal (GI) tract operations, ventilator therapy > 48 h, prosthetic implants, transplant surgery (immunosuppressive agents) and human immunodeficiency virus (HIV) infection. These factors are associated with invasive infection from organisms usually considered to have low virulence including *Candida*, other fungi, coagulase-negative staphylococci, enterococci and cytomegalovirus. The clinical scenario accompanying infection with these organisms is the previous administration of multiple antibiotics (prophylactic or more commonly therapeutic) to moderately ill patients who have sustained some deficit in host defenses. The administration of multiple antibiotics results in the growth of resistant organisms with widespread colonization. Depressed host defenses allow for the invasion into and/or proliferation within body tissues. To date, cytomegalovirus infection appears to require severe immunosuppression as a result of immunosuppressive therapy or HIV infection, but invasive disease secondary to the other organisms listed does not require profound depression of host defenses.

As discussed in Chapter 5, Gastrointestinal dysfunction section, the upper intestinal tract (stomach and proximal small intestine) may serve as a reservoir for several endogenous and ICU-related organisms. Here the organisms may proliferate (due to the use of multiple antibiotics which kill other flora or medications which decrease stomach acid) and result in invasive infection (e.g. pneumonia from aspiration, bacteremia/fungemia from translocation). Once a patient exhibits evidence of colonization and/or invasion with one organism, characteristically present in the upper GI tract, the clinician should be alert to the possibility that other organisms located in this region will become problematic. For instance, positive blood cultures for fungus in critically ill surgical patients are associated with up to a 40% incidence of blood cultures positive for coagulase-negative staphylococci.

**Fungal infection**
Fungal infection, particularly with *Candida* and related species, is one of the most common of these infections. *Candida* is a normal GI tract organism (mouth to anus) and proliferates when bacterial growth is suppressed by antibacterial antibiotics. Total body colonization allows for invasion from a variety of potential sites, such as the GI tract, skin via venous catheters and urinary tract.

Transient fungemia may occur without destructive tissue invasion; likewise, destructive tissue invasion may occur without positive blood cultures. The diagnosis of destructive tissue invasion is based on the following criteria:

(1) Culture of organism from tissue (kidney, heart valve);

(2) Endophthalmitis;

(3) Burn wound invasion;

(4) Peritoneal fluid culture (sick patient, bacteria will be treated);

(5) Culture from three separate sites (i.e. sputum, urine, blood; sputum, wound, urine);

(6) Two positive blood cultures 24 h apart without a central venous catheter;

(7) Two positive blood cultures with second culture > 24 h after removal of a central venous catheter.

Importantly, evidence of burn wound invasion and peritoneal contamination in a critically ill patient should be considered as sufficient to make a diagnosis of invasive disease.

Destructive tissue infection from these organisms demands the same therapeutic principles applied to invasion by any microorganisms: drainage and debridement when possible, plus the administration of systemic therapy. Fluconazole (400 mg/day) is usually sufficient systemic therapy and demonstrates little toxicity at this dosage. Patients suffering severe organ malfunction from invasive fungal infection may require amphotericin B, usually 0.5 mg/kg for 14 days. Renal toxicity is the main risk, but when renal failure is secondary to invasive fungal infection, renal function may improve following amphotericin administration.

Early recognition of the patient at risk for severe fungal infection may allow steps to be taken to prevent destructive tissue invasion, namely prophylaxis (prevention of colonization and subsequent invasion) and early presumptive therapy (recognition of colonization and initiation of therapy before invasive disease develops). Neither prophylaxis nor early presumptive therapy have been studied widely. Mycostatin (applied topically to the GI tract and burns) and ketoconazole (200 mg/day via the GI tract) have been used for prophylaxis. Mycostatin appears to be effective if used very early (i.e. day of admission) and before or at the same time as the first antibiotics have been administered. Ketoconazole appears to be effective later, even after antibiotics have been used. Ketoconazole, a thromboxane synthesis inhibitor, has also been shown to reduce the risk of acute respiratory distress syndrome in critically ill patients.

With early presumptive therapy, a patient at risk for destructive tissue invasion receives fluconazole (200–400 mg/day) after significant colonization with a sensitive organism has been demonstrated (i.e. >100 000 organisms/ml urine) but before clear evidence of severe infection has developed. Since fluconazole exhibits little toxicity, this concept of using a non-toxic drug before tissue invasion develops but after significant colonization has developed may offer two distinct advantages: (1) avoidance of the sequelae of destructive tissue invasion, and (2) knowledge from culture results that the organism is likely to be sensitive to fluconazole. Using this scheme fluconazole is not administered for prophylaxis but is instead administered only after evidence that a sensitive organism is colonizing a patient at risk for invasion. This strategy, as compared with providing prophylaxis before colonization, should diminish concern that over use of fluconazole will result in resistant fungal species colonizing the ICU environment.

### Coagulase-negative staphylococci

Positive blood cultures for coagulase-negative staphylococci (S. epidermidis, S. hemolyticus) are considered secondary to skin contamination or related to indwelling vascular devices which when removed, eliminate the infection. However, in a pattern similar to that for fungal infections, coagulase-negative staphylococci may become invasive in critically ill surgical patients and require aggressive antibiotic therapy. At least as difficult as the clinical determination of invasive fungal infection is a firm diagnosis of invasive infection from coagulase-negative staphylococci. Criteria for invasive *S. epidermidis* sepsis include:

(1) Positive blood culture with positive tissue or abscess culture;

(2) Two or more positive blood cultures with other foci positive (e.g. wound, urine, sputum, drain sites);

(3) Two or more positive blood cultures with an intravascular prosthesis or a damaged heart valve in place.

The slime produced by *S. epidermidis* appears to be an important factor both for the adherence of the organism to intravascular devices and antibiotic resistance patterns. Invasive coagulase-negative staphylococci infection is usually secondary to nosocomial organisms resistant to many antibiotics. Often vancomycin is the antibiotic of choice, with therapy for at least 7–10 days.

## Enterococcus

Coincident with the widespread use of cephalosporin antibiotics for prophylaxis and therapy in surgical patients, enterococci are now commonly isolated from surgical patients, especially from wounds, urinary tract, intraabdominal collections and the bloodstream. Enterococcus has become the third most common pathogen associated with bloodstream infections and a frequent cause of superinfection in critically ill surgical patients.

Recognized as a significant pathogen in endocarditis and meningitis, the pathogenicity and resultant morbidity and mortality from other enterococcal infection is controversial. For instance, the treatment of enterococcal bacteremia in surgical patients does not clearly affect mortality. While the clinician would not commonly ignore positive blood cultures for bacteria, the common setting of enterococcal bacteremia with associated Gram-negative infection may require the treatment of only the Gram-negative organisms without specific therapy against the enterococcus. Guidelines for the management of enterococcal infection are similar to those for coagulase-negative staphylococci. When the enterococcus appears to be predominant and/or when there is a potentially infected intravascular prosthesis or heart valve, aggressive therapy is warranted. When the enterococcus appears as part of a polymicrobial, and especially Gram-negative, infectious process, treating the associated Gram-negative organisms may be all that is necessary.

Antibiotic resistance is becoming more prevalent with enterococcus than with coagulase-negative staphylococci. Therefore, before administering progressively potent antibiotics, it is necessary to consider carefully which patients will benefit from therapy directed at the enterococcus. Other methods, such as effective infection control precautions, may be more effective than are antibiotics in controlling serious infection from these organisms.

## Cytomegalovirus

Serious illness from cytomegalovirus infection is seen in severely immunosuppressed patients, such as organ transplant recipients and patients with HIV infection. Symptoms usually occur 4–6 weeks after exposure (sometimes from the donated organ), with viremia associated with fever, malaise, myalgias, maculopapular rash, arthralgias and hepatosplenomegaly. Leukopenia is the most common laboratory finding. Progression of disease may result in interstitial pneumonitis, gastrointestinal hemorrhage, gastrointestinal perforation, pancreatitis and hepatitis.

Cytomegalovirus may be present for many years and following immunosuppression may result in a secondary infection, which may not be as morbid. Serious illness is most often from a primary infection. Primary infection may be diagnosed by demonstrating a two or more dilution increase in cytomegalovirus antibody titer over a 2-week interval, or shedding of virus at several sites (saliva, urine, cervix) or viremia.

Acyclovir has been effective for prophylaxis after bone marrow transplantation and cadaveric renal transplantation. For treatment ganciclovir is more effective than acyclovir.

## ANTIBIOTICS

Depending on the disease process, antibiotics may or may not have a significant role in preventing or treating serious infection. Clearly, antibiotics are the most effective and frequently the only therapy for infectious diseases which are rarely treated with surgery (e.g. pneumonia, meningitis, pyelonephritis, cellulitis without an abscess). Short-term antibiotics have also been shown repeatedly to be effective in surgical prophylaxis. More difficult to define is the necessity and duration of antibiotics when surgery is the prime mode of therapy (i.e. drainage of an abscess, removal of an infected gallbladder).

As stated above, prolonged antibiotics use is associated with infections with resistant organisms. Striking the proper balance between treatment and promotion of microorganism overgrowth is a clinical problem not yet well clarified. As a general rule, however, when antibiotics are used as an adjuvant to surgical therapy the clinician should provide the shortest possible course with the least number of antibiotics. Endpoints such as resolution of fever and return to normal white blood cell count have been associated with little risk of recurrent or undertreated infection.

### Basic antibiotic pharmacology
The seven main variables that determine antibiotic tissue concentration are:

(1) Blood flow to tissue;

(2) Serum concentration;

(3) Binding to serum proteins;

(4) Binding to tissue (intracellular);

(5) Membrane transport barriers (endothelial and cellular);

(6) Cell wall transport mechanisms;

(7) Effects of disease on binding and transport barriers.

Administration of any drug results in a volume of distribution incorporating various body spaces and tissues, as well as the clearance of the drug by excretion and/or metabolism. Both the volume of distribution and clearance are time- and concentration-dependent. The half-life of a drug depends on both distribution and clearance. Factors that enhance tissue drug concentration are high tissue binding and high blood flow, and those that diminish drug concentration are prompt clearance, protein binding, membrane inhibition and low blood flow. The partition ratio is the ratio of tissue levels to serum levels. Drugs with high partition ratios for a given tissue are more likely to produce toxicity; those with a low partition ratio are more likely to be ineffective. For instance, all tissues have high affinity for aminoglycosides, and with time these will accumulate to a high intracellular concentration. The kidneys can have a partition ratio of one or greater. Cephalosporins do not penetrate the blood–brain barrier and have a low partition ratio for cerebrospinal fluid. The complexity of interactions determining tissue toxicity illustrates the potential hazards of relying simply on peak and trough levels for dosing antibiotics.

### Antibiotic adjustments in renal failure
The most common reason for monitoring and adjusting antibiotic administration in surgical patients is acute or chronic renal failure. Table 2 lists the

recommended dosage for patients in mild-to-severe renal failure, which can be supplemented by antibiotic level determinations. Factors that a clinician should review before determining an antibiotic dosage are:

(1) Quantification of renal impairment;

(2) Characterization of serum half-life;

(3) Mode of metabolism–excretion with normal kidney function;

(4) Degree of serum binding;

(5) Influence of peritoneal or hemodialysis.

Creatinine clearance (CRCL) is the most accurate clinical method of assessing glomerular filtration rate (GFR). For best accuracy a 24-h urine sample should be obtained with two serum creatinine values spaced 12 h

**TABLE 2   ANTIBIOTIC ADJUSTMENTS IN RENAL FAILURE (TAKEN FROM APPEL)**

| Antibiotic | Mild failure (GFR 30–50 ml/min) | Severe failure (GFR <30 ml/min) |
|---|---|---|
| Amikacin | 7.5 mg/kg/9 × Cr | |
| Amoxycillin | NC | 250–500 mg/16–24 h |
| Amphotericin | 0.5 mg/kg/48 h | |
| Ampicillin | NC | 0.5–1.0 g/8 h |
| Carbenicillin | 3 g/4 h | 2 g/12 h |
| Cephazolin | 0.5 g/12–16 h | 0.5 g/24 h |
| Cefoxitin | NC | 1 g/12–24 h |
| Chloramphenicol | NC | 10% decrease |
| Clindamycin | NC | 300 mg/8 h |
| Dicloxacillin | NC | NC |
| Erythromycin | NC | NC |
| Gentamicin | 1 mg/kg/8 × Cr | |
| Methicillin | NC | avoid |
| Nafcillin | NC | NC |
| Oxacillin | NC | 1 g/6 h |
| Penicillin G | NC | $1 \times 10^6$ U/6 h |
| Ticarcillin | 2 g/24 h | 2 g/12 h |
| Tobramycin | 1 mg/kg/6 × Cr | |
| Trimethoprim | 40 mg/12 h | 40 mg/24 h |
| Vancomycin | 1 g/day | 1 g/7 days |

GFR, glomerular filtration rate; Cr, creatinine; NC, no change apart. A 12-h collection with serum values at 6-h intervals may suffice. While awaiting the clearance determination, CRCL may be estimated using the Siersbaek-Nielsen nomogram. One should remember that the relationship between serum creatinine and functioning nephrons is hyperbolic so that prior to damage small elevations in creatinine denote marked functional loss, whereas subsequent to further damage larger creatinine elevations will be seen with lesser increments in malfunction. Serum creatinine is also influenced by the factors in Table 3.

Once an estimate of CRCL is obtained, the clinician can estimate the amount and dosing of an antibiotic according to standard tables. However, while not a perfect measure of tissue levels, serum levels to determine peak and trough values or, better still, serum half-life will help avoid toxicity as well as inadequate therapy.

### Commonly used antibiotics

Table 4 lists commonly used antibiotics in surgery, along with the spectrum of action, toxicity and major indications. Allergy in this listing refers to all types of reactions that imply allergy, from rash to anaphylaxis and the associated potential for organ injury, usually renal (see Chapter 5, The renal system; Renal failure and selected metabolic disturbances). Second- and third-generation cephalosporins are particularly confusing, and commonly used agents are listed in Table 5. Penicillins and penicillin derivatives have a $\beta$-lactam ring which if disrupted inactivates the antibiotic. Many resistant microorganisms employ $\beta$-lactamase. Antibiotics which have resistant $\beta$-lactam rings or which employ an inhibitor of $\beta$-lactamase are listed in Table 6.


### TABLE 3  FACTORS THAT INFLUENCE CREATININE

*Creatinine clearance*

*Production of creatinine*
Increased with muscle injury
Decreased in elderly

*Higher than normal GFR (slight reduction in serum creatinine means much higher GFR)*
Pregnancy
Volume expansion

GFR, glomerular filtration rate

**TABLE 4  COMMONLY USED ANTIBIOTICS IN SURGERY**

| Antibiotic | Spectrum | Major problems | Indications |
|---|---|---|---|
| Ampicillin, Amoxycillin | penicillin-sensitive organisms, Gram positives, good vs. enterococcus, meningococcus, gonococcus, *Proteus mirabilis, Hemophilus influenza, Clostridia*, anaerobic cocci | allergy, nephritis, colitis | treatment of diarrhea, susceptible infections, not *Escherichia coli* prophylaxis |
| Ticarcillin | Penicillin-sensitive | allergy | treatment of susceptible infections, not prophylaxis |
| Carbenicillin | Gram positives, poor vs. enterococcus, meningococcus, gonococcus, *E. coli, P. mirabilis, Pseudomonas, H. influenza, Bacteroides fragilis, Clostridia*, anaerobic cocci | nephritis | usually not used alone for *Pseudomonas* |
| Piperacillin, mezlocillin | Penicillin-sensitive organisms, Gram positives, poor vs. enterococcus, meningococcus, gonococcus, *E. coli, P. mirabilis, Pseudomonas, H. influenza, Klebsiella, Enterobacter, B. fragilis, Clostridia*, anaerobic cocci | allergy, nephritis | treatment of susceptible infections, not prophylaxis, usually not used alone for *Pseudomonas* |
| Oxacillin, nafcillin, dicloxacillin | penicillinase-resistant, Gram positives | allergy, nephritis | treatment of susceptible infections, not prophylaxis, except for clean cases |

*(Continued)*

295

**TABLE 4  (CONTINUED)**

| Antibiotic | Spectrum | Major problems | Indications |
|---|---|---|---|
| Cephazolin | penicillin-sensitive and penicillin-resistant, Gram positives, E. coli, some Klebsiella, H. influenza, P. mirabilis | allergy, alkaline phosphatase increase | prophylaxis, treatment of susceptible infection |
| Gentamicin, tobramycin, amikacin | Gram negative aerobes especially Pseudomonas and enterococcus | renal toxicity, neuromuscular blockade | susceptible organisms, synergistic for staphylococci and enterococcus, especially gentamicin |
| Chloramphenicol | Gram positives and Gram negatives, B. fragilis | hematologic | susceptible organisms |
| Clindamycin | staphylococci, streptococci, B. fragilis | Diarrhea, Clostridium difficile | susceptible organisms |
| Erythromycin | Gram positives, B. fragilis, Legionella | allergy, hepatic toxicity | susceptible gastrointestinal surgery prophylaxis, PO |
| Vancomycin | staphylococci, enterococcus | renal toxicity | susceptible organisms resistant to other treatment or because of allergy |
| Trimethroprim | Gram positives | allergy | susceptible organisms |
| Sulfamethoxazole | not enterococcus, Gram negatives, Pneumocystis | | |

(Continued)

## TABLE 4 (CONTINUED)

| Antibiotic | Spectrum | Major problems | Indications |
|---|---|---|---|
| Metronidazole | anaerobes | gastrointestinal upset | susceptible organisms, gastrointestinal surgery prophylaxis |

PO, oral administration.

## TABLE 5 SECOND- AND THIRD-GENERATION CEPHALOSPORINS

| | Spectrum | Major problems | Indications |
|---|---|---|---|
| *Second generation* | | | |
| Cefoxitin | Gram positives, not enterococcus, Gram negatives, especially *Bacteroides fragilis*, but not *Pseudomonas* or *Enterobacter* | allergy | GI surgery prophylaxis, susceptible organisms |
| Cefotetan | same as cefoxitin | allergy | GI surgery prophylaxis, susceptible organisms |
| Cefuroxime | group B streptococci, otherwise like cefoxitin | allergy | susceptible organisms |
| *Third generation* | | | |
| Ceftazidime | Gram negatives, Enterobacteriaceae, *Pseudomonas aeruginosa* | allergy | susceptible organisms |
| Cefotaxime | similar to ceftazidime except few *Pseudomonas* | allergy | susceptible organisms |
| Cefoperazone | similar to ceftazidime | allergy | susceptible organisms |

GI, gastrointestinal.

**TABLE 6   CARBAPENEMS, MONOBACTAMS AND COMBINATIONS WITH β-LACTAMASE INHIBITORS**

| Antibiotic | Spectrum | Major problems | Indications |
|---|---|---|---|
| *Carbapenem* | | | |
| Imipenem and cilastatin | Gram positives, not MRSA, not *Staphylococcus epidermidis*, Gram negatives | emergence of resistant *Pseudomonas*, initial broad-spectrum | susceptible organisms |
| *Monobactam* | | | |
| Aztreonam | Gram negatives | allergy | susceptible organisms |
| *Combination with β-lactamase inhibitor* | | | |
| Ticarcillin and clavulanate | Gram positives, not MRSA, Gram negative anaerobes | allergy | susceptible organisms |

MRSA, methicillin-resistant *Staphylococcus aureus*

# 11

# SYNOPSIS

As stated in Chapter 1, the evaluation and management of the critically ill surgical patient proceeds through a series of three questions: (1) where is the hole? (2) how do I plug the hole? and (3) why is the hole there? This iterative process must begin, however, with the recognition that a hole is present. The surgical patient may exhibit a variety of subtle and not so subtle clues that an opening is present or developing (Table 1). When evidence of disease is not subtle, the holes that must be recognized and plugged quickly are the deficits related to the ABCs of resuscitation. Usually, problems with the airway and breathing can be improved rapidly by methods such as intubation, mechanical ventilation and chest tube insertion. More vexing is the rapid restoration of the circulation. As presented in Chapter 2, The circulation, the etiology of circulation deficits may be difficult to discern. Vigorous effort to ascertain a circulatory diagnosis is imperative, as is rapid restoration and sometimes enhancement of global blood flow.

## TABLE 1    CLUES OF ILLNESS IN SURGICAL PATIENTS

*Not subtle*
Hypotension
Tachycardia
Severe dyspnea
High fever/hypothermia
Obtundation/coma
Severe oliguria
Hypoxemia
Disseminated intravascular coagulation
Leukopenia

*More subtle*
Increasing fluid sequestration
Tachypnea
Delirium
Increasing white blood cell count
Increasing creatinine
Increasing bilirubin
Decreasing ionized calcium
Metabolic acidosis
Decreased platelet count
Prolonged ileus

Once the ABCs of resuscitation are in progress, the clinician can begin to ask, 'why is the hole there?'. The primary principle for this clinical guide has been the linking of deficits in the circulation (both global and regional) with non-physiological or pathological inflammation. For most critically ill surgical patients, improving the circulation and locating and treating pathological inflammation will be the key to a successful outcome. Vigorous attention to one without the other ignores the intimate pathophysiology of these insults to cell function. Therefore, the clinician confronted with either non-subtle or subtle evidence of organ malfunction should follow a path highlighted by vigilant recognition of this link. This path should provide an excellent circulation and locate and treat pathological inflammation. Following this path with *The Clinical Handbook for Surgical Critical Care* will hopefully help the clinician to find the hole, plug the hole effectively and make the hole disappear.

# BIBLIOGRAPHY

## 1. BASIC PRINCIPLES

Alexander J, MacMillan B, Stinnett J, *et al*. Beneficial effects of aggressive protein feeding in severely burned children. *Ann Surg* 1980;192:505–19

Barr L, Dunn G, Brennan M. Essential fatty acid deficiency. *Ann Surg* 1981;193:304–11

Brinson R, Pitts M. Enteral nutrition in the critically ill patient. *Crit Care Med* 1989;17:367–70

Brown P, McClave S, Hoy N, *et al*. The Acute Physiology and Chronic Health Evaluation II classification system. *Crit Care Med* 1993;21:363

Buzby G. Overview of randomized clinical trials. *World J Surg* 1993;17: 173–7

Cannon WB. *Traumatic Shock*. New York, London: D. Appleton and Company, 1923

Cerra F, McPerson J, Konstantinides FN, *et al*. Enteral nutrition. *Surgery* 1988;104:727–33

Curtis SE, Cain SM. Regional and systemic oxygen delivery/uptake relations and lactate flux in hyperdynamic, endotoxin-treated dogs. *Am Rev Respir Dis* 1992;145:348–54

DeBiasse M, Wilmore D. What is optimal nutritional support? *New Horizons* 1994;2:122–30

Evans JA, Darlington DN, Gann DS. A circulating factor(s) mediates cell depolarization in hemorrhagic shock. *Ann Surg* 1991;213:549–57

Grankenfield D, Wiles C, Bagley S, *et al*. Relationships between resting and total energy expenditure. *Crit Care Med* 1994;22:1796–804

Grant J. Nutritional support in critically ill patients. *Ann Surg* 1994;5: 610–16

Hayek M, Eisenberg P. Severe hypophosphatemia. *Arch Surg* 1989;124: 1325–8

Heyland D, Cook D, Guyatt G. Does the formulation of enteral feeding products influence infectious morbidity of the critically ill patient? *Crit Care Med* 1994;22:1192–202

Hosoda N, Nishi M, Nakagawa M, *et al*. Structural and functional alterations in the gut. *J Surg Res* 1987;47:129–33

Hwang T, Hwang S, Chen M. The use of indirect calorimetry. *J Trauma* 1993;34:247–51

Jeejeebhoy K. How should we monitor nutritional support: structure or function? *New Horizons* 1994;2:131–8

Kay R, Tasman-Jones C, Pybus J, *et al*. A syndrome of acute zinc deficiency. *Ann Surg* 1976;183:331–40

LeVoyer T, Cioffi W, Pratt L, *et al*. Alterations in intestinal permeability. *Arch Surg* 1992;127:26–30

Lowry S, Thompson W. Nutrient modification of inflammatory mediator production. *New Horizons* 1994;2:164–74

Mainous M, Block E, Deitch E. Nutritional support of the gut: how and why. *New Horizons* 1994;2:193–201

McClave S, Snider H. Use of indirect calorimetry. *Nutr Clin Pract* 1992;7:207–21

Meguid M, Campos A, Hammond W. Nutritional support in surgical practice. 1. *Am J Surg* 1990;159:345–58

Minard G, Kudsk K. Is early feeding beneficial? How early is early? *New Horizons* 1994;2:156–63

Mochizuki H, Trocki O, Dominioni L, *et al*. Mechanism of prevention of postburn hypermetabolism and catabolism. *Ann Surg* 1989;200:297–310

Moore E, Jones T. Benefits of immediate jejunostomy feeding. *J Trauma* 1986;26:874–81

Moore F, Feliciano D, Andrassy R, *et al*. Early enteral feeding, compared with parenteral, reduces postoperative septic complications. *Ann Surg* 1992;216:172–83

Moore F, Moore E, Kudsk K, *et al*. Clinical benefits of an immune-enhancing diet. *J Trauma* 1994;37:607–14

Peterson V, Moore E, Jones T, *et al*. Total enteral nutrition versus total parenteral nutrition. *Surgery* 1988;104:199–207

Shizgal H. The effect of malnutrition on body composition. *Surg Gynecol Obstet* 1981;152:22–6

Shizgal H, Milne C, Spanier A. The effect of nitrogen-sparing. *Surgery* 1979;85:496–503

Streat S, Beddoe A, Hill G. Aggressive nutritional support. *J Trauma* 1987; 27:262–6

Streat S, Hill G. Nutritional support. *World J Surg* 1987;11:194–201

Tellado J, Garcia-Sabrido J, Hanley J, *et al*. Predicting mortality based on body composition analysis. *Ann Surg* 1989;209:81–7

Wiggers CJ. *Physiology of Shock*. New York: The Commonwealth Fund, 1950

Wolfe R, Jahoor F, Hartl W. Protein and amino acid metabolism. *Diabetes/Metab Rev* 1989;5:149–64

Veterans Affairs Total Parenteral Nutrition Cooperative Study Group. Perioperative total parenteral nutrition. *N Engl J Med* 1991;325:525–32

## 2. THE CIRCULATION

Abou-Khalil B, Scalea TT, Trooskin SZ, *et al*. Hemodynamic responses to shock in young trauma patients: need for invasive monitoring. *Crit Care Med* 1994;22:633–9

Abraham SA, Coles NA, Coley CM, *et al*. Coronary risk of noncardiac surgery. *Prog Cardiovasc Dis* 1991;34:205–34

Abramson D, Scalea TM, Hitchcock R, *et al*. Lactate clearance and survival following injury. J Trauma 1993;35:584

Barroso-Aranda J, Chavez-Chavez RH, Schmid-Schönbein GW. Spontaneous neutrophil activation and the outcome of hemorrhagic shock in rabbits. *Circ Shock* 1992;36:185–90

Bulkley GB. The role of oxygen free radicals in human disease processes. *Surgery* 1983;94:407

Burchard KW, Gann DS, Colliton J, *et al*. Ionized calcium, parathormone, and mortality in critically ill surgical patients. *Ann Surg* 1990;212:543–50

Califf RM, Bengtson JR. Cardiogenic shock. *N Engl J Med* 1994;330: 1724–30

Calvin JE, Driedger AA, Sibbald WJ. Does the pulmonary capillary wedge pressure predict left ventricular preload in critically ill patients? *Crit Care Med* 1981;9:437

Celoria G, Steingrub JS, Vickers-Lahti M, et al. Clinical assessment of hemodynamic values in two surgical intensive care units. Arch Surg 1990; 125:1036–9

Cross JS, Gruber DP, Burchard KW, et al. Hypertonic saline fluid therapy following surgery: a prospective study. J Trauma 1989;29:817

Edwards JD. Practical application of oxygen transport principles. Crit Care Med 1990;18:S45

Fleming A, Bishop M, Shoemaker W, et al. Prospective trial of supranormal values as goals of resuscitation in severe trauma. Arch Surg 1992; 127:1175–81

Forrester JS, Diamond G, Chatterjee K, et al. Medical therapy of acute myocardial infarction by application of hemodynamic subsets (Part 1). N Engl J Med 1976;295:1356–62

Forrester JS, Diamond G, Chatterjee K, et al. Medical therapy of acute myocardial infarction by application of hemodynamic subsets (Part 2). N Engl J Med 1976;295:1404

Francis GS, Archer SL. Diagnosis and management of acute congestive heart failure in the intensive care unit. J Intensive Care Med 1989;4:84–92

Gattinoni L, Brazzi L, Pelosi P, et al. A trial of goal-oriented hemodynamic therapy in critically ill patients. N Engl J Med 1995;333:1025–32

Grossman W. Diastolic dysfunction in congestive heart failure. N Engl J Med 1991;325:1557–64

Gutierrez G, Bismar H, Dantzker DR, et al. Comparison of gastric intramucosal pH with measures of oxygen transport and consumption in critically ill patients. Crit Care Med 1992;20:451–7

Guyton AC, Jones CE, Coleman TG. Circulatory Physiology: Cardiac Output and its Regulation. Philadelphia: W.B. Saunders Company, 1973

Harkin AH. Lactic acidosis. Surg Gynecol Obstet 1976;142:593

Harms BA, Kramer GC, Bodai BI, et al. Effect of hypoproteinemia on pulmonary and soft tissue edema formation. Crit Care Med 1981;9:503

Iberti TJ, Kelly KM, Gentili DR, et al. A simple technique to accurately determine intra-abdominal pressure. Crit Care Med 1987;15:1140

Krausz MM. Controversies in shock research: hypertonic resuscitation – pros and cons. Shock 1995;3:69–72

Kvilekval KHV, Mason RA, Newton GB, *et al.* Complications of percutaneous intra-aortic balloon pump use in patients with peripheral vascular disease. *Arch Surg* 1991;126:621–3

Loeb HS, Bredakis J, Gunnar RM. Superiority of dobutamine over dopamine for augmentation of cardiac output in patients with chronic low output cardiac failure. *Circulation* 1977;375–8

Mangano DT, Goldman L. Preoperative assessment of patients with known or suspected coronary disease. *N Engl J Med* 1995;333:1750–6

Mann DL, Young JB. Basic mechanisms in congestive heart failure. *Chest* 1994;105:897–904

Maynard N, Bihari D, Beale R, *et al.* Assessment of splanchnic oxygenation by gastric tonometry in patients with acute circulatory failure. *J Am Med Assoc* 1993;270:1203–10

Mimoz O, Rauss A, Rekik N, *et al.* Pulmonary artery catheterization in critically ill patients: a prospective analysis of outcome changes associated with catheter-prompted changes in therapy. *Crit Care Med* 1994;22:573–9

Pauca AL, Wallenhaupt SL, Kon ND, *et al.* Does radial artery pressure accurately reflect aortic pressure? *Chest* 1992;102:1193–8

Pricolo VE, Burchard KW, Singh AK, *et al.* Trendelenburg versus PASG application – hemodynamic response in man. *J Trauma* 1986;26:718

Rajacich N, Burchard KW, Hasan F, *et al.* Esophageal pressure monitoring: a practical adjuvant to hemodynamic monitoring with positive end-expiratory pressure. *J Crit Care* 1988;17:483–88

Rajacich N, Burchard KW, Hasan FM, *et al.* Central venous pressure and pulmonary capillary wedge pressure as estimates of left atrial pressure: effects of positive end-expiratory pressure and catheter tip malposition. *Crit Care Med* 1989;17:7

Raper R, Sibbald WJ. Right ventricular function in the surgical patient. *World J Surg* 1987;11:154–60

Shoemaker WC. A new approach to physiology, monitoring, and therapy of shock states. *World J Surg* 1987;11:133–46

Sibbald WJ. Myocardial function in the critically ill. *Surg Clin North Am* 1985;65:867

Shibutani K, Komatsu T, Kubal K, et al. Critical level of oxygen delivery in anesthetized man. Crit Care Med 1983;11:640

Velanovich V. Crystalloid versus colloid fluid resuscitation: a meta-analysis of mortality. Surgery 1989;105:65–71

Voyce SJ, Rippe JM. Pulmonary artery catheters: an update. J Intensive Care Med 1990;5:175–92

Weisel RD, Berger RL, Hechtman HB. Current concepts measurement of cardiac output by thermodilution. N Engl J Med 1975;292:682–4

## 3. INFLAMMATION

Abraham E. T- and B-cell function and their roles in resistance to infection. New Horizons 1993;1:28–36

Alverdy JC, Aoys E, Moss GS. Total parenteral nutrition promotes bacterial translocation from the gut. Surgery 1988;104:185–90

Baue AE. Multiple organ failure, multiple organ dysfunction syndrome, and the systemic inflammatory response syndrome – where do we stand?, Shock 1994;2:385–97

Bellomo R, Tipping P, Boyce N. Continuous veno-venous hemofiltration with dialysis removes cytokines from the circulation of septic patients. Crit Care Med 1993;21:522–6

Beutler B. Endotoxin, tumor necrosis factor, and related mediators: new approaches to shock. New Horizons 1993;1:3–12

Bone RC. Toward a theory regarding the pathogenesis of the systemic inflammatory response syndrome: what we do and do not know about cytokine regulation. Crit Care Med 1996;24:163–72

Briegel J, Kellermann W, Forst H, et al. Low-dose hydrocortisone infusion attenuates the systemic inflammatory response syndrome. Clin Invest 1994;72:782–7

Burrell R. Human responses to bacterial endotoxin. Circ Shock 1994; 43:137–53

Christou NV, Meakins JL, Gordon J, et al. The delayed hypersensitivity response and host resistance in surgical patients. Ann Surg 1995;222: 534–48

Cerra FB. Hypermetabolism, organ failure, and metabolic support. *Surgery* 1987;101:1–14

Cronin L, Cook DJ, Carlet J, *et al*. Corticosteroid treatment for sepsis: a critical appraisal and meta-analysis of the literature. *Crit Care Med* 1995; 23:1430–9

Deitch EA. Multiple organ failure. *Ann Surg* 1992;216:117–34

DiPietro LA. Wound healing: the role of the macrophage and other immune cells. *Shock* 1995;4:233–40

Downey GP, Fialkow L, Fukushima T. Initial interaction of leukocytes within the microvasculature: deformability adhesion and transmigration. *New Horizons* 1995;3:219–28

Eastridge BJ, Darlington DN, Evans JA, *et al*. A circulating shock protein depolarizes cells in hemorrhage and sepsis. *Ann Surg* 1994;219:298–305

Endres S, Sinha B, Fulle HJ. Amrinone suppresses the synthesis of tumor necrosis factor-$\alpha$ in human mononuclear cells. *Shock* 1994;1:377–80

Fink MP. Gastrointestinal mucosal injury in experimental models of shock, trauma and sepsis. *Crit Care Med* 1991;19:627

Ganz T. Macrophage function. *New Horizons* 1993;1:23–7

Golub R, Sorrento JJ, Cantu R Jr, *et al*. Efficacy of albumin supplementation in the surgical intensive care unit: a prospective, randomized study. *Crit Care Med* 1994;22:613–19

Gramm J, Smith S, Gamelli RL, *et al*. Effect of transfusion on oxygen transport in critically ill patients. *Shock* 1996;5:190–3

Howard RJ, Simmons RL (eds). *Surgical Infectious Diseases*, 2nd edn. Connecticut: Appleton and Lange, 1988

Livingston DH, Mosenthal AC, Deitsch EA. Sepsis and multiple organ dysfunction syndrome: a clinical-mechanistic overview. *New Horizons* 1995;3:257–66

McMillen MA, Huribal M, Sumpio B. Common pathway of endothelial–leukocyte interaction in shock, ischemia, and reperfusion. *Am J Surg* 1993;166:557–62

Noda H, Noshima S, Nakazawa H, *et al*. Left ventricular dysfunction and acute lung injury induced by continuous administration of endotoxin in sheep. *Shock* 1994;1:291–8

Pannen BHJ, Robotham JL. The acute-phase response. *New Horizons* 1995;3:183–97

Richmond JM, Sibbald WJ, Linton AM, *et al.* Patterns of urinary protein excretion in patients with sepsis. *Nephron* 1982;31:219–23

Rodeberg DA, Chaet MS, Bass RC, *et al.* Nitric oxide: an overview. *Am J Surg* 1995;170:292–303

Schiller HJ, Reilly PM, Bulkley GB. Antioxidant therapy. *Crit Care Med* 1993;21:S92–S102

Simms HH. Polymorphonuclear leukocytes: their role as central cellular elements in shock pathogenesis. *Shock* 1995;4:225–31

Souba WW, Herskowitz K, Klimberg S, *et al.* The effects of sepsis and endotoxemia on gut glutamine metabolism. *Ann Surg* 1990;211:543–50

Stoner HB. Metabolism after trauma and in sepsis. *Circ Shock* 1986;19: 75–87

St John RC, Dorinsky PM. Immunologic therapy for ARDS, septic shock and multiple-organ failure. *Chest* 1993;103:932–43

Todd JC, Mollitt DL. Effect of sepsis on erythrocyte intracellular calcium homeostasis. *Crit Care Med* 1995;23:459–65

Vadas P, Pruzanski W. Induction of group II phospholipase A2 expression and pathogenesis of the sepsis syndrome. *Circ Shock* 1993;39:160–7

Vary TC, Sigel JH, Nakatani T, *et al.* Effect of sepsis on activity of pyruvate dehydrogenase complex in skeletal muscle and liver. *Am J Physiol* 1986; 250:634–40

## 4. THE PULMONARY SYSTEM

Allen SJ, Drake RE, Williams JP, *et al.* Recent advances in pulmonary edema. *Crit Care Med* 1987;15:963–70

Bates DV, Macklem PT, Christie RV. *Respiratory Function in Disease.* Philadelphia: W.B. Saunders Company, 1971

Bernard GR, Luce JM, Sprung CL, *et al.* High-dose corticosteroids in patients with the adult respiratory distress syndrome. *N Engl J Med* 1987; 317:1565–70

Bongard FS, Matthay M, Mackersie RC, *et al.* Morphologic and physiologic correlates of increased extravascular lung water. *Surgery* 1984; 96:395–402

Bonten MJM, Gaillard CA, Wouters EFM, *et al.* Problems in diagnosing nosocomial pneumonia in mechanically ventilated patients: a review. *Crit Care Med* 1994;22:1683–91

Boyson PG, Block AJ, Moulder PV. Relationship between preoperative pulmonary function tests and complications after thoracotomy. *Surg Gynecol Obstet* 1981;152:813–815

Caldini P. Pulmonary hemodynamics and arterial oxygen saturation in pulmonary embolism. *J Appl Physiol* 1965;20:184–90

Claggett GP, Anderson FA Jr, Heit J, *et al.* Prevention of venous thromboembolism. *Chest* 1995;108(Suppl):312–34

Coates NE, Weigelt JA. Weaning from mechanical ventilation. *Surg Crit Care* 1991;71:859

Comroe JH Jr. *Physiology of Respiration.* Chicago: Year Book Medical Publishers, Inc., 1965

Demling RH. Current concepts on the adult respiratory distress syndrome. *Circ Shock* 1990;30:297–309

Dries DJ. Permissive hypercapnia. *J Trauma* 1995;39:984–9

Dupuis YG. *Ventilators: Theory and Clinical Application.* St Louis: Mosby Year Book, 1986

Gooch JL, Suchyta MR, Balbierz JM, *et al.* Prolonged paralysis after treatment with neuromuscular junction blocking agents. *Crit Care Med* 1991;19:1125

Guyton AC, Lindsey AW. Effect of elevated left atrial pressure and decreased plasma protein concentration on the development of pulmonary edema. *Circ Res* 1959;7:649–57

Huemer G, Kolev N, Kurz A, *et al.* Influence of positive end-expiratory pressure on right and left ventricular performance assessed by Doppler two-dimensional echocardiography. *Chest* 1994;106:67–73

Jenkinson SG. Oxygen toxicity. *J Intensive Care Med* 1988;3:137–52

Kearney DJ, Lee TH, Reilly JJ, *et al.* Assessment of operative risk in patients undergoing lung resection. *Chest* 1994;105:753–9

Kollef MH, Schuster DP. The acute respiratory distress syndrome. *Med Prog* 1995;332:27–37

Lain DC, Di Bennedetto R, Morris SL, *et al*. Pressure control inverse ratio ventilation as a method to reduce peak inspiratory pressure and provide adequate ventilation and oxygenation. *Chest* 1989;95:108–88

Lava J, Rice CL, Moss GS, *et al*. Pulmonary dysfunction in sepsis: is pulmonary edema the culprit? *J Trauma* 1982;22:280–4

MacIntyre NR. Clinically available new strategies for mechanical ventilatory support. *Chest* 1993;104:560–5

Manning HL, Schwartzstein RM. Pathophysiology of dyspnea. *N Engl J Med* 1995;333:1547–53

Marcy TW. Barotrauma: detection, recognition, and management. *Chest* 1993;104:578–84

Marcy TW, Marini JJ. Inverse ratio ventilation in ARDS: rationale and implementation. *Chest* 1991;100:494–504

Meduri GU, Chinn A. Fibroproliferation in late adult respiratory distress syndrome. *Chest* 1994;105:127S–9S

Mock CN, Burchard KW, Hasan F, *et al*. Surgical intensive care unit pneumonia. *Surgery* 1988;104:494–9

Ognibene FP, Martin SE, Parker MM. Adult respiratory distress syndrome in patients with severe neutropenia. *N Engl J Med* 1986;315:547–51

Plotkin JS, Shah JB, Lofland GK, *et al*. Extracorporeal membrane oxygenation in the successful treatment of adult respiratory distress syndrome: case report and review. *J Trauma* 1994;37:127–30

Rappaport SH, Shpiner R, Yoshihara G, *et al*. Randomized, prospective trial of pressure-limited versus volume controlled ventilation in severe respiratory failure. *Crit Care Med* 1994;22:22–32

Rivkind AI, Siegel JH, Guadalupi P, *et al*. Sequential patterns of eicosanoid, platelet, and neutrophil interactions in the evolution of the fulminant post-traumatic adult respiratory distress syndrome. *Ann Surg* 1989;210:355–73

Rochon RB, Mozingo DW, Weigelt JA. New modes of mechanical ventilation. *Surg Clin North Am* 1991;71:843–57

Rossaint R, Falke KJ, Lopez F, *et al*. Inhaled nitric oxide for the adult respiratory distress syndrome. *N Engl J Med* 1993;328:399–405

Sauaia A, Moore FA, Moore EE, *et al.* Diagnosing pneumonia in mechanically ventilated trauma patients: endotracheal aspirate versus bronchoalveolar lavage. *J Trauma* 1993;35:512–17

Shires III GT, Peitzman AB, Albert SA, *et al.* Response of extravascular lung water to intraoperative fluids. *Ann Surg* 1983;197:515–19

Slutsky AS. Mechanical ventilation. *Chest* 1993;104:1833–59

Stein PD, Hull RD, Saltzman HA, *et al.* Strategy for diagnosis of patients with suspected acute pulmonary embolism. *Chest* 1993;103:1553–9

Teplitz C. The core pathobiology and integrated medical science of adult acute respiratory insufficiency. *Surg Clin North Am* 1976;56:1091–133

West JB, Dollery CT, Naimark A. Distribution of blood flow in isolated lungs: relation to vascular and alveolar pressures. *J Appl Physiol* 1964;19: 713–24

West JB. *Pulmonary Pathophysiology – the Essentials*, 2nd edn. Baltimore: Williams and Wilkins, 1982

Wheeler AP. Sedation, analgesia, and paralysis in the intensive care unit. *Chest* 1993;104:566–77

Wilson DO, Rogers RM. The role of nutrition in weaning from mechanical ventilation. *J Intensive Care Med* 1989;4:124–33

Yu M, Tomasa G. A double-blind, prospective, randomized trial of ketoconazole, a thromboxane synthetase inhibitor, in the prophylaxis of the adult respiratory distress syndrome. *Crit Care Med* 1993;21:1635–42

## 5. THE RENAL SYSTEM

Arieff AI, Ayus JC. Pathogenesis of hyponatremic encephalopathy. *Chest* 1993;103:607–10

Bellomo R. Continuous hemofiltration as blood purification in sepsis. *New Horizons* 1995;3:732–7

Bellomo R, Tipping P, Boyce N. Continuous veno-venous hemofiltration with dialysis removes cytokines from the circulation of septic patients. *Crit Care Med* 1993;21:522–6

Bersten AD, Holt AW. Vasoactive drugs and the importance of renal perfusion pressure. *New Horizons* 1995;3:650–61

Broner CW, Stidham GL, Westenkirchner DF, *et al.* Hypermagnesemia and hypocalcemia as predictors of high mortality in critically ill pediatric patients. *Crit Care Med* 1990;18:921

Claussen MS, Landercasper J, Cogbill TH. Acute adrenal insufficiency presenting as shock after trauma and surgery: three cases and review of the literature. *J Trauma* 1992;32:94–100

Corwin HL, Korbet SM, Schwartz MM. Clinical correlates of eosinophiluria. *Arch Intern Med* 1985;145:1097–9

Epstein M, Perez G, Oster JR. Management of renal complications of liver disease. *J Intensive Care Med* 1988;3:71–86

Fraser CL, Arieff AI. Metabolic encephalopathy as a complication of renal failure: mechanisms and mediators. *New Horizons* 1994;2:518–26

Friedman BS, Lumb PD. Prevention and management of metabolic alkalosis. *J Intensive Care Med* 1990;5(Suppl):22–7

Galat JA, Robinson AV, Rhodes RS. Oxygen free radical mediated renal dysfunction. *J Surg Res* 1989;46:520–5

Harman PK, Kron IL, McLachlan HD, *et al.* Elevated intra-abdominal pressure and renal function. *Ann Surg* 1982;196:594–7

Hotchkiss RS, Karl IE. Calcium: a regulator of the inflammatory response in endotoxemia and sepsis. *New Horizons* 1996;4:58–71

Johnson JP, Rokaw MD. Sepsis or ischemia in experimental acute renal failure: what have we learned? *New Horizons* 1995;3:608–14

Koch SM, Taylor RW. Chloride ion in intensive care medicine. *Crit Care Med* 1992;20:227–40

Kingston ME, Al-Siba'i MB, Skooge WC. Clinical manifestations of hypomagnesemia. *Crit Care Med* 1986;14:950

Kron IL, Harman PK, Nolan SP. The measurement of intra-abdominal pressure as a criterion for abdominal re-exploration. *Ann Surg* 1984;199: 28–30

Lang S, Küchle C, Fricke H, *et al.* Biocompatible intermittent hemodialysis. *New Horizons* 1995;3:680–7

Lucas CE, Zito JG, Carter KM, *et al.* Questionable value of furosemide in preventing renal failure. *Surgery* 1977;3:314–20

Makhoul RG, Gewertz BL. Renal prostaglandins. *J Surg Res* 1986;40: 181–92

Meleney FL. Hemolytic streptococcal gangrene. *Arch Surg* 1924;9:317–64

Munck A, Guyre P, Holbrook NJ. Physiological functions of glucocorticoids in stress and their relation to pharmacological actions. *Endoc Rev* 1984;5:25–44

Myers BD, Moran SM. Hemodynamically mediated acute renal failure. *N Engl J Med* 1986;314:97–105

Neuschwander-Tetri BA. Organ interactions in the hepatorenal syndrome. *New Horizons* 1994;2:527–44

Oh MS, Carroll HJ. Disorders of sodium metabolism: hypernatremia and hyponatremia. *Crit Care Med* 1992;20:94

Oken DE. On the differential diagnosis of acute renal failure. *Am J Med* 1981;71:916–20

Parker S, Carlon GC, Isaacs M, *et al.* Dopamine administration in oliguria and oliguric renal failure. *Crit Care Med* 1981;9:630–2

Racusen LC. The histopathology of acute renal failure. *New Horizons* 1995;3:662–8

Reed RL, Wu A, Miller-Crotchett P, *et al.* Pharmacokinetic monitoring of nephrotoxic antibiotics in surgical intensive care patients. *J Trauma* 1989; 29:1462–70

Reeder RF, Harbaugh RE. Administration of intravenous urea and normal saline for the treatment of hyponatremia in neurosurgical patients. *J Neurosurg* 1989;70:201–6

Rhee KH, Toro LO, McDonald GG, *et al.* Carbicarb, sodium bicarbonate, and sodium chloride in hypoxic lactic acidosis. *Chest* 1993;104:913–18

Rubeiz GJ, Thill-Baharozian M, Hardie D, *et al.* Association of hypomagnesemia and mortality in acutely ill medical patients. *Crit Care Med* 1993; 21:203–9

Salem M, Tainish RE Jr, Bromberg J, *et al.* Perioperative glucocorticoid coverage. *Ann Surg* 1994;219:416–25

Schein RMH, Sprung CL, Marcial E, *et al.* Plasma cortisol levels in patients with septic shock. *Crit Care Med* 1990;18:259

Schwartz LB, Gewertz BL. The renal response to low dose dopamine. *J Surg Res* 1988;45:574–88

Soni A, Pepper GM, Wyrwinski PM, *et al*. Adrenal insufficiency occurring during septic shock: incidence, outcome and relationship to peripheral cytokine levels. *Am J Med* 1995;98:265–71

Sterns RH. Severe hyponatremia: the case for conservative management. *Crit Care Med* 1992;20:534–8

Thadhani R, Pascual M, Bonventure JV. Acute renal failure. *N Engl J Med* 1996;334:1448–60

## 6. THE GASTROINTESTINAL/NUTRITIONAL SYSTEM

Alexander JW, Macmillan BG, Stinnett JD, *et al*. Beneficial effects of aggressive protein feeding in severely burned children. *Ann Surg* 1980; 192:505–19

Barr LH, Dunn GD, Brennan MF. Essential fatty acid deficiency during total parenteral nutrition. *Ann Surg* 1981;193:304–11

Bessey PQ. Metabolic response to critical illness. *Care in the ICU*, Scientific American, 1994

Brinson RR, Pitts WM. Enteral nutrition in the critically ill patient: role of hypoalbuminemia. *Crit Care Med* 1989;17:367–70

Brooks GS, Zimbler AG, Bodenheimer HC Jr, *et al*. Patterns of liver test abnormalities in patients with surgical sepsis. *Am Surg* 1991;57:656–62

Brown PE, McClave SA, Hoy NW, *et al*. The Acute Physiology and Chronic Health Evaluation II classification system is a valid marker for physiologic stress in the critically ill patient. *Crit Care Med* 1993;21:363–7

Buzby GP. Overview of randomized clinical trials of total parenteral nutrition for malnourished surgical patients. *World J Surg* 1993;17:173–7

Cerra FB, McPherson JP, Konstantinides FN, *et al*. Enteral nutrition does not prevent multiple organ failure syndrome (MOFS) after sepsis. *Surgery* 1988;104:727–33

Champion HR, Jones RT, Trump BF, *et al*. A clinicopathologic study of hepatic dysfunction following shock. *Surgery* 1976;142:657–63

Chang MC, Cheatham ML, Nelson LD, *et al.* Gastric tonometry supplements information provided by systemic indicators of oxygen transport. *J Trauma* 1994;37:488–94

Cook DJ, Fuller HD, Guyatt GH, *et al.* Risk factors for gastrointestinal bleeding in critically ill patients. *N Engl J Med* 1994;330:377–81

DeBiasse MA, Wilmore DW. What is optimal nutritional support? *New Horizons* 1994;2:122–30

Doglio GR, Pusajo JF, Egurrola MA, *et al.* Gastric mucosal pH as a prognostic index of mortality in critically ill patients. *Crit Care Med* 1991; 19:1037

Epstein M. Renal sodium retention in liver disease. *Hosp Pract* 1995;33–42

Fernandez-Del Castillo C, Harringer W, Warshaw AL, *et al.* Risk factors for pancreatic cellular injury after cardiopulmonary bypass. *N Engl J Med* 1991;325:382–7

Fink MP, Kaups KL, Wang H, *et al.* Maintenance of superior mesenteric arterial perfusion prevents increased intestinal mucosal permeability in endotoxic pigs. *Surgery* 1991;110:154–61

Frankenfeld DC, Wiles CE III, Bagley S, *et al.* Relationships between resting and total energy expenditure in injured and septic patients. *Crit Care Med* 1994;22:1796–804

Grant JP. Nutritional support in critically ill patients. *Ann Surg* 1994; 220:610–16

Hagland U. Systemic mediators released from the gut in critical illness. *Crit Care Med* 1993;21:S15–18

Hayek ME, Eisenberg PG. Severe hypophosphatemia following the institution of enteral feedings. *Arch Surg* 1989;124:1325–8

Heyland DK, Cook DJ, Guyatt GH. Does the formulation of enteral feeding products influence infectious morbidity and mortality rates in the critically ill patient? A critical review of the evidence. *Crit Care Med* 1994;22:1192–202

Heyland DK, Cook DJ, Jaeschke R, *et al.* Selective decontamination of the digestive tract. *Chest* 1994;105:1221–9

Horton JW, Burnweit CA. Hemodynamic function in acute pancreatitis. *Surgery* 1988;103:538–46

Hosoda N, Nishi M, Nakagawa M, *et al.* Structural and functional alterations in the gut of parenterally or enterally fed rats. *J Surg Res* 1989; 47:129–33

Hwang T-L, Huang S-L, Chen M-F. The use of indirect calorimetry in critically ill patients – the relationship of measured energy expenditure to injury severity score, septic severity score, and APACHE II score. *J Trauma* 1993;34:247–51

Imperiale TF, Teran JC, McCullough AJ. A meta-analysis of somatostatin versus vasopressin in the management of acute esophageal variceal hemorrhage. *Gastroenterology* 1995;109:1289–94

Jeejeebhoy KN. How should we monitor nutritional support: structure or function? *New Horizons* 1994;2:131–8

Kay RG, Tasman-Jones C, Pybus J, *et al.* A syndrome of acute zinc deficiency during total parenteral alimentation in man. *Ann Surg* 1976;183: 331–40

Kelly CP, Pothoulakis C, LaMont JT. *Clostridium difficile* colitis. *N Engl J Med* 1994;330:257–62

Lee H, Hawker FH, Selby W, *et al.* Intensive care treatment of patients with bleeding esophageal varices: results, predictors of mortality, and predictors of the adult respiratory distress syndrome. *Crit Care Med* 1992; 20:1555–63

Levine R, Fromm RE Jr, Mojtahedzadeh M, *et al.* Equivalence of litmus paper and intragastric pH probes for intragastric pH monitoring in the intensive care unit. *Crit Care Med* 1994;22:945–8

LeVoyer T, Cioffi WG Jr, Pratt L, *et al.* Alterations in intestinal permeability after thermal injury. *Arch Surg* 1992;127:26–30

Lowry SF, Thompson WA. Nutrient modification of inflammatory mediator production. *New Horizons* 1994;2:164–74

Mainous MR, Block EFJ, Deitch EA. Nutritional support of the gut: how and why. *New Horizons* 1994;2:193–201

Malcynski JT, Iwanow IC, Burchard KW. Severe pancreatitis: determinants of mortality in a tertiary referral center. *Arch Surg* 1996;131:242–6

Marshall JC, Christou NV, Meakins JL. The gastrointestinal tract: the 'undrained abscess' of multiple organ failure. *Ann Surg* 1993;218:111–19

Maton PN. Omeprazole. *N Engl J Med* 1991;324:965–75

McCarthy DM. Sucralfate. *N Engl J Med* 1991;325:1017–25

McClave SA, Snider HL. Use of indirect calorimetry in clinical nutrition. *Nutr Clin Pract* 1992;7:207–21

Medich DS, Lee TK, Melham MF, *et al*. Pathogenesis of pancreatic sepsis. *Am J Surg* 1993;165:46–52

Meguid MM, Campos AC, Hammond WG. Nutritional support in surgical practice: part 1. *Am J Surg* 1990;159:345–58

Minard G, Kudsk KA. Is early feeding beneficial? How early is early? *New Horizons* 1994;2:156–63

Mochizuki H, Trocki O, Dominioni L. Mechanism of prevention of postburn hypermetabolism and catabolism by early enteral feeding. *Ann Surg* 1989;200:297–310

Moore EE, Jones TN. Benefits of immediate jejunostomy feeding after major abdominal trauma – a prospective, randomized study. *J Trauma* 1986;26:874–81

Moore FA, Moore EE, Jones TN, *et al*. TEN versus TPN following major abdominal trauma – reduced septic morbidity. *J Trauma* 1989;29:916–23

Moore FA, Moore EE, Kudsk KA, *et al*. Clinical benefits of an immune-enhancing diet for early postinjury enteral feeding. *J Trauma* 1994; 37:604–14

Moore FA, Feliciano DV, Andrassy RJ, *et al*. Early enteral feeding, compared with parenteral, reduces postoperative septic complications. *Ann Surg* 1992;216:172–83

Moore K, Wendon J, Frazer M, *et al*. Plasma endothelin immunoreactivity in liver disease and the hepatorenal syndrome. *N Engl J Med* 1992;327: 1774–8

Mullen KD, Gacad R. Pathogenetic mechanisms of acute hepatic encephalopathy. *New Horizons* 1994;2:505–11

Neuschwander-Tetri BA. Organ interactions in the hepatorenal syndrome. *New Horizons* 1994;2:527–44

Pesola GE, Hogg JE, Yonnios T, *et al*. Isotonic nasogastric tube feedings: do they cause diarrhea? *Crit Care Med* 1989;17:1151

Peterson VM, Moore EE, Jones TN, *et al*. Total enteral nutrition versus total parenteral nutrition after major torso injury: attenuation of hepatic protein reprioritization. *Surgery* 1988;104:199–207

Ranson JHC. The role of surgery in the management of acute pancreatitis. *Ann Surg* 1990;211:382–93

Ranson JC, Berman RS. Long peritoneal lavage decreases pancreatic sepsis in acute pancreatitis. *Ann Surg* 1990;211:708–18

Raunest J, Imhof M, Rauen U, *et al*. Acute cholecystitis: a complication in severely injured intensive care patients. *J Trauma* 1992;32:433–40

Reed L, Martin M, Manglano R, *et al*. Bacterial translocation following abdominal trauma in humans. *Circ Shock* 1994;42:1–6

Rombeau JL, Rolandelli XH, Wilmore DW. Nutritional support. *Care in the ICU*. Scientific American, 1994

Rossle M, Haag K, Ochs A, *et al*. The transjugular intrahepatic porto-systemic stent–shunt procedure for variceal bleeding. *N Engl J Med* 1994; 330:165–71

Runyon BA. Care of patients with ascites. *Curr Concept* 1994;330:337–42

Ryan CM, Yarmush ML, Burke JF, *et al*. Increased gut permeability early after burns correlates with the extent of burn injury. *Crit Care Med* 1992; 20:1508–12

Shizgal HM. The effect of malnutrition on body composition. *Surg Gynecol Obstet* 1981;152:22–6

Shizgal HM, Milne CA, Spanier AH. The effect of nitrogen-sparing, intravenously administered fluids on postoperative body composition. *Surgery* 1979;85:496–503

Souba WS, Klimberg S, Plumley DA, *et al*. The role of glutamine in maintaining a healthy gut and supporting the metabolic response in injury and infection. *J Surg Res* 1990;48:383–91

Streat SJ, Beddoe AH, Hill GL. Aggressive nutritional support does not prevent protein loss despite fat gain in septic intensive care patients. *J Trauma* 1987;27:262–6

Streat SJ, Hill GL. Nutritional support in the management of critically ill patients in surgical intensive care. *World J Surg* 1987;11:194–201

Szabo S. Mechanisms of gastric mucosal injury and protection. *J Clin Gastroenterol* 1991;13(Suppl 2):21–4

Tellado JM, Garcia-Sabrido JL, Hanley JA, *et al*. Predicting mortality based on body composition analysis. *Ann Surg* 1989;209:81–7

Theuer CJ, Wilson MA, Steeb GD, *et al*. Microvascular vasoconstriction and mucosal hypoperfusion of the rat small intestine during bacteremia. *Circ Shock* 1993;40:61–8

Tryba M. Sucralfate versus antacids or $H_2$-antagonist for stress ulcer prophylaxis: a meta-analysis of efficacy and pneumonia rate. *Crit Care Med* 1991;19:942

Wang P, Ba ZF, Chaundry IH. Hepatic extraction of indocyanine green is depressed early in sepsis despite increased hepatic flow and cardiac output. *Arch Surg* 1991;126;219–24

Warren BL. Small vessel occlusion in acute acalculous cholecystitis. *Surgery* 1992;111:163–8

Werbel GB, Nahrworld DL, Joehl RJ, *et al*. Percutaneous cholecystostomy in the diagnosis and treatment of acute cholecystitis in the high-risk patient. *Arch Surg* 1989;124:782–6

Wilmore DW, Smith RJ, O'Dwyer ST, *et al*. The gut: a central organ after surgical stress. *Surgery* 1988;104:917–23

Wolfe RR, Jahoor F, Hartl WH. Protein and amino acid metabolism after injury. *Diabetes Metab Rev* 1989;5:149–64

Perioperative total parenteral nutrition in surgical patients. *N Engl J Med* 1991;325:525–32

## 7. THE CENTRAL NERVOUS SYSTEM

Bouma GJ, Muizelaar JP. Cerebral blood flow in severe clinical head injury. *New Horizons* 1995;3:384–94

Bowton DL, Betels NH, Prough DS, *et al*. Cerebral blood flow is reduced in patients with sepsis. *Crit Care Med* 1989;17:399

Bullock R. Mannitol and other diuretics in severe neurotrauma. *New Horizons* 1995;3:448–52

Changaris DG, McGraw CP, Richardson JD, *et al*. Correlation of cerebral perfusion pressure and Glasgow Coma Scale to outcome. *J Trauma* 1987;27:1007–13

Chesnut RM. Secondary brain insults after head injury: clinical perspectives. *New Horizons* 1995;3:366–75

Chesnut RM, Marshall LF, Klauber MR, *et al.* Role of secondary brain injury in determining outcome from severe head injury. *J Trauma* 1993;34: 216–22

Chiles BW, Cooper PR. Acute spinal injury. *N Engl J Med* 1996;334:514–20

Cruz J, Jaggi JL, Hoffstad OJ. Cerebral blood flow, vascular resistance, and oxygen metabolism in acute brain trauma: redefining the role of cerebral perfusion pressure? *Crit Care Med* 1995;23:1412–17

DeMaria EJ, Reichman W, Kenney PR, *et al.* Septic complications of corticosteroid administration after central nervous system trauma. *Ann Surg* 1985;202:248–52

DeWitt D, Jenkins LS, Prough DW. Enhanced vulnerability to secondary ischemic insults after experimental traumatic brain injury. *New Horizons* 1995;3:376–83

Fukamachi A, Kohno K, Nagaseki Y, *et al.* Incidence of delayed traumatic intracerebral hematoma with extradural hemorrhages. *J Trauma* 1985;25: 145–9

Galandiuk S, Raque G, Appel S, *et al.* The two-edged sword of large-dose steroids for spinal cord trauma. *Ann Surg* 1993;218:419–27

Hariri RJ, Ghajar JB, Pomerantz KB, *et al.* Human glial cell production of lipoxygenase-generated eicosanoids: a potential role in the pathophysiology of vascular changes following traumatic brain injury. *J Trauma* 1989;29:1203–10

Sprung CL, Peduzzi PN, Shatney CH, *et al.* Impact of encephalopathy on mortality in the sepsis syndrome. The Veterans Administration Systemic Sepsis Cooperative Study Group. *Crit Care Med* 1990;18:801–6

Kong DL, Prough DS, Whitley JM, *et al.* Hemorrhage and intracranial hypertension in combination increase cerebral production of thromboxane $A_2$. *Crit Care Med* 1991;19:532

Lang EW, Chesnut RM. Intracranial pressure and cerebral perfusion pressure in severe head injury. *New Horizons* 1995;3:400–9

Levitt MA, Fleischer AS, Meislin HW. Acute post-traumatic diabetes insipidus: treatment with continuous intravenous vasopressin. *J Trauma* 1984;24:532–5

Marion DW, Firlik A, McLaughlin MR. Hyperventilation therapy for severe traumatic brain injury. *New Horizons* 1995;3:439–47

Ohar JM, Fowler AA, Selhorst JB, *et al*. Intravenous nitroglycerin-induced intracranial hypertension. *Crit Care Med* 1985;13:867–8

Pietropaoli JA, Rogers FB, Shackford SR, *et al*. Deleterious effects of intraoperative hypotension on outcome in patients with severe head injuries. *J Trauma* 1992;33:403–7

Plum F, Posner JB. *The Diagnosis of Stupor and Coma*. Philadelphia: F.A. Davis Company, 1972

Prall JA, Nichols JS, Brennan R, *et al*. Early definitive abdominal evaluation in the triage of unconscious normotensive blunt trauma patients. *J Trauma* 1994;37:792–7

Robertson CS, Cormio M. Cerebral metabolic management. *New Horizons* 1995;3:410–22

Rosner MJ, Rosner SD, Johnson AH. Cerebral perfusion pressure: management protocol and clinical results. *J Neurosurg* 1995;83:949–62

Schmoker JD, Zhuang J, Shackford SR. Hypertonic fluid resuscitation improves cerebral oxygen delivery and reduces intracranial pressure after hemorrhagic shock. *J Trauma* 1991;31:1607–13

Schmoker JD, Zhuang J, Shackford SR. Hemorrhagic hypotension after brain injury causes an early and sustained reduction in cerebral oxygen delivery despite normalization of systemic oxygen delivery. *J Trauma* 1992;32:714–22

Shackford SR. Fluid resuscitation in head injury. *J Intensive Care Med* 1990;5:59–68

Sieber FE, Traystman RJ. Special issues: glucose and the brain. *Crit Care Med* 1992;20:104

Sprung CL, Peduzzi PN, Shatney CH, *et al*. Impact of encephalopathy on mortality in the sepsis syndrome. *Crit Care Med* 1990;18:801

Waxman K, Sundine MJ, Young RF. Is early prediction of outcome in severe head injury possible? *Arch Surg* 1991;126:1237–42

White RJ, Likavec MJ. The diagnosis and initial management of head injury. *N Engl J Med* 1992;327:1507–11

Winchell RJ, Simons RK, Hoyt DB. Transient systolic hypotension: a serious problem in the management of head injury. *Arch Surg* 1996;131: 533–9

Zhuang J, Shackford SR, Schmoker JD. The association of leukocytes with secondary brain injury. *J Trauma* 1993;35:415–22

## 8. THE INTEGUMENT/BURNS

Alexander F, Mathieson M, Teoh KHT, *et al.* Arachidonic acid metabolites mediate early burn edema. *J Trauma* 1984;24:709–12

Artz CP, Moncrief JA, Pruitt BA. *Burns: A Team Approach.* Philadelphia: WB Saunders & Co, 1979

Caldwell FT Jr, Wallace BH, Cone JB, *et al.* Control of the hypermetabolic response to burn injury using environmental factors. *Ann Surg* 1992;215: 485–90

Chibber-Chandra N, Siu CO, Munster AM. Clinical predictors of myocardial damage after high voltage electrical injury. *Crit Care Med* 1990;18:293–97

Cioffi WG, Vaughan GM, Heironimus JD, *et al.* Dissociation of blood volume and flow in regulation of salt and water balance in burn patients. *Ann Surg* 1991;214:213–8

Clayton JM, Russell HE, Hartford CE, *et al.* Sequential circulatory changes in the circumferentially burned limb. *Ann Surg* 1977;185:391–6

Demling RH, Kramer GC, Gunther R, *et al.* Effect of nonprotein colloid on postburn edema formation in soft tissues and lung. *Surgery* 1984;95:593–602

Goodwin CW, Dorethy J, Lam V, *et al.* Randomized trial of efficacy of crystalloid and colloid resuscitation of hemodynamic response and lung water following thermal injury. *Ann Surg* 1983;197:520–30

Gunn ML, Hansbrough JF, Davis JW, *et al.* Prospective, randomized trial of hypertonic sodium lactate versus lactated Ringer's solution for burn shock resuscitation. *J Trauma* 1989;29:1261–7

Hansbrough JF. Burn wound sepsis. *J Intensive Care Med* 1987;2:313–27

Holliman CJ, Meuleman TR, Larsen KR, *et al.* The effect of ketanserin, a specific serotonin antagonist on  burn shock hemodynamic parameters in a porcine burn model. *J Trauma* 1983;23:867–71

Huang PP, Stucky FS, Dimick AR, *et al.* Hypertonic sodium resuscitation is associated with renal failure and death. *Ann Surg* 1995;221:543–54

Knox J, Demling R, Wilmore D, *et al.* Increased survival after major thermal injury: the effect of growth hormone therapy in adults. *J Trauma* 1995;39:526–30

Kowal-Vern A, Gamelli RL, Walenga JM, *et al.* The effect of burn wound size on hemostasis: a correlation of the hemostatic changes to the clinical state. *J Trauma* 1992;33:50–6

Lund T, Bert JL, Onarheim H, *et al.* Microvascular exchange during burn injury. 1: a review. *Circ Shock* 1989;28:179–97

Mackie DP, van Hertum WAJ, Schumburg T, *et al.* Prevention of infection in burns: preliminary experience with selective decontamination of the digestive tract in patients with extensive injuries. *J Trauma* 1992;32:570–5

Masanes M, Legendre C, Lioret N, *et al.* Fiberoptic bronchoscopy for the early diagnosis of subglottal inhalation injury: comparative value in the assessment of prognosis. *J Trauma* 1994;36:59–67

Monafo WW, Halverson JD, Schechtman K. The role of concentrated sodium solutions in the resuscitation of patients with severe burns. *Surgery* 1984;95:129–34

McDonald WS, Sharp CW, Deitch EA. Immediate enteral feeding in burn patients is safe and effective. *Ann Surg* 1991;213:177–83

Moore DB, Rainey WC, Caldwell FT, *et al.* The effect of rapid resuscitation upon cardiac index following thermal trauma in a porcine model. *J Trauma* 1987;27:141–6

Ogura H, Saitoh D, Johnson AA, *et al.* The effect of inhaled nitric oxide on pulmonary ventilation–perfusion matching following smoke inhalation injury. *J Trauma* 1994;37:893–8

Parshley PF, Kilgore J, Pulito JF, *et al.* Aggressive approach to the extremity damaged by electric current. *Am J Surg* 1985;150:78–82

Robson MC, Burns BF, Smith DJ. Acute management of the burned patient. *Plast Reconst Surg* 1992;89:1155–68

Rodriguez JL, Miller CG, Garner WL, *et al.* Correlation of the local and systemic cytokine response with clinical outcome following thermal injury. *J Trauma* 1993;34:684–94

Rue LL, Cioffi WG, Mason AD, et al. Improved survival of burned patients with inhalation injury. Arch Surg 1993;128:772–80

Saez JC, Ward PH, Gunther B, et al. Superoxide radical involvement in the pathogenesis of burn shock. Circ Shock 1984;12:229–39

Saffle JR, Medina E, Raymond J, et al. Use of indirect calorimetry in the nutritional management of burned patients. J Trauma 1985;25:32–9

Saffle JR, Sullivan JJ, Tuohig GM, et al. Multiple organ failure in patients with thermal injury. Crit Care Med 1993;21:1673–83

Sartorelli KH, Silver GM, Gamelli RL. The effect of granulocyte colony-stimulating factor (G-CSF) upon burn-induced defective neutrophil chemotaxis. J Trauma 1991;31:523–30

Shimazaki S, Yukioka T, Matuda H. Fluid distribution and pulmonary dysfunction following burn shock. J Trauma 1991;31:623–8

Sittig K, Deitsch EA. Effect of bacteremia on mortality after thermal injury. Arch Surg 1988;123:1367–70

Smith DL, Cairns BA, Ramadan F, et al. Effect of inhalation injury, burn size, and age on mortality: a study of 1447 consecutive burn patients. J Trauma 1994;37:655–9

Stratta RJ, Warden GD, Ninnemann JL, et al. Immunologic parameters in burned patients: effect of therapeutic interventions. J Trauma 1986;26: 7–16

Tchervenkov JI, Epstein MD, Silberstein EB, et al. Early burn wound excision and skin grafting postburn trauma restores in vivo neutrophil delivery to inflammatory lesions. Arch Surg 1988;123:1477–81

Teodorczyk-Injeyan JA, Sparkes BG, Falk RE, et al. Interleukin-2 secretion and transmembrane signalling in burned patients. J Trauma 1988;28: 152–7

Tranbaugh RF, Elings VB, Christensen JM, et al. Effect of inhalation injury on lung water accumulation. J Trauma 1983;23:597–604

Tredget EE, Yu Y. The metabolic effects of thermal injury. World J Surg 1992;16:68–79

Turner WW, Ireton CS, Hunt JL, et al. Predicting energy expenditures in burned patients. J Trauma 1985;25:11–16

Walsh M, Miller SL, Kagen LJ. Myoglobinemia in severely burned patients: correlations with severity and survival. *J Trauma* 1982;22:6–10

Warden GD, Stratta RJ, Saffle JR, *et al*. Plasma exchange therapy in patients failing to resuscitate from burn shock. *J Trauma* 1983;23:945–51

## 9. THE HEMATOPOIETIC SYSTEM

Baughman RP, Lower EE, Flessa HC, *et al*. Thrombocytopenia in the intensive care unit. *Chest* 1993;104:1243–7

Boldt J, Menges T, Wollbruck M, *et al*. Platelet function in critically ill patients. *Chest* 1994;106:899–903

Capon SM, Sacher RA. Hemolytic transfusion reactions: a review of mechanisms, sequelae, and management. *J Intensive Care Med* 1989;4: 100–11

Collins JA. Recent developments in the area of massive transfusion. *World J Surg* 1987;11:75–81

Danzl DF, Pozos RS. Accidental hypothermia. *N Engl J Med* 1994;331: 1756–60

Gentilello LL, Cobean RA, Offner PJ, *et al*. Continuous arteriovenous rewarming: rapid reversal of hypothermia in critically ill patients. *J Trauma* 1992;32:316–27

Gubler KK, Gentilello LM, Hassantash SA, *et al*. The impact of hypothermia on dilutional coagulopathy. *J Trauma* 1994;36:847–51

Harrigan C, Lucas CE, Ledgerwood AM. The effect of hemorrhagic shock on the clotting cascade in injured patients. *J Trauma* 1989;29:1416–22

Horst HM, Dlugos S, Fath JJ, *et al*. Coagulopathy and intraoperative blood salvage (IBS). *J Trauma* 1992;32:646–52

Iberti TJ, Rand JH, Benjamin E, *et al*. Thrombocytopenia following peritonitis in surgical patients. *Ann Surg* 1986;204:341–5

Kelton JG, Sheridan D, Santos A, *et al*. Heparin-induced thrombocyto-penia: laboratory studies. *Blood* 1988;3:925–30

Letsou GV, Kopf GS, Elefteriades JA, *et al*. Is cardiopulmonary bypass effective for treatment of hypothermic arrest due to drowning or exposure? *Arch Surg* 1992;127:525–8

Luna GK, Maier RV, Pavlin EG, et al. Incidence and effect of hypothermia in seriously injured patients. J Trauma 1987;27:1014–18

Ozmen V, McSwain NE Jr, Nichols RL, et al. Autotransfusion of potentially culture-positive blood (CPB) in abdominal trauma: preliminary data from a prospective study. J Trauma 1992;32:36–9

Reed RL II, Johnston TD, Hudson JD, et al. The disparity between hypothermic coagulopathy and clotting studies. J Trauma 1992;33:465–70

Reed RL II, Ciavarella D, Heimbach DM, et al. Prophylactic platelet administration during massive transfusion. Ann Surg 1986;203:40–8

Rohrer MJ, Natale AM. Effect of hypothermia on the coagulation cascade. Crit Care Med 1992;20:1402–5

Slotman GJ, Jed EH, Burchard KW. Adverse effects of hypothermia in postoperative patients. Am J Surg 1985;149:495–501

Taylor FB Jr. The inflammatory-coagulant axis in the host response to Gram-negative sepsis: regulatory roles of proteins and inhibitors of tissue factor. New Horizons 1994;2:555–65

Valeri CR, MacGregor H, Cassidy G, et al. Effects of temperature on bleeding time and clotting time in normal male and female volunteers. Crit Care Med 1995;23:698–704

Wudel JH, Morris JA Jr, Yates K, et al. Massive transfusion: outcome in blunt trauma patients. J Trauma 1991;31:1–7

## 10.   INTENSIVE CARE UNIT INFECTIOUS DISEASE

Alden SM, Frank E, Flancbaum L. Abdominal candidiasis in surgical patients. Am Surg 1989;55:45–9

Appel GB, Neu HC. The nephrotoxicity of antimicrobial agents. N Engl J Med 1977;296:663–7

Barie PS, Christou NV, Dellinger EP, et al. Pathogenicity of the enterococcus in surgical infections. Ann Surg 1990;212:155–9

Barrall DT, Kenney PR, Slotman GJ, et al. Enterococcal bacteremia in surgical patients. Arch Surg 1985;120:57–63

Burchard KW, Minor LB, Slotman GJ, et al. Fungal sepsis in surgical patients. Arch Surg 1983;118:217–21

Burchard KW, Minor LB, Slotman GJ, et al. Staphylococcus epidermis sepsis in surgical patients. Arch Surg 1984;119:96–100

Carlson MA, Condon RE. Nephrotoxicity of amphotericin B. J Am Coll Surg 1994;179:361–81

Cobb DK, High KP, Sawyer RG, et al. A controlled trial of scheduled replacement of central venous and pulmonary-artery catheters. N Engl J Med 1992;327:1062–8

Como JA, Dismukes WE. Oral azole drugs as systemic antifungal therapy. N Engl J Med 1994;330:263–72

Cornwell EE III, Belzberg H, Berne TV, et al. The pattern of fungal infections in critically ill surgical patients. Am Surg 1995;61:847–50

Dean DA, Burchard KW. Fungal infection in surgical patients. Am J Surg 1996;171:374–82

Desai MH, Rutan RL, Heggers JP, et al. Candida infection with and without nystatin prophylaxis. Arch Surg 1992;127:159–62

de Vera ME, Simmons RL. Antibiotic-resistant enterococci and the changing face of surgical infections. Arch Surg 1996;131:338–42

Dunn DL, Najarian JS. New approaches to the diagnosis, prevention, and treatment of cytomegalovirus infection after transplantation. Am J Surg 1991;161:250–4

Garrison RN, Fry DE, Berberich S, et al. Enterococcal bacteremia: clinical implications and determinants of death. Ann Surg 1982;196:43–7

Henderson VJ, Hirvela ER. Emerging and reemerging microbial threats. Arch Surg 1995;131:330–7

Hilton E, Haslett TM, Borenstein MT, et al. Central catheter infections: single- versus triple-lumen catheters. Am J Med 1988;84:667–72

Kauffman CA, Bradley SF, Ross SC, et al. Hepatosplenic candidiasis: successful treatment with fluconazole. Am J Med 1991;91:137–41

Large M, Stubbs E, Benn R, et al. A study of coagulase-negative staphylococci isolated from clinically significant infections at an Australian teaching hospital. Pathology 1989;21:19–22

Lee RB, Buckner M, Sharp KW. Do multi-lumen catheters increase central venous catheter sepsis compared to single-lumen catheters? J Trauma 1988;28:1472–4

Lennard ES, Dellinger EP, Wertz MJ, et al. Implications of leukocytosis and fever at conclusion of antibiotic therapy for intra-abdominal sepsis. Ann Surg 1982;195:19–24

Low DE, Willey BM, McGreer AJ. Multidrug-resistant enterococci: a threat to the surgical patient. Am J Surg 1995;169:8S–12S

Marshall JC, Christou NV, Meakins JL. The gastrointestinal tract: the 'undrained abscess' of multiple organ failure. Ann Surg 1993;218:111–19

Mayoral JL, Loeffler CM, Fasola CG, et al. Diagnosis and treatment of cytomegalovirus disease in transplant patients based on gastrointestinal tract manifestations. Arch Surg 1991;126:202–6

Nassoura Z, Ivatury RR, Simon RJ, et al. Candiduria as an early marker of disseminated infection in critically ill surgical patients: the role of fluconazole therapy. J Trauma 1993;35:290–5

Pittet D, Monod M, Suter PM, et al. Candida colonization and subsequent infections in critically ill surgical patients. Ann Surg 1994;220:751–8

Reese RE, Betts RF. Handbook of Antibiotics. Boston: Little, Brown and Company, 1993:

Rex JH, Bennett JE, Sugar AM, et al. A randomized trial comparing fluconazole with amphotericin B for the treatment of candidemia in patients without neutropenia. N Engl J Med 1994;331:1325–30

Slotman GJ, Burchard KW. Ketoconazole prevents Candida sepsis in critically ill surgical patients. Arch Surg 1987;122:147–51

Solomkin JS, Flohr A, Simmons RL. Candida infections in surgical patients: dose requirements and toxicity of amphotericin B. Ann Surg 1982;195:177–85

Solomkin JS, Flohr AM, Simmons RL. Indications for therapy for fungemia in postoperative patients. Arch Surg 1982;117:1272–5

Stratta RJ, Shaefer MS, Markin RS, et al. Clinical patterns of cytomegalovirus disease after liver transplantation. Arch Surg 1989;124:1443–50

## 11. OVERVIEW AND GUIDELINES

Bakker J, Gris P, Coffernils M, et al. Serial blood lactate levels can predict the development of multiple organ failure following septic shock. Am J Surg 1996;171:221–6

Baue AE. The horror autotoxicus and multiple-organ failure. *Arch Surg* 1992;127:1451–62

Botha AJ, Moore FA, Moore EE, *et al.* Early neutrophil sequestration after injury: a pathogenic mechanism for multiple organ failure. *J Trauma* 1995; 39:411

Marshall JC, Cook DJ, Christou NV, *et al.* Multiple organ dysfunction score: a reliable descriptor of a complex clinical outcome. *Crit Care Med* 1995;23:1638–52

Sauaia A, Moore FA, Moore EE, *et al.* Early predictors of postinjury multiple organ failure. *Arch Surg* 1994;129:39–45

# INDEX

.